MEMBRANE ALTERATIONS IN CANCER

GANN Monograph on Cancer Research

The Japanese Cancer Association supports two series of publications. GANN is an official organ of the Association, and is published bimonthly. The "GANN Monograph on Cancer Research" series consists of collected contributions on current topics in cancer problems and allied research fields. This semiannual series was initiated in 1966 by the late Dr. Tomizo Yoshida (1903–1973), and is now published jointly by Japan Scientific Societies Press, Tokyo / Plenum Press, New York and London. The publication of this monograph owes much to the financial support given by the late Professor Kazushige Higuchi of Jikei University.

The planning to publish a monograph is made by the Board of Executive Directors of the Japanese Cancer Association, with the final approval of the Board of Directors. It is hoped that the series will serve as an important source of information in cancer research.

Japanese Cancer Association

JAPANESE CANCER ASSOCIATION
GANN Monograph on Cancer Research No.29

MEMBRANE ALTERATIONS IN CANCER

Edited by AKIRA MAKITA
SHIGERU TSUIKI
SETSURO FUJII
LEONARD WARREN

JAPAN SCIENTIFIC SOCIETIES PRESS, Tokyo
PLENUM PRESS, New York and London

Published jointly by
JAPAN SCIENTIFIC SOCIETIES PRESS, Tokyo
ISBN 4-7622-6374-5
         and
PLENUM PRESS, New York and London
ISBN 0-306-41565-8

Distributed in all areas outside Japan and Asia between Pakistan and Korea by PLENUM PRESS, New York and London.

Printed in Japan

PREFACE

In recent years much attention has been paid to cell membrane alterations associated with transformation and malignancy. Alterations of tumor cell membrane have been demonstrated in terms of cell biology, such as increased agglutinability of tumor cells with lectins and elevation of sugar transport across the membrane. Changes in the carbohydrate chains of cell surface glycoproteins and glycolipids probably ascribable to quantitative and qualitative shifts of synthetic and possibly degradative enzymes have been extensively studied. Some enzymes which are localized on the cell surface are shed into the circulation of cancer patients, and are of potential clinical value.

While it is clear that new insights into a number of problems have been generated, we still do not understand the mechanisms by which changes at the level of the genome bring about membrane changes and how these in turn are the basis for the cancer phenotype: autonomous growth, metastasis, and altered differentiation and function.

This monograph has been edited from materials presented at the Second Symposium of Sapporo Cancer Seminar which was held in July 1982. The object of this publication is to discuss biochemical problems related to surface changes of malignant cells from a number of different areas of biochemistry. Membrane involvement in carcinogenesis, metastasis and differentiation is discussed in Parts I, II, and III. Parts IV and V integrate informationon alterations of membrane glycoconjugates and their metabolism that accompany transformation and malignancy. Part VI deals with molecular variations of membrane-bound enzymes in malignancy and their clinical relevance. We hope that the work presented here will help to promote future research.

Finally, we are grateful to Dr. Takeo Yamazaki, Dr. Hiroshi Kobayashi and N. Taniguchi, and to our colleagues for their invaluable help in organizing the Symposium.

June 1983

Akira MAKITA
Shigeru TSUIKI
Setsuro FUJII
Leonard WARREN

CONTENTS

V. ENZYMES OF GLYCOCONJUGATE METABOLISM IN CANCER

VI. MEMBRANE ENZYMES IN CANCER

I. CARCINOGENESIS AND MEMBRANES

EFFECT OF TUMOR PROMOTERS IN RELATION TO THE CELL MEMBRANE

Takashi Sugimura and Hirota Fujiki

National Cancer Center Research Institute*

Since tumor promoters are important in human carcinogenesis, we tried to find other tumor promoters than 12-O-tetradecanoylphorbol-13-acetate (TPA) in our environment. For this purpose we developed a simple and practical short term method consisting of three tests: tests of irritation of mouse ear, induction of ornithine decarboxylase (ODC) in skin of the back of mice, and adhesion of HL-60 cells. We also carried out an *in vivo* two-stage carcinogenesis experiment. With these tests we examined about 300 compounds from various sources and found two new classes of tumor promoters, indole alkaloids and polyacetates, which are structurally unrelated to TPA. The indole alkaloids included dihydroteleocidin B, teleocidin and lyngbyatoxin A and the polyacetates included aplysiatoxin and debromoaplysiatoxin. Three indole alkaloids and aplysiatoxin showed tumor promoting activity as potent as TPA, whereas debromoaplysiatoxin, a debrominated form of aplysiatoxin was a weaker tumor promoter than TPA. We found that all these compounds inhibited the specific binding of ^{3}H-TPA to a mouse particulate fraction, indicating that they have the same receptor as TPA.

By comparison of the tumor promoting activities of aplysiatoxin and debromoaplysiatoxin, we classified various biological effects induced by tumor promoters into effects less relevant (category A) and more relevant (category B) to tumor promotion. Effects of category B, such as cell adhesion of HL-60 cells and differentiation of HL-60 cells, aggregation of NL-3 cells, inhibition of differentiation of Friend erythroleukemia cells, and induction of early antigen (EA) positive cells were mediated through many steps in the cell. Effects of category B were correlated relatively well with tumor promoting activity *in vivo*.

Finally, in this paper, the fact that tumor promoters have not only epigenetic but also genetic effects is discussed.

Carcinogenesis is a very complicated process. Animal experiments have shown the existence of two steps, initiation and promotion (*3, 36*). Agents that promote the carcinogenic process in initiated cells are called tumor promoters. Certain tumor promoters apparently act by binding to specific cell surface receptors causing alteration in membrane structure and function. The most extensively studied tumor promoter is 12-O-tetradecanoylphorbol-13-acetate (TPA), which was isolated from croton oil, obtained from seeds of *Croton tiglium* L. (Euphorbiaceae) as the most active principle. The structure of TPA was determined independently by Hecker and Van Duuren in

---

* Tsukiji 5-1-1, Chuo-ku, Tokyo 104, Japan (杉村　隆, 藤木博太).

the 1960's (*20, 58*). TPA or croton oil had been almost the only available tumor promoter in the last forty years.

We are convinced that there must be other potent tumor promoters than TPA in our environment and thus we thought it important to screen for tumor promoters with a view to preventing human cancers. Fortunately we have now discovered new indole alkaloids and polyacetates as potent tumor promoters. The indole alkaloids are dihydroteleocidin B, teleocidin and lyngbyatoxin A and the polyacetates include aplysiatoxin and debromoaplysiatoxin. The specific activities of these five tumor promoters in *in vivo* and *in vitro* systems are almost the same as that of TPA. Although the structures of indole alkaloids and polyacetates are entirely different from that of TPA, these two new classes of tumor promoters appear to share a similar mechanism of action to TPA through the same cell surface receptor. Moreover, they exert many biological effects in common with TPA *in vivo* and *in vitro* in cultured cells. Since some of the effects are membrane-associated, we will report our new results on tumor promoters with emphasis on the cell membrane.

Structures of New Tumor Promoters

Teleocidin, which was isolated from *Streptomyces mediocidicus*, is a mixture of teleocidin A and teleocidin B (*53*). Recently we found that teleocidin A consists of two isomers and teleocidin B of four isomers (*15*). In Fig. 1, the carbon atoms of teleocidins shown in circles are achiral carbons. Teleocidin A has a molecular weight of 437 daltons, and teleocidin B has one of 451. Dihydroteleocidin B is a catalytically hydrogenated derivative of one of the four isomers of teleocidin B (*54*). It has been reported that the crystalline form can easily be obtained by hydrogenation of teleocidin (*17*).

While we were studying the biological effects of dihydroteleocidin B and teleocidin, an exciting paper entitled "Seaweed dermatitis: Structure of lyngbyatoxin A" in *Science* (*4*) attracted our attention, because the similarity in structure of the indole alkaloids, dihydroteleocidin B, teleocidin and lyngbyatoxin A was apparent. Lyngbyatoxin A was isolated from the blue-green alga *Lyngbya majuscula*, which is known to be a causative agent of swimmer's itch in Hawaii. Moore at the University of Hawaii had determined

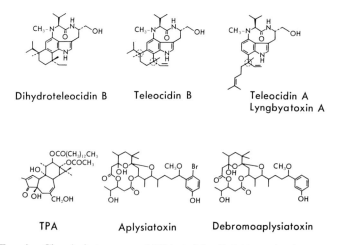

FIG. 1.   Chemical structures of TPA, indole alkaloids, and polyacetates.

its gross structure from chemical and spectral data (*4*). Recently, we found that lyng-byatoxin A corresponds to one isomer of teleocidin A (*16*).

From information on lyngbyatoxin A, we paid special attention to information on outbreaks of swimmer's itch and found another new class of tumor promoters, polyace-tates. Aplysiatoxin and debromoaplysiatoxin were shown to be causative agents of swim-mer's itch in Hawaii in 1980. Moore isolated these two compounds from another variety of *L. majuscula* (*35*). Interestingly, these two compounds had first been found in the digestive tract of the sea hare, *Stylocheilus longicauda* by Kato and Scheuer at the University of Hawaii. Their chemical structures were determined by them (*33*). The two compounds have the same structure except that aplysiatoxin contains a bromine residue while debromoaplysiatoxin does not. We also found aplysiatoxin and debromoaply-siatoxin in the blue-gree alga of Okinawa, where seaweed dermatitis is often reported in summer (*18*).

Three-step Screening Test

In screening for tumor promoters, we developed a practical and simple short term method consisting of three tests (Table I) (*11, 12*). The first test is on irritation of mouse ear. Irritancy is estimated 24 hr after application of the test compound and is expressed as the ID_{50}^{24} value, which is the amount causing redness of the ear of 50% of the mice (*21*). The second test is on induction of ornithine decarboxylase (ODC) in the skin of the back of mice. ODC activity is determined 4 hr after application of the compound (*11, 41*). The third test is on adhesion of human promyelocytic leukemia cells (HL-60) (*30, 43*). Cell adhesion is measured by determining the number of cells not attached to the bottom of a flask 48 hr after addition of the test compound to the medium. The concentrations of test compounds required for 50% cell adhesion are used to compare their potencies (*39*).

We tested over 300 compounds from various sources. Of these, 43 caused redness

TABLE I. Various Effects of Tumor Promoters

	TPA	Dihydro-teleocidin B	Teleocidin	Lyngbya-toxin A	Aplysia-toxin	Debromo-aplysiatoxin
Irritant test ID_{50}^{24} (nmol/ear)	0.016	0.017	0.008	0.011	0.005	0.005
Induction of ODC (nmol CO_2/5.0 μg compound)	1.45	1.55	1.89	2.05	2.15	2.05
Adhesion of HL-60 cells ED_{50} (ng/ml)	1.5	0.3	4.0	7.0	2.0	180
Phagocytosis of HL-60 cells ED_{30} (ng/ml)	2.5	1.4	3.6	2.5	1.7	100
Aggregation of NL-3 cells ED_{50} (ng/ml)	11.2	6.5	3.1	2.4	2.1	180
Inhibition of differentiation of Friend erythroleukemia cells ED_{50} (ng/ml)	1.0	0.2	2.0	0.4	n.d.	150
Inhibition of specific binding of ^{3}H-PDBu ED_{50} (ng/ml)	3.0	n.d.	5.0	8.0	4.0	52
Tumor promoting activity in week 30 (%)	100	90	100	80	93	53

n. d., not determined.

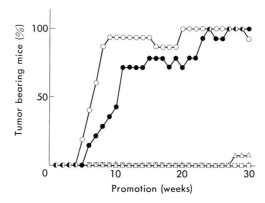

FIG. 2. Effects of teleocidin and TPA in tumor formation. Percentages of tumor bearing mice treated with DMBA plus teleocidin (●), and DMBA plus TPA (○). No tumors were observed in the groups treated with teleocidin alone, or DMBA alone (□). Only one mouse in the group treated with TPA had a tumor (△).

of mouse ear and 15 of these 43 induced ODC activity significantly. Some of the 15 compounds caused adhesion of HL-60 cells. Now five compounds have been found to show tumor promoting activity in *in vivo* carcinogenesis experiments; the names of these five compounds are given in the previous paragraph.

Two-step Carcinogenesis Experiment with New Tumor Promoter

In vivo animal experiments were carried out with a two-step protocol. Carcinogenesis was initiated in the skin of the back of 8-week-old female CD-1 mice by application of 100 μg of 7,12-dimethylbenz(a)anthracene (DMBA). From one week later, either 2.5 μg of dihydroteleocidin B, or 2.5 μg of teleocidin, or 3.0 μg of lyngbyatoxin A was applied topically twice weekly. Aplysiatoxin or debromoaplysiatoxin was given at a dose of 0.5 μg for 8 weeks and then of 1.25 μg until week 30. For comparison, 2.5 μg of TPA was applied to the skin twice weekly as a positive control. Figure 2 shows the tumor formation with teleocidin. The number of tumors 1 mm or more in diameter were counted weekly and tumor promoting activity was expressed as the percentage of tumor bearing mice. The tumor promoting activity in week 30 in the groups treated with DMBA and these new compounds, dihydroteleocidin B, teleocidin, lyngbyatoxin A, aplysiatoxin, and debromoaplysiatoxin, are summarized in Table I. Dihydroteleocidin B, teleocidin, lyngbyatoxin A, and aplysiatoxin are very strong tumor promoters like TPA, whereas debromoaplysiatoxin is a weak promoter (*12–14, 49–52*).

Similarity of the Effects of TPA and the New Tumor Promoters on Membrane Receptors

Recent evidence has suggested that TPA binds to specific receptors on the cell surface and that this leads to rapid biochemical alterations in the composition of membrane phospholipids. These changes in the cell membrane probably produce secondary messengers which cause various biological effects in the cytoplasm, and also chromosomal alterations (*7, 47, 60*).

It was of great interest to find out how TPA and the new tumor promoters, three indole alkaloids and aplysiatoxin, all exert strong tumor promoting activity on mouse skin, although the two new classes of tumor promoters are structurally unrelated to TPA. Studies on the following different systems indicated that the action of TPA, indole alkaloid and polyacetate may be mediated by the same receptor system.

Induction of early antigen (EA) and/or virus capsid antigen (VCA) in the Epstein-Barr virus (EBV) genome-carrying cell lines C-6 and P3HR-1 cells was observed by teleocidin or TPA (28, 63). Teleocidin or TPA enhanced both EA and VCA synthesis in P3HR-1 cells additively with 3 mM n-butyrate, but not with TPA or teleocidin (61). These results suggested that teleocidin and TPA may enhance synthesis of EBV antigens by a common mechanism which differs from that of n-butyrate.

Collins and Rozengurt observed stimulation of DNA synthesis in Swiss 3T3 cells by teleocidin with a wide range of purified growth factors. As in the case of TPA, teleocidin has a synergistic action with insulin, but not with vasopressin, suggesting that teleocidin acts through the same mitogenic pathway as TPA (5, 6).

HL-60 cells were induced to differentiate into macrophage-like cells in a dose-dependent manner by teleocidin or TPA. Huberman et al. isolated a cell variant that is resistant to induction of differentiation by TPA (designated as R-59 cells) and showed that teleocidin can induce macrophage-like cell differentiation in the parent HL-60 cells, but not in R-59 cells (29). Similar results have been obtained with Friend erythroleukemia cells (Marks et al., unpublished results), and nematodes (Caenorhabditis elegans) (Miwa et al., unpublished results).

Driedger and Blumberg demonstrated the specific and saturable binding of ^{3}H-phorbol-12,13-dibutyrate (^{3}H-PDBu), which has a shorter fatty acid chain than TPA (7). Horowitz et al. studied the binding of ^{3}H-PDBu to its specific receptor in cloned rat embryo fibroblasts (CREF), an established line derived from Fisher rats. These cells contain two classes of binding sites, a high affinity site with a K_D of nM at 1.6×10^5 sites/cell and a low affinity site with a K_D of 710 nM at 3×10^6 sites/cell (26). Umezawa et al. examined the inhibition of binding of ^{3}H-PDBu to CREF cells by TPA and teleocidin; 50% inhibition (ED_{50}) was achieved with 6 nM TPA and 11 nM teleocidin (57). We carried out similar experiments with dihydroteleocidin B, lyngbyatoxin A, aplysiatoxin, and debromoaplysiatoxin in collaboration with Dr. Weinstein's group, finding that the ED_{50} value of dihydroteleocidin B was 26 nM, that of lyngbyatoxin A was 8 nM and those of aplysiatoxin and debromoaplysiatoxin were 14 nM and 94 nM, respectively (25).

Specific binding of ^{3}H-phorbol-12,13-dipropionate (^{3}H-PDPr) to a particulate fraction of mouse skin was inhibited by several tumor promoters. From these results, Schmidt et al. classified tumor promoters into three types: group A, which exhibits positive correlations between the potencies of irritation, promoting activity and inhibition of specific binding; group B, which shows strong irritant and inhibitor activities, but little or no promoting activity, and group C, which shows strong irritant activity with little or no inhibitory activity and little or no promoting activity (45). The inhibition coefficient (K_i) of TPA was 1.7 nM, that of dihydroteleocidin B was 11 nM, that of teleocidin was 3.1 nM, that of lyngbyatoxin A was 4.4 nM and that of debromoaplysia-toxin was 70 nM (45). The three indole alkaloids and aplysiatoxin seem to belong to group A and debromoaplysiatoxin may belong to group B rather than group C, because there was only a 10-fold difference in the K_i values of the two polyacetates, aplysiatoxin, and debromoaplysiatoxin.

Recently, a method for direct measurement of specific binding of ^{3}H-TPA to a mouse particulate fraction using cold acetone was developed independently by two research groups (2, 22). The abilities of aplysiatoxin and debromoaplysiatoxin to inhibit the specific binding of ^{3}H-TPA were tested by this method. We found that the ED_{50} value of aplysiatoxin was 6.6 nM and that of debromoaplysiatoxin was 8.0 nM (Tahira, Suganuma, Fujiki, Moore, and Sugimura, in preparation).

It is noteworthy that three indole alkaloids and aplysiatoxin in the class of polyacetates, which are structurally unrelated to phorbol ester, showed very potent tumor promoting activity like TPA. We found that the molecules of these promoters all possess both hydrophobic and hydrophilic domains. Furthermore, structure studies by Dr. Weinstein's group in collaboration with our group on these three classes of tumor promoter by computer graphics showed that some functional groups, such as a carbonyl group and a hydroxyl group are located in similar positions in the molecules (25).

In Vivo and in Vitro Biological Effects of Tumor Promoters

TPA has various biological and biochemical effects *in vivo* and *in vitro* in cultured cells. Like TPA, indole alkaloids, and polyacetates induce redness of mouse ear, ODC in mouse skin and adhesion and differentiation of HL-60 cells. These three effects were examined in the three-step screening test, as described above. In addition, these compounds enhance aggregation of human lymphoblastoid cells (NL-3) (27) and inhibit terminal differentiation of Friend erythroleukemia cells (Table I) (11, 12). It is still uncertain which of these effects are specific and relevant to tumor promotion. Many investigators have attempted to demonstrate a positive correlation between the tumor promoting activity of various phorbol esters and effects in their own *in vivo* or *in vitro* assay systems. Table II shows 26 effects *in vitro* that were induced by both TPA and

TABLE II. *In Vitro* Effects Induced by TPA and Teleocidin

Cell adhesion of HL-60 cells (39)	Inhibtion of creatine kinase isoenzyme transition in normal human myoblast cultures (10)
Aggregation of NL-3 cells (27)	
Increase of hexose transport (57)	
Release of arachidonic acid (44, 57)	Colony formation of EBV-infected cord blood lymphocytes (28)
Formation of prostaglandins (44, 57)	
Release of choline (44, 57)	Induction of EBV (EA and VCA) (8, 28, 61)
Increase of ^{32}P-incorporation into phospholipids (40)	
	Inhibition of EGF binding (57)
Increase of membrane lipid fluidity (9, 15)	Inhibition of specific ^{3}H-PDPr, ^{3}H-PDBu binding (25, 45, 57)
Increase of 32,000-dalton protein (24)	
Inhibition of metabolic cooperation (31)	Inhibition of specific ^{3}H-TPA binding (15)
Inhibition of pseudoemperiopolesis (32)	Induction of specific ganglioside changes (48)
Production of superoxide anion radical (O_2^-) (56)	Induction of cell binding phenotype (CBP) (8)
Induction of differentiation of HL-60 cells (39)	Induction of changes in the cytoskeleton (15, 42)
Inhibition of differentiation in Friend erythroleukemia cells (11, 12)	Enhancement of malignant cell transformation induced by methylcholanthrene or ultraviolet radiation in A31-1-1 mouse cells (23)
Inhibition of melanogenesis in B-16 cells (10, 46)	
	Enhancement of adenovirus type 5 transformation of CREF cells (10)

TABLE III. Classification of Various Effects of Tumor Promoters

Category A
    1. Irritation of mouse ear
    2. Induction of ODC
    3. Release of arachidonic acid and formation of prostaglandins
    4. Release of choline
    5. Induction of dark keratinocytes
    6. Induction of CBP
    7. Inhibition of EGF binding
    8. Inhibition of specific bindings of ^{3}H-PDPr, ^{3}H-PDBu, and ^{3}H-TPA

Category B
    1. Adhesion and induction of differentiation of HL-60
    2. Aggregation of NL-3 cells
    3. Inhibition of differentiation of Friend erythroleukemia cells
    4. Increase of membrane lipid fluidity
    5. Increase of ^{32}P-incorporation into phospholipids
    6. Increase in 32,000-dalton protein
    7. Induction of EBV (EA and VCA)

indole alkaloids. However, these studies have not led to a clear understanding of which biological effects are relevant to tumor promotion.

Recently we found that the presence of one bromine residue in the phenol group changes the weak tumor promoting activity of debromoaplysiatoxin to the strong activity of aplysiatoxin (14). As Table I shows, there were remarkable differences in the effects of aplysiatoxin and debromoaplysiatoxin on various biological parameters. These qualitative and quantitative differences prompted us to reconsider the significance of various biological effects. By comparison of the effects of these two polyacetates, we classified the various biological effects induced by tumor promoters into two categories, category A being less relevant, and category B being more relevant to tumor promotion (Table III). Effects of category A were induced by both aplysiatoxin and debromoaplysiatoxin at the same concentration, whereas those of category B were induced only by strong promoters such as aplysiatoxin. For induction of the effects in category B, such as adhesion of HL-60 cells and aggregation of NL-3 cells, a 100 times higher concentration of the weak promoter debromoaplysiatoxin than of the strong promoter aplysiatoxin was required. Therefore, we suppose, at this moment, that the effects of category B reflect more specific phenotypic changes associated with tumor promotion (14).

1. Category A of biological effects of tumor promoters
1) Irritation test on mouse ear

Compounds were tested on the ear of 8-week-old female CD-1 mice. This test was originally used by Hecker for purification of TPA from croton oil (21). As Table I shows, TPA, dihydroteleocidin B, teleocidin, lyngbyatoxin A, aplysiatoxin, and debromoaplysiatoxin were very strong skin irritants, their ID_{50}^{24} values being 0.005–0.017 nmol per ear (14).

2) Induction of ODC activity

Test compounds were applied as solutions in 0.2 ml of acetone. ODC activity was determined by measuring release of CO_2, as described by O'Brien et al. (41). These six compounds at doses of 5.0 μg caused similar extents of induction of ODC in mouse skin, and the amounts of $^{14}CO_2$ released were 1.45–2.15 nmol CO_2/mg protein (*14*). Their effects in induction of ODC were all inhibited by 13-*cis*-retinoic acid.

3) Release of arachidonic acid and formation of prostaglandins

C3H 10T1/2 cells were prelabeled with ^{3}H-arachidonic acid under conditions in which over 95% of the arachidonic acid was incorporated into phospholipids. Addition of TPA, dihydroteleocidin B, or teleocidin to these cultures induced rapid release of ^{3}H-arachidonic acid into the medium, reflecting increased phospholipid degradation (*37, 57*). Similar results were obtained with CREF cells and HeLa cells under the same conditions (*25, 44*). It was especially remarkable that the dose producing 50% of maximal effect (ED_{50}) value of aplysiatoxin was 5.9 nM and that of debromoaplysiatoxin was 5.5 nM (*25*). The release of arachidonic acid induced by these six tumor promoters was associated with increased synthesis of prostaglandins (*57*).

4) Release of choline

When HeLa cells were prelabeled with ^{14}C-choline, TPA, dihydroteleocidin B, and lyngbyatoxin A stimulated release of radioactivity from the cells (*43*). Aplysiatoxin and debromoaplysiatoxin were also shown to cause release of ^{3}H-choline from CREF cells. The ED_{50} value of aplysiatoxin was 4 nM and that of debromoaplysiatoxin was 3.7 nM (*25*).

5) Induction of dark keratinocytes

Klein-Szanto *et al.* reported a good correlation between tumor promoting activity and induction of dark keratinocytes in the epidermis of mice (*34*). The number of dark keratinocytes was determined 48 hr after application of test compounds. TPA induced 37.1 dark keratinocytes per 1,000 basal cells, teleocidin induced 40.9, and lyngbyatoxin A induced 44.8, whereas the weak promoter debromoaplysiatoxin induced 36.7. Acetone alone induced only 10.2 dark keratinocytes (*1*).

6) Induction of the cell binding phenotype (CBP)

TPA and several phorbol esters induce morphological changes and aggregation of human lymphocytes, which is named the "cell binding phenotype" (*8*). Both strong and weak promoters induce cell-to-cell binding; the percentages of aggregated cells were almost the same with concentrations of over 7.5 ng/ml of all these compounds (*8*).

7) Inhibition of epidermal growth factor (EGF) binding

Addition of TPA, dihydroteleocidin B, or teleocidin to the culture medium led to marked inhibition of ^{125}I-EGF binding to C3H 10T1/2 cells, CREF cells, and HeLa cells (*25, 57*). The inhibition occurred through a secondary change resulting from binding of promoter to the cell surface receptor. The ED_{50} value of aplysiatoxin was 5.1 nM and that of debromoaplysiatoxin was 55 nM in CREF cells (*25*). Thus there was only a 5- to 10-fold difference in the ED_{50} values of these two polyacetates.

8) Inhibition of specific bindings of ^{3}H-PDPr, ^{3}H-PDBu, and ^{3}H-TPA

Aplysiatoxin inhibited specific binding of ^{3}H-PDPr, ^{3}H-PDBu, and ^{3}H-TPA to a mouse particulate fraction as effectively as debromoaplysiatoxin, as described previously. Since aplysiatoxin is a strong promoter and debromoaplysiatoxin is weak, the results of binding tests on these compounds were not well correlated with those on their potencies of tumor promotion in mouse skin (*45*).

2. Category B of biological effects of tumor promoters

1) Adhesion and induction of differentiation of HL-60 cells

Huberman and Callaham found a good correlation between the tumor promoting activities of phorbol esters and their abilities to induce terminal differentiation of HL-60 cells (30). Three indole alkaloids and two polyacetates induced cell adhesion of HL-60 cells, and differentiation of HL-60 cells, measured as increase in phagocytic activity. A concentration of debromoaplysiatoxin 100 times those of the other five compounds was required to achieve the same effects, as shown in Table I (14).

2) *Aggregation of NL-3 cells*

TPA, dihydroteleocidin B, teleocidin, and lyngbyatoxin A induced remarkable aggregation of NL-3 cells after incubation for 6 hr. NL-3 cells are a human lymphoblastoid cell line transformed by EBV (55). As Table I shows, a 100-time higher concentration of debromoaplysiatoxin than of aplysiatoxin was required to achieve the same effect (14).

3) *Inhibition of differentiation of Friend erythroleukemia cells*

Terminal differentiation of Friend erythroleukemia cells induced by dimethyl sulfoxide was inhibited by tumor promoters (62). The concentrations of TPA, dihydroteleocidin B, teleocidin, and lyngbyatoxin A required for 50% reduction of benzidine-reactive cells were 1.0 ng/ml, 0.2 ng/ml, 2.0 ng/ml, and 0.4 ng/ml, respectively, whereas that of debromoaplysiatoxin was 150 ng/ml (11, 12).

4) *Increase of membrane lipid fluidity*

The dynamics of membrane lipid in Friend erythroleukemia cells was examined by fluorescence polarization of 1,6-diphenyl-1,3,5-hexatriene (9). Fisher *et al*. reported that TPA-resistant clones showed higher fluorescence anisotropy values, indicating decreased membrane lipid fluidity (9). Concentration of 100 ng/ml of TPA, teleocidin, and aplysiatoxin decreased the fluorescence polarization of the membranes of C3H 10T1/2 cells, whereas debromoaplysiatoxin was inactive at up to 1,000 ng/ml (Tran, Horowitz, Fujiki, Schachter, Sugimura, Castagna, and Weinstein, unpublished results).

5) *Increase of ^{32}P-incorporation into phospholipids*

Tumor promoters increase the incorporation of radioactive inorganic phosphate (^{32}P$_i$) into phospholipids, which reflects alteration in phospholipid metabolism (40). Debromoaplysiatoxin was efficient only at about 100 times higher concentration than TPA, dihydroteleocidin B, teleocidin, lyngbyatoxin A, and aplysiatoxin in HeLa cells (40).

6) *Increased synthesis of 32,000-dalton protein*

The synthesis of 32,000-dalton protein in BALB/c3T3 cells nearly doubled in 2 hr after addition of TPA (24). Concentrations of 20 ng/ml of TPA, dihydroteleocidin B, teleocidin, lyngbyatoxin A, and aplysiatoxin increased the synthesis of this protein to the same extent, but debromoaplysiatoxin stimulated the synthesis of this protein only at higher concentration (>200 ng/ml) (Hiwasa, Fujiki, Sugimura, and Sakiyama, manuscript submitted).

7) *Induction of EBV (EA and VCA)*

As described under "Similarity of the Effects of TPA and the New Tumor Promoters on Membrane Receptors," TPA or teleocidin enhanced EA and/or VCA synthesis in P3HR-1 cells additively with 3 mM *n*-butyrate. Maximal induction of EA synthesis was achieved by strong tumor promoters at concentrations of 5 to 10 ng/ml, whereas a concentration of 250 ng/ml of debromoaplysiatoxin was required to achieve the same effect (8).

DISCUSSION

During the past twenty years TPA and phorbol esters have been widely used in *in vivo* and *in vitro* systems as the only available potent tumor promoters. Based on the two-step concept of experimental carcinogenesis we paid special attention to the existence of potent tumor promoters in the environment in relation to human carcinogenesis. We found three indole alkaloids, dihydroteleocidin B, teleocidin, and lyngbyatoxin A, which are all potent tumor promoters although they differ structurally from TPA. In addition, a strong promoter, aplysiatoxin, and a weak promoter, debromoaplysiatoxin, were found in blue-green alga.

The finding that three classes of tumor promoter, phorbol esters, indole alkaloids, and polyacetates bind to the same receptor on the cell surface increased our interest in the mechanism of action of these potent tumor promoters. It was of especial interest to find that the addition of one bromine residue to the phenol group of aplysiatoxin results in change from weak to strong tumor promoting activity. In addition to these two polyacetates, several derivatives of these compounds, such as 19-bromoaplysiatoxin, oscillatoxin A, 21-bromooscillatoxin A, and 19,21-dibromooscillatoxin A, were found in a mixture of *Oscillatoria nigroviridis* and *Schizothrix calcicola* from Enewetak (*38*). These derivatives are representatives of a new class of tumor promoters differing from phorbol esters and indole alkaloids.

By comparison of the biological effects of a strong promoter, aplysiatoxin, and a weak promoter, debromoaplysiatoxin, we classified the effects into two categories: effects less relevant (category A) and more relevant (category B) to tumor promotion. The effects in category A were exerted very quickly after the administration of the compounds, whereas the effects in category B, such as cell adhesion and differentiation of HL-60 cells, aggregation of NL-3 cells and induction of EA-positive cells were mediated through many steps in the cell. We suppose that the relative potencies of tumor promoters for effects in category B correspond relatively well with their tumor promoting activities in animal experiments *in vivo*.

It is worthy to mention that dihydroteleocidin B is unusually potent in enhancing 3-methylcholanthren (MCA)-induced malignant transformation in A31-1-1 mouse cells (*23*). The effective concentration of dihydroteleocidin B is only one-hundredth than that of TPA, whereas both promoters possessed almost equal potencies to induce several biological effects shown in Table II.

Since some biological effects induced by tumor promoters are membrane-associated phenomena, specific changes in gangliosides should be briefly discussed. Srinivas and Colburn showed that treatment of JB6 mouse epidermal cells with TPA produced a specific decrease in D-(1-^{14}C) glucosamine incorporation into trisialoganglioside G_T and an increase in its incorporation into disialoganglioside G_{DIb} and an unknown gangglioside G_x. These ganglioside responses were antagonized by retinoic acid. These results strongly suggest that alterations in ganglioside levels may be involved in promotion of transformation (*48*). Similarly, Saito reported that teleocidin induced changes of gangliosides of the cell membrane (HL-60) (Saito, personal communication).

Recently, Varshavsky found that TPA enhances amplification by methotrexate of the dihydrofolate reductase gene in cultured mouse cells (*59*). From this result we realized that tumor promoters have not only epigenetic but also genetic effects in the cells. Hayashi in our laboratory showed that tumor promoters of three classes, TPA, dihydroteleocidin B, and aplysiatoxin, enhanced the appearance of CdCl$_2$-resistant Chinese hamster lung cells and that these cadmium-resistant cells showed over-production of metallothionein I mRNA and amplification of the metallothionein I gene (*19*). An important aspect of this finding is that tumor promoting activity was well correlated with the ability to induce cadmium-resistant cells (*19*). Since, the advanced stage of promotion in mouse skin is not reversible, such genetic changes probably play a crucial role in the multistep process of tumor promotion.

Acknowledgments

This work was supported in part by Grants-in-Aid for Cancer Research from the Ministry of Education, Science and Culture and the Ministry of Health and Welfare of Japan, and the Princess Takamatsu Cancer Research Fund. Work on the isolations of lyngbyatoxin A, aplysiatoxin, and debromoaplysiatoxin used in this study was supported by Grant CA 12623-09 to Dr. R. E. Moore at the University of Hawaii from the National Cancer Institute, Health and Human Services, USA. We thank Dr. R. E. Moore and Dr. I. B. Weinstein for valuable collaborations.

REFERENCES

1. Arai, M., Hibino, T., Fujiki, H., Sugimura, T., and Ito, N. *In* "Proc. Japan. Cancer Assoc. 40th Annu. Meet.," p. 49 (1981) (in Japanese).
2. Ashendel, C. L. and Boutwell, R. K. *Biochem. Biophys. Res. Commun.*, **99**, 543–549 (1981).
3. Berenblum, I. *Cancer Res.*, **1**, 44–48 (1941).
4. Cardellina, J. H., II, Marner, F.-J., and Moore, R. E. *Science*, **204**, 193–195 (1979).
5. Collins, M. and Rozengurt, E. *Biochem. Biophys. Res. Commun.*, **104**, 1159–1166 (1982).
6. Dicker, P. and Rozengurt, E. *Nature*, **287**, 607–612 (1980).
7. Driedger, P. E. and Blumberg, P. M. *Proc. Natl. Acad. Sci. U.S.*, **77**, 567–571 (1980).
8. Eliasson, L., Kallin, B., Patarroyo, M., Klein, G., Fujiki, H., and Sugimura, T. *Int. J. Cancer*, **31**, 7–11 (1983).
9. Fisher, P. B., Cogan, U., Horowitz, A. D., Schachter, D., and Weinstein, I. B. *Biochem. Biophys. Res. Commun.*, **100**, 370–376 (1981).
10. Fisher, P. B., Miranda, A. F., Mufson, R. A., Weinstein, L. S., Fujiki, H., Sugimura, T., and Weinstein, I. B. *Cancer Res.*, **42**, 2829–2835 (1982).
11. Fujiki, H., Mori, M., Nakayasu, M., Terada, M., and Sugimura, T. *Biochem. Biophys. Res. Commun.*, **90**, 976–983 (1979).
12. Fujiki, H., Mori, M., Nakayasu, M., Terada, M., Sugimura, T., and Moore, R. E. *Proc. Natl. Acad. Sci. U.S.*, **78**, 3872–3876 (1981).
13. Fujiki, H., Suganuma, M., Matsukura, N., Sugimura, T., and Takayama, S. *Carcinogenesis*, **3**, 895–898 (1982).
14. Fujiki, H., Suganuma, M., Nakayasu, M., Hoshino, H., Moore, R. E., and Sugimura, T. *Gann*, **73**, 495–497 (1982).
15. Fujiki, H. and Sugimura, T. *In* "Genes and Proteins in Oncogenesis," ed. I. B. Weinstein and H. Vogel. Columbia University Press, New York, in press.
16. Fujiki, H., Sugimura, T., and Moore, R. E. *Environ. Health Perspect.*, **50**, in press.
17. Harada, H., Sakabe, N., Hirata, Y., Tomiie, Y., and Nitta, I. *Bull. Chem. Soc. Japan.*, **39**, 1773–1775 (1966).
18. Hashimoto, Y., Kamiya, H., Yamazato, K., and Nozawa, K. *In* "Animal, Plant and Microbial Toxins," Vol. 1, ed. A. Ohsaka, K. Hayashi, and Y. Sawai, pp. 333–338 (1976). Plenum Press, New York.
19. Hayashi, K., Fujiki, H., and Sugimura, T. *In* "Proc. Japan. Cancer Assoc. 41st Annu. Meet.," p. 188 (1982) (in Japanese).

20. Hecker, E. *Naturwissenschaften*, **54**, 282–284 (1967).
21. Hecker, E. *In* "Methods in Cancer Research," Vol. 6, ed. H. Busch, pp. 439–484 (1971). Academic Press, New York and London.
22. Hergenhahn, M. and Hecker, E. *Carcinogenesis*, **2**, 1277–1281 (1981).
23. Hirakawa, T., Kakunaga, T., Fujiki, H., and Sugimura, T. *Science*, **216**, 527–529 (1982).
24. Hiwasa, T., Fujimura, S., and Sakiyama, S. *Proc. Natl. Acad. Sci. U.S.*, **79**, 1800–1804 (1982).
25. Horowitz, A. D., Fujiki, H., Weinstein, I. B., Jeffrey, A., Okin, E., Moore, R. E., and Sugimura, T. *Cancer Res.*, **43**, 1529–1535 (1983).
26. Horowitz, A. D., Greenebaum, E., and Weinstein, I. B. *Proc. Natl. Acad. Sci. U.S.*, **78**, 2315–2319 (1981).
27. Hoshino, H., Miwa, M., Fujiki, H., and Sugimura, T. *Biochem. Biophys. Res. Commun.*, **95**, 842–848 (1980).
28. Hoshino, H., Miwa, M., Fujiki, H., Sugimura, T., Yamamoto, H., Katsuki, T., and Hinuma, Y. *Cancer Lett.*, **13**, 275–280 (1981).
29. Huberman, E., Braslawsky, G. R., Callaham, M., and Fujiki, H. *Carcinogenesis*, **3**, 111–114 (1982).
30. Huberman, E. and Callaham, M. F. *Proc. Natl. Acad. Sci. U.S.*, **76**, 1293–1297 (1979).
31. Jone, C. M., Trosko, J. E., Chang, C.-C., Fujiki, H., and Sugimura, T. *Gann*, **73**, 874–878 (1982).
32. Kaneshima, H., Hiai, H., Fujiki, H., Iijima, S., Sugimura, T., and Nishizuka, Y. *Leukemia Res.*, in press.
33. Kato, Y. and Scheuer, P. J. *J. Am. Chem. Soc.*, **96**, 2245–2246 (1974).
34. Klein-Szanto, A.J.P., Major, S. K., and Slaga, T. J. *Carcinogenesis*, **1**, 399–406 (1980).
35. Moore, R. E. *Pure Appl. Chem.*, **54**, 1919–1934 (1982).
36. Mottram, J. C. *J. Pathol. Bacteriol.*, **56**, 181–187 (1944).
37. Mufson, R. A., DeFeo, D., and Weinstein, I. B. *Mol. Pharmacol.*, **16**, 569–578 (1979).
38. Mynderse, J. S. and Moore, R. E. *J. Org. Chem.*, **43**, 2301–2303 (1978).
39. Nakayasu, M., Fujiki, H., Mori, M., Sugimura, T., and Moore, R. E. *Cancer Lett.*, **12**, 271–277 (1981).
40. Nishino, H., Fujiki, H., Terada, M., and Sato, S. *Carcinogenesis*, **4**, 107–110 (1983).
41. O'Brien, T. G., Simsiman, R. C., and Boutwell, R. K. *Cancer Res.*, **35**, 1662–1670 (1975).
42. Rifkin, D. B., Crowe, R. M., and Pollack, R. *Cell*, **18**, 361–368 (1979).
43. Rovera, G., Santoli, D., and Damsky, C. *Proc. Natl. Acad. Sci. U.S.*, **76**, 2779–2783 (1979).
44. Sakamoto, H., Terada, M., Fujiki, H., Mori, M., Nakayasu, M., Sugimura, T., and Weinstein, I. B. *Biochem. Biophys. Res. Commun.*, **102**, 100–107 (1981).
45. Schmidt, R., Adolf, W., Marston, A., Roeser, H., Sorg, B., Fujiki, H., Sugimura, T., Moore, R. E., and Hecker, E. *Carcinogenesis*, **4**, 77–81 (1983).
46. Sekiguchi, T., Tosu, M., Yoshida, M. C., Oikawa, A., Ishihara, K., Fujiki, H., Tumuraya, M., and Kameya, T. *Somat. Cell. Genet.*, **8**, 605–622 (1982).
47. Shoyab, M. and Todaro, G. J. *Nature*, **288**, 451–455 (1980).
48. Srinivas, L. and Colburn, N. H. *J. Natl. Cancer Inst.*, **68**, 469–473 (1982).
49. Sugimura, T. *In* "Environmental Mutagens and Carcinogens," ed. T. Sugimura, S. Kondo, and H. Takebe, pp. 3–20 (1982). University of Tokyo Press, Tokyo.
50. Sugimura, T. *Cancer*, **49**, 1970–1984 (1982).
51. Sugimura, T. *Gann*, **73**, 499–507 (1982).
52. Sugimura, T., Fujiki, H., Mori, M., Nakayasu, M., Terada, M., Umezawa, K., and Moore, R. E. *In* "Carcinogenesis—A Comprehensive Survey," Vol. 7, ed. E. Hecker, N. E. Fusenig, W. Kunz, F. Marks, and H. W. Thielmann, pp. 69–73 (1982). Raven Press, New York.

53. Takashima, M. and Sakai, H. *Bull. Agric. Chem. Soc. Japan*, **24**, 652–655 (1960).
54. Takashima, M., Sakai, H., and Arima, K. *Agric. Biol. Chem.*, **26**, 660–668 (1962).
55. Tohda, H., Oikawa, A., Katsuki, T., Hinuma, Y., and Seiji, M. *Cancer Res.*, **38**, 253–256 (1978).
56. Troll, W., Witz, G., Goldstein, B., Stone, D., and Sugimura, T. *In* "Carcinogenesis—A Comprehensive Survey," Vol. 7, ed. by E. Hecker, N. E. Fusenig, W. Kunz, F. Marks, and H. W. Thielmann, pp. 593–597 (1982). Raven Press, New York.
57. Umezawa, K., Weinstein, I. B., Horowitz, A., Fujiki, H., Matsushima, T., and Sugimura, T. *Nature*, **290**, 411–413 (1981).
58. Van Duuren, B. L. *Prog. Exp. Tumor Res.*, **11**, 31–68 (1969).
59. Varshavsky, A. *Cell*, **25**, 561–572 (1981).
60. Weinstein, I. B., Mufson, R. A., Lee, L., Fisher, P. B., Laskin, J., Horowitz, A. D., and Ivanovic, V. *In* "Carcinogenesis: Fundamental Mechanisms and Environmental Effects," ed. B. Pullman, P.O.P. Ts'o, and H. Gelboin, pp. 543–563 (1980). R. Reidel Publishing Co., Amsterdam.
61. Yamamoto, H., Katsuki, T., Hinuma, Y., Hoshino, H., Miwa, M., Fujiki, H., and Sugimura, T. *Int. J. Cancer*, **28**, 125–129 (1981).
62. Yamazaki, H., Fibach, E., Nudel, U., Weinstein, I. B., Rifkind, R. A., and Marks, P. *Proc. Natl. Acad. Sci. U.S.*, **74**, 3451–3455 (1977).
63. Zur Hausen, H., Bornkamm, G. W., Schmidt, R., and Hecker, E. *Proc. Natl. Acad. Sci. U.S.*, **76**, 782–785 (1979).

MEMBRANE ASSOCIATION OF VIRUS-CODED PROTEIN IN CELLS TRANSFORMED BY SIMIAN VIRUS 40

Donald F. H. WALLACH

*Division of Radiobiology, Tufts-New England Medical Center**

Neoplastic conversion by simian virus 40 (SV40) requires expression of one or more protein(s) encoded in overlapping sequences of the early virus DNA. Available evidence suggests that at least one such protein, surface-associated T-antigen, is associated with the plasma membrane of transformed cells. An amino acid sequence for T*, a SV40-coded, membrane-associated protein has been derived from analyses of early mRNAs. I present a model for the membrane association of T*, correlating new information on protein insertion into membranes, surface labeling, glycosylation and peptide mapping with the amino acid sequence postulated for T*.

Two very closely related DNA viruses SV40 and polyoma (Py) can neoplastically convert cells of susceptible species (*24*). As the DNAs of both viruses have been sequenced (*13, 14, 22*) and the gene products expressed by virus transformed cells have been largely identified, characterization of these gene products offers important insights into mechanisms of carcinogenesis.

The DNAs of SV40 and Py consist of about 5,200 base pairs (bp). About half of the DNA, starting near the origin of replication, codes for functions expressed early in lytic infections. These include gene products that initiate and maintain neoplastic transformation in cells which are not permissive of replication and integrate virus DNA into their genome. DNA coding for late functions is not integrated, or not expressed. It does not contribute to transformation.

Py and SV40 Early-Gene Products

Three virus-coded proteins are produced by Py-transformed cells, namely t-, mT-, and T-antigens, with molecular weights (M_rs) near, 20,000, 56,000–58,000, and 100,000, respectively. These proteins are coded for by overlapping sequences within the early DNA (*22*). Of three possible reading frames, only frame 1 is open for extensive translation in the early region. It allows translation of 211 codons between initiation and the first termination codon and accounts for t-antigen. Further translation occurs by a shift of 1 nucleotide into frame 2. This provides for consecutive translation of 264 codons. The frame 1 and frame 2 transcripts are spliced and translated into a protein with a frame 1 N- and a frame-2 C-terminus, namely mT-antigen. The third protein, T-antigen, shares the N-terminal sequences of t- and mT-antigens (frame-1), but its C-terminal region arises from mRNA splicing and a shift to frame 3. Py T-antigen, a nuclear phos-

---

* Boston, Massachusetts 02110, U.S.A.

phoprotein that acts at the initiation site of the viral DNA, supports integration and thereby enhances transformation. Neither it nor t-antigen are required to initiate or maintain the neoplastic state (5, 10). mT-antigen, however, appears essential for neoplastic conversion and seems to exert this action as a plasma membrane anchored protein (5, 10). Membrane insertion is believed to occur via a hydrophobic C-terminal sequence (frame 2) not present in t- or T-antigens.

Until recently, only two coding sequences had been identified in the early SV40 DNA (13, 14), a 2,600 bp stretch starting at the initiation site. The gene products are the M_r 90,000–100,000 SV40 T-antigen and the M_r 17,000 t-antigen, both very similar to the corresponding Py products. The T-antigen is a nuclear phosphoprotein acting at the initiation site. It is translated from mRNA that lacks a sequence of 346 nucleotides present in the DNA. The gap is spliced and T-antigen is thus coded for by 708 codons that are not contiguous in the early DNA. t-antigen is translated from 174 codons that are contiguous in the DNA and precede a splice in the t-antigen mRNA.

The apparent lack of a third coding sequence, corresponding to that for Py mT-antigen, has appeared puzzling because of (a) the close relationship of SV40 to Py, including DNA sequence homologies and immunological crossreactivity of gene products, and (b) extensive evidence for a SV40-specific protein related to T-antigen and located at the plasma membranes of transformed cells. This protein was originally defined as a SV40-specific "tumor-specific transplantation antigen" (TSTA) and/or surface antigen (TSSA). A close relationship has been established between SV40 T-antigen and TSTA/TSSA by (a) copurification of these entities during biochemical fractionation (12); (b) similar subcellular distribution of the two groups of antigens (3, 21); (c) their concordant expression at permissive and nonpermissive temperature in cells transformed by nondefective tsA mutants (1, 23); (d) induction of an in vivo TSTA response by purified T-antigen (4); (e) discovery that a M_r 94,000 protein immunochemically closely related to nuclear T-antigen reacts at plasma membranes of SV40 transformed cells (15, 20, 21). Also peptide homology exists between nuclear T-antigen and a SV40-specific, pI 4.7/M_r 94,000 plasma membrane glycoprotein, T_M (20).

A host cell-coded membrane phosphoprotein (M_r 53,000–55,000) occurs in close association with the SV40-coded protein but can be discriminated from the latter by immunological techniques (6, 9, 12) and peptide mapping (20). A similar protein also appears upon oncogenic transformation with agents other than SV40.

Is T* a Third SV40 Early Gene Product?

Information about the expression of early SV40 DNA has been placed into perspective by Mark and Berg (13) who have demonstrated a third early SV40 mRNA with a splice of about 50 nucleotides located about 180 nucleotides from the 3′ end. This species makes up about 25% of the total early mRNA and is predicted to code for a third early protein, called T*. It is proposed that T* results from the splicing out of 17–21 nucleotides, shifting translation phase into a frame that allows translation past the termination codon of T-antigen for an additional 19 codons. The base sequences predict a protein identical to T-antigen from the N- nearly all the way to the C-terminus and differing in length by only two amino acids. The C-terminal region (Fig. 1) would correspond to that of T-antigen for two residues past an unusual D_4-E-D sequence, to T-antigen residue 660, but would then replace a 68-residue hydrophilic sequence with a 70-residue hydro-

-G-M-L-N-A-L-I-H-S-P-K-A-H-F-R-P-L-S-P-H-S-L-P-M-I-I-I -S-H-T-T-F-V-E-V-L-L-A-L-K   1

-N-L-P-H-L-P-L-N-L-K-H-K-M-N-A-I-V-V-V-N-L-F-I-A-A-Y-N-G-Y-K----C-terminus.   41

FIG. 1. Carboxyl-terminal sequence of putative T* SV40 antigen. One letter amino acid code (A, Ala; D, Asp; E, Glu; F, Phe; G, Gly; H, His; I, Ile; K, Lys; M, Met; N, Asn; P, Pro; Q, Gln; R, Arg; S, Ser; T, Thr; V, Val; W, Trp; Y, Tyr). The first residue of the sequence (G) is numbered 1. Hydrophobic residues underscored.

phobic sequence. The proposed sequence shows remarkable similarities to the frame-shifted segment of Py mT-antigen. There one also finds a run of six dicarboxylic acids (E_6) followed by an unusually hydrophobic carboxyl-terminal domain.

Possible Membrane Associations of T*

How might the T* sequence insert into the plasma membranes of SV40- converted cells? Inspection of the full sequence of early SV40 DNA shows (13, 14), that no protein encoded in this region has a hydrophobic N-terminal sequence for membrane insertion. Indeed, T- and t-antigens do not have any hydrophobic stretches of significant extent, and in T* the hydrophobic segment is near the C-terminus. This implies that t- and T-antigens cannot associate firmly with membranes and that T* can do so only *via* its unique C-terminal sequence.

It is established that, while the direct translation products of some membrane proteins have hydrophobic leaders, such are not prerequisites for membrane insertion or association (18). Insertion may not begin until translation is far beyond the N-terminus (8). Even with a hydrophobic N-terminal leader, permanent association can be restricted to a small sequence at the C-terminus. Information about the insertion of proteins into membranes (2, 8, 18) and mechanisms involved (8, 18), indicates that insertion starts cotranslationally, but not necessarily at the N-terminus, *via* "hairpin" loops with trans-membrane helical segments. 3_{10}-Helices, which form in apolar media, are considered more probable than α-helices (18). These require hydrophobic stretches of 11–25 residues to cross the membrane core. The helices would need to be linked by three or more re-latively polar residues (2, 18). Permanent associations occur *via* one or more transmem-brane helices (2, 8, 18).

The data in (18) allows one to predict the membrane topology of a peptide with the sequence of T* (Fig. 2):

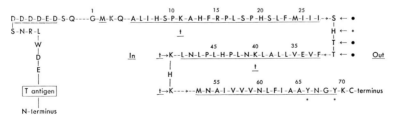

FIG. 2. Hypothetical membrane disposition of T*. Single letter amino acid code as in Fig. 1. Numbering as in Fig. 1. Double underscoring indicates acidic sequence in amino terminal direction. This is in common with T-antigen. Single underscoring indicates postulated transmembrane helices. * possible iodination sites; ● possible glycosylation site; t, presumed trypsin cleavage sites.

In the direction of the N-terminus, membrane insertion is limited by a cluster of six acidic side chains (D_4-E-D). (E_3-G-F-E limits the N-terminal portion of the IgM transmembrane u_m-chain segment;). The T* sequence *per se* begins at residue G^1. It includes three hydrophobic segments separated by short hydrophilic stretches. Going towards the C-terminus, the first hydrophobic segment extends from residue 5 to residue 27. Four polar residues are followed by the second hydrophobic stretch (residues 32–49). A third hydrophobic segment begins after 3 polar residues and runs almost to the C-terminus (residues 53–69). Each of the three hydrophobic segments has the length needed to span the membrane in 3_{10}-helical array and all exhibit amino acid composition comparable to known transmembrane peptide segments. These considerations are compatible with the topology schematized in Fig. 1. This model suggests the following:

(a) T* is anchored into the membrane by three transmembrane helices; (b) the T* sequences in common with T-antigen lie in the cytoplasmic space; (c) only small T* peptide segments extend to the outer membrane surface.

One must determine whether the proposed model is compatible with information about the exposure of SV40-coded protein at the external surfaces of transformed cells:

(a) Immunological work by Santos and Butel (15) and peptide mapping by ourselves (20) indicate that SV40-coded proteins have iodinatable groups exposed at the outer membrane surface. This is compatible with the sequence postulated in Ref. 13 and Fig. 1, placing one histidine and one or two tyrosines at the external surface where they might be labeled by the peroxidase technique.

(b) Peptide mapping after lactoperoxidase-catalyzed radioiodination (20) reveals two iodinated peptides unique to T_M. One can be assigned to the 54–70 stretch, containing tyrosines 67 and 69. As there are no other tyrosines, and as histidine can be iodinated, the second peptide can only be assigned to the 12–39 stretch bearing histidine 29 (cleavage at R^{15} is blocked by p^{16}).

(c) The SV40-coded pI 4.7/M_r 94,000 membrane protein is glycosylated (18–20). This is compatible with the fact that only one of the two peptides labeled by lactoperoxidase-catalyzed radioiodination is marked also after metabolic sugar labeling. This is the peptide assigned to the 12–40 sequence containing S-H-T-T. The data are compatible with the localization of this sequence at the external plasma membrane face.

According to work with other systems (2, 8, 18), sugars ending up at the external plasma membrane face are attached, mostly cotranslationally in rough endoplasmic reticulum cisternae, including nuclear envelope. Initiated oligosaccharides are often completed in the Golgi apparatus before being externalized at the cell surface. The data are compatible with O-glycosylation (16) of serine and/or threonine and can account for the demonstration of the SV40-specific pI 4.7/M_r 94,000 protein in association with nuclear envelope, by direct fractionation (17), and in the perinculear and Golgi regions by immune fluorescence (11).

It is important to define the mechanisms responsible for membrane anomalies in oncogenesis. Available data are compatible with the proposal of Mark and Berg (13) but do not prove it. However this hypothesis, the model derived therefrom (Fig. 1) and postulated mechanisms of membrane insertion can be tested unambiguously by the following:

(a) Analysis of SV40-specific tryptic peptides derived from plasma membranes of transformed cells after surface radioiodination or sugar-labeling, using thermolysin cleavage, peptide mapping and amino acid sequencing. (b) Chymotrypsin treatment of

[35]S-labeled plasma membranes from the cytoplasmic side, cleaving at Trp[647], to release most of the sequence common to T and T*, leaving the D_4-E-D sequence attached and recoverable as N-S-D_4-E-D-S-Q-G-M-K-. (c) Demonstration of the body of T*, the sequences in common with T, at the cytoplasmic faces of rough endoplasmic reticulum, nuclear envelope and Golgi membranes, and unique iodinatable/glycosylated T* peptides at the cisternal faces of these organelles. (d) Cell-free translation of early SV40 mRNA in a system (2) that supports and monitors membrane protein insertion and glycosylation and analysis of the peptide disposition of inserted protein. These studies are in progress.

REFERENCES

1. Anderson, J. L., Chang, C., Mora, P. T., and Martin, R. G. *J. Virol.*, **21**, 459–467 (1976).
2. Braell, N. A. and Lodish, H. F. *Cell*, **28**, 23–31 (1982).
3. Chang, C., Pancake, S. J., Luborsky, S. W., and Mora, P. T. *Int. J. Cancer*, **19**, 258–266 (1977).
4. Chang, C., Martin, R. G., Livingston, D. M., Luborsky, S. W., Hu, C.-P., and Mora, P. T. *J. Virol.*, **29**, 69–75 (1979).
5. Crawford, L. V. *Trends Biochem. Sci.* **5**, 39–42 (1980).
6. Crawford, L. V., Pim, D. C., Goodfellow, P., and Taylor-Papadimitrou, J. *Proc. Natl. Acad. Sci. U.S.*, **78**, 41–45 (1981).
7. Engelman, D. M., Henderson, R., McLachlan, A. D., and Wallace, B. A. *Proc. Natl. Acad. Sci. U.S.*, **77**, 2023–2027 (1980).
8. Engelman, D. M. and Steitz, T. A. *Cell*, **23**, 411–422 (1981).
9. Harlow, Ed., Crawford, L. V., Pim, D. C., and Williamson, N. M. *J. Virol.*, **37**, 861–869 (1981).
10. Ito, Y. and Spurr, N. *Cold Spring Harbor Symp. Quant. Biol.*, **44**, 149–157 (1979).
11. Lin, P.-S., Schmidt-Ullrich, R., Thompson, W. S., and Wallach, D.F.H. *Proc. Natl. Acad. Sci. U.S.*, **74**, 2495–2499 (1977).
12. Luborsky, S. W., Chang, C., Pancake, S. J., and Mora, P. T. *Cancer Res.*, **38**, 2367–2371 (1978).
13. Mark, D. F. and Berg, H. P. *Cold Spring Harbor Symp. Quant. Biol.*, **44**, 55–62 (1979).
14. Reddy, V. B., Ghosh, P. K., Lebowitz, P., Piatak, M., and Weisman, S. M. *J. Virol.*, **30**, 279–296 (1979).
15. Santos, M. and Butel, J. S. *Virology*, **120**, 1–17 (1982).
16. Schachter, H. and Williams, D. *In* "Mucus in Health and Disease," ed. E. N. Chantler, J. B. Elder, and M. Elstein, pp. 3–27 (1982). Plenum Publishing, New York.
17. Schmidt-Ullrich, R., Thompson, W. S., Lin, P.-S., and Wallach, D.F.H. *Proc. Natl. Acad. Sci. U.S.*, **74**. 5069–5072 (1977).
18. Schmidt-Ullrich, R., Thompson, W. S., and Wallach, D.F.H. *Biochem. Biophys. Res. Commun.*, **88**, 887–894 (1979).
19. Schmidt-Ullrich, R., Kahn, S. J., Thompson, W. S., and Wallach, D.F.H. *J. Natl. Cancer Inst.*, **65**, 585–593 (1980).
20. Schmidt-Ullrich, R., Kahn, S., Thompson, W. S., Monroe, M. T., and Wallach, D.F.H. *J. Natl. Cancer Inst.*, **69**, 839–849 (1982).
21. Soule, H. R. and Butel, J. S. *J. Virol.*, **30**, 523–532 (1979).
22. Soeda, E. J., Arrand, R., Smolar, N., and Griffin, B. E. *Cell*, **17**, 357–365 (1979).
23. Tenen, D. G., Martin, R. G., Anderson, J., and Livingston, D. M. *J. Virol.*, **22**, 210–218 (1978).

24. Tooze, J. (ed.). "DNA Tumor Viruses," 2nd Ed., Vol. 2 (1980). Cold Spring Harbor
     Laboratory, Cold Spring Harbor.

PROPERTIES OF MOLECULAR FORMS OF γ-GLUTAMYL TRANSPEPTIDASE AND URIDINE DIPHOSPHATE-GLUCURONYLTRANSFERASE AS HEPATIC PRENEOPLASTIC MARKER ENZYMES

Kiyomi SATO,[*1] Shigeki TSUCHIDA,[*1,*2] Fusako WARAGAI,[*1]
Zongzhu YIN,[*1,*3] and Tetsunori EBINA[*1]

Second Department of Biochemistry[*1] *and First Department of Internal Medicine,*[*2] *Hirosaki University School of Medicine*

Molecular forms and their properties of γ-glutamyl transpeptidase (γGTP) (bound to plasma membrane) and uridine diphosphate-glucuronyltransferase (UDP-GT) (bound to microsomal membrane) induced during rat chemical hepatocarcinogenesis are reviewed from the viewpoint of preneoplastic marker enzymes. Their altered patterns are compared along with those of other marker enzymes.

The activity of γGTP, a glycoprotein, increases markedly with the appearance of preneoplastic foci and hyperplastic nodules during chemical hepatocarcinogenesis. A comparison of subunit structures, immunological properties, isoelectric points before and after neuraminidase treatment and the affinity for concanavalin A (Con A)-Sepharose between γGTPs from the nodules and primary and transplantable hepatomas and those from normal adult kidney and from fetal liver, suggests that the molecular form of γGTP may alter during hepatocarcinogenesis not in the protein portion but in the sugar portion. There may be variability among hepatomas. A similar investigation on human hepatoma supported the above conclusion.

The activity of the late fetal form (enzyme 1) of UDP-GT assayed with *o*-aminophenol (*o*-GT) is increased in hyperplastic nodules and in well differentiated hepatomas but is decreased in poorly differentiated hepatomas, while the activity of the neonatal form (enzyme 2), assayed with phenolphthalein (*p*-GT), changes little or decreases from the nodule during hepatocarcinogenesis. *o*-GT and *p*-GT, inducible by a hepatocarcinogen, diethylnitrosamine or phenobarbital, differed from each other in induction pattern, molecular weight, pI, and kinetic properties but were similar immunologically.

Chemical carcinogenesis in the liver as well as in other tissues is supposed to proceed through at least two stages, initiation and promotion, as first proposed by Berenblum (*1*) on skin carcinogenesis. During the promotion stage in chemical hepatocarcinogenesis, specific cell populations such as enzyme-altered foci and hyperplastic nodules are observed and considered as preneoplastic cell populations (*5*). Hyperplastic nodules can be observed macroscopically, while enzyme-altered foci are detectable microscopi-

[*1,*2] Zaifucho 5, Hirosaki 036, Japan (佐藤清美, 土田成紀, 藁谷房子, 尹　宗柱, 蝦名鉄徳).
[*3] Present address: Yanbian Medical College, Yanji, The People's Republic of China.

K. SATO ET AL.

TABLE I. Marker Enzymes for Preneoplastic Hepatic Cells[a]

  (I) Enzymes with decreased activity
     G6Pase (microsome) (and other hepatic marker enzymes)
     Ca^{2+}, Mg^{2+}-ATPase (canalicular membrane)
     Glycogen phosphorylase (resulting in glycogen storage)
     Cytochrome P-450 (microsome)
     Aryl hydrocarbon hydroxylase (AHH) (microsome)
     β-Glucuronidase (lysosomal membrane)
  (II) Enzymes with increased activity (fetal or prototypic isozymes)
     γGTP (plasma membrane)
     Butyrylesterase (L-1) (microsome)
     EH (same as preoplastic antigen?) (microsome)
     UDP-GT (microsome): o-GT (fetal form)
     GST (cytosol): A-form

[a] Modified from the review by Farber and Cameron (5).

cally by histochemical staining of certain enzymes known as preneoplastic marker enzymes. Many enzymes have been considered as such marker enzymes (5) (Table I). They are divided into two groups: enzymes with decreased activity are in one group and many hepatic marker enzymes such as glucose-6-phosphatase (G6Pase) are included. Enzymes with increased activity are included in the other group and have more or less fetal characteristics. It should be noted that most of these enzymes are bound to membranes such as plasma-, microsomal-, and lysosomal-membranes.

Among these enzymes, γ-glutamyl transpeptidase (γGTP) is known as one of the most useful hepatic marker enzymes; some drug-metabolizing enzymes such as cytochrome P-450 in group I and epoxide hydrase (EH) in group II are also included.

We have been investigating enzyme alteration during rat chemical hepatocarcinogenesis to detect new marker enzyme forms for hepatic preneoplastic cell populations among drug-metabolizing enzymes, especially detoxicating enzymes related to chemical carcinogenesis. Chemical hepatocarcinogenesis may depend on a balance between activation and detoxication reactions of chemical carcinogens in vivo. We have found that the fetal form of uridine diphosphate-glucuronyltransferase (UDP-GT) and the A-form of glutathione (GSH) S-transferase (GST) (in cytosol) are new molecular forms of marker enzymes (Table I).

In this paper, properties of molecular forms of two membrane-bound enzymes, γGTP (bound to plasma membrane) and UDP-GT (bound to microsomal membrane) which we have characterized as hepatic preneoplastic marker enzymes are reviewed.

γGTP

1. The induction pattern of γGTP during hepatocarcinogenesis

It is well known that γGTP activity markedly increases during chemical hepatocarcinogenesis with the appearance of preneoplastic hepatic cell populations such as enzyme-altered foci and hyperplastic nodules (5, 15, 21). The increase is considered one of the most useful markers for the histochemical detection of these cell populations, although it is reported that the enzyme is absent and can not be a marker enzyme in the nodules and hepatomas induced by some chemicals (13). The increased activity is retained in hepatomas with no apparent relation to the degree of tissue differentiation or to the rate of growth of the hepatoma (15) (see also Fig. 3).

2. Properties of γGTP in hyperplastic nodules and hepatomas

It is also known that γGTP is a glycoprotein and has oncofetal properties (6, 20, 21). γGTP activity in fetal liver increases at the termination of gestation but after birth it decreases rapidly to a very low level in the adult liver. This activity re-elevates with aging in certain rat strains (9). However, it is not known whether there are true isozymes of this enzyme consisting of different peptide chains in hepatomas or in normal tissues. γGTP is a membrane-bound enzyme, and two forms have been purified: one is the detergent-solubilized form (D-form) and the other is the protease (bromelain or papain)-solubilized form (P-form). We demonstrated (21) and others confirmed (26) that P-forms purified from hyperplastic nodules and hepatomas are immunologically identical in activity inhibition and in double diffusion tests to the form from kidney, which has the highest activity among normal adult rat tissues. Furthermore, they have subunit structures consisting of heavy (H) and light (L) chains (subunits) similar to those of the kidney enzyme as seen by sodium dodecylsulfate-polyacrylamide gel electrophoresis (SDS-PAGE), though H-subunits of D-forms from nodules and hepatomas were slightly larger than that of the kidney enzyme (23). The H- and L-subunits of P-form from hepatoma are also identical to those of the kidney enzyme, as shown by double immunodiffusion (21). However, γGTP (P-forms) purified from hyperplastic nodules and primary hepatomas, differed from the kidney enzyme in their isoelectric point (pI) on isoelectric focusing in polyacrylamide gel, apparently because of different contents of sialic acid (21). As also seen by isoelectric focusing using cellulose acetate membrane (Fig. 1), kidney γGTP (P-form) shows a microheterogeneity, while γGTPs from hyperplastic nodules and primary hepatomas as well as from fetal liver, except for AH 13, have almost single

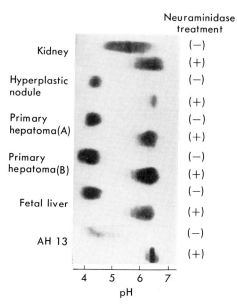

FIG. 1. Isoelectric focusing of γGTPs (P-form) on cellulose acetate membrane.

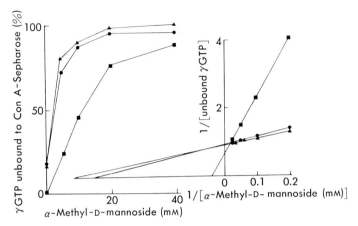

FIG. 2. Affinity of γGTPs from kidney, primary and transplantable hepatomas for
Con A-Sepharose in the absence or presence of α-methyl-D-mannoside at various
concentrations. The procedure was carried out as described in Ref. 8. ▲ primary
hepatoma; ● kidney; ■ AH 13.

forms which are more acidic than any forms of kidney enzyme. After neuraminidase
treatment the differences between kidney and other γGTPs were reduced, though mi-
croheterogeneities were still or newly observed. Furthermore, H- and L-subunits of
kidney P-form showed multiple forms, having more alkaline pIs than those of hepatomas
(unpublished data). According to these results and other data, we have suggested that
γGTPs from nodules and hepatomas may differ not in the protein portion but in the
sugar portion from the kidney enzyme and may be similar to fetal liver enzyme (21).
Sialic acid may be one of the factors causing multimolecular forms of this enzyme.

As γGTPs in hyperplastic nodules and hepatomas are immunologically indistinguishable from the kidney enzyme, we have devised a method for purification of P-forms
and D-forms of γGTPs from the nodules and hepatomas as well as from the kidney by
immunoaffinity column chromatography using Sepharose 4B coupled with the antibody
against the P-form of kidney γGTP (23). After solubilization with Triton-X 100 and
treatment without and with papain, both D- and P-forms could be purified very effectively using this antibody column (23). This method is especially useful for the purification of γGTP from tissues with low activities.

γGTP from an ascites hepatoma AH 13, which had the maximum activity of all
γGTP hepatomas that we have examined, showed a heterogeneity on isoelectric focusing
without neuraminidase treatment (Fig. 1). γGTP from AH 13 also differed not only from
kidney enzymes but also those from primary hepatoma in that it had a higher affinity for
concanavalin A (Con A)-Sepharose than did the others, as shown in Fig. 2. These results
together with those reported by others (26) indicate that the sugar portion differs between primary (solid) and ascites (free cell) hepatomas and that ascites hepatomas such
as AH 13 exhibit much deviated phenotypes even in the sugar portion. However, it
should be also considered that phenotypes in the sugar portion of hepatomas may vary
according to their growing situations, i.e., dependent on a solid or ascites state.

3. *Comparison of γGTP from human hepatoma and non-hepatoma tissue*
    To investigate changes in molecular forms of γGTP during hepatocarcinogenesis,

TABLE II. A Comparison of γGTP Properties of Human Hepatoma and
Non-hepatoma Tissues of the Liver

	Hepatoma	Non-hepatoma
Activity		
1. Homogenate		
units/g tissue	4.00	3.65
units/mg protein	0.027	0.024
2. Purified P-form		
units/mg protein	403	440
Properties of P-form		
1. Molecular weight		
L-chain	26,000	26,000
H-chain	64,000	64,000
2. pI		
Before neuraminidase treatment	3.7–3.9	3.7–3.9
After neuraminidase treatment	5.7	5.7
3. Mobility on PAGE	Same	
4. Amino acid composition	Same	
5. Glucosamine (nmol/mg protein)	362	125
6. Amounts bound to lectins		
to Con A	Lower	Higher
WGA	Higher	Lower
PHA	Higher	Lower
CB	Higher	Lower

WGA, wheat germ agglutinin; PHA, phytohemagglutinin; CB, castor bean lectin (RCA-120).

γGTPs from hyperplastic nodules and hepatomas should be compared more precisely in their protein and sugar structures with γGTP from normal liver, because recently it was reported that γGTP from rat pancreas is immunologically indistinguishable from kidney γGTP but differs from the latter in amino acid composition (19). Though γGTP activity is very low in normal adult rat liver, in normal adult human liver it is significantly high; accordingly we compared γGTP from primary human hepatoma with that from non-hepatoma tissue in the same liver and from apparently normal liver. Results are summarized in Table II. It is noticed that γGTP activity in the non-hepatoma tissue as well as in normal human liver (data not shown) is very high and comparable to the activity in hepatoma. γGTP from hepatoma and non-hepatoma did not show any significant differences in molecular weight, pIs before and after neuraminidase treatment, mobility on PAGE, or amino acid composition. But they showed significant differences in glucosamine content and in the amounts bound to lectins, again suggesting that the molecular alteration of γGTP may occur not in the protein portion but in the sugar portion even in human hepatocarcinogenesis.

Clinically, multiple forms of γGTP are observed in human serum and a novel γGTP isozyme has been reported in sera of patients bearing primary hepatomas (17). According to our investigation (22), multiple forms in human serum are due to differences in molecular size and in charge but are immunologically indistinguishable from the kidney γGTP, though the apparent immunological properties differ according to their molecular size. Sawabu et al. (16) have also reported that the novel γGTP isozyme is immunologically indistinguishable from human kidney γGTP.

The function of γGTP induced during chemical hepatocarcinogenesis has not yet been clarified. As mentioned above, γGTP activity increases with appearance of pre-neoplastic cell populations. However, it has also been reported that γGTP activity is not increased in spontaneous C3H mouse hepatomas but is increased in hepatomas induced by the administration of phenobarbital (PB) to the mice (*10*). Therefore, the increasing activity of γGTP during chemical hepatocarcinogenesis seems to be due to the induction by drugs, including carcinogens administered to animals. Meister (*12*) proposed that γGTP may participate in amino acid incorporation into cells as one of the enzymes in the γ-glutamyl cycle in the kidney. However, this possibility is unlikely in transplantable hepatoma (*7*). It is known, on the other hands, that γGTP participates in the formation of mercapturic acid (*3*). This pathway is initiated by the conjugation reaction between GSH and electrophilic compounds catalyzed by GST, whose activity is also increased in hyperplastic nodules and in well differentiated hepatomas (*11, 14*). Thus, γGTP in preneoplastic cells and hepatomas should be investigated more precisely as one of the drug-metabolizing enzymes.

UDP-GT

1. Developmental patterns of UDP-GTs in rat liver

It has been suggested that there are at least two molecular species of UDP-GT in the liver (*4*). One is the late fetal form or enzyme 1, which increases at the terminal stage of gestation and is known to be induced by 3-methylcholanthrene (3-MC). The other is the neonatal form or enzyme 2, inducible by PB, as was confirmed by us (*25*) with *o*-aminophenol as substrate for enzyme 1 and with phenolphthalein for enzyme 2. The UDP-GT activity towards *o*-aminophenol (*o*-GT) increases with development of fetal liver, displays maximum activity at the termination of gestation and then declines rapidly but remains at a significant level in the adult liver. The activity of the enzyme towards phenolphthalein (*p*-GT) increases after the birth of rats and approaches maximum at 2 to 3 weeks, then declines slowly to the adult level (*25*).

2. Changes in molecular forms of UDP-GT in hepatocarcinogenesis

Changes in molecular forms of UDP-GT were examined during the induction of enzyme-altered foci or hyperplastic nodules by the system of Solt and Farber (*18*). A clear relationship exists between increased *o*-GT activity and the increased number of foci in individual samples (*25*). However, there is no relationship between *p*-GT activity and the number of foci, though the activity is elevated in livers from all rats treated by various procedures. Furthermore, as shown in Fig. 3, even in isolated large hyperplastic nodules and well differentiated hepatomas, *o*-GT activity is markedly increased, whereas *p*-GT activity tends to fall below the level of normal liver. It should be noted that no carcinogen such as diethylnitrosamine (DEN) or N-2-fluorenylacetamide (FAA), which directly affects the level of UDP-GT activity, was given to the rats when they were killed to obtain these nodules and hepatomas.

3. Properties of UDP-GTs

Although two forms of UDP-GT inducible by 3-MC or PB were purified by Bock *et al.* (*2*), we also purified the two forms, especially *o*-GT from the liver from DEN-injected rats using a hydrophobic column, amino-hexyl Sepharose 4B after solubilizing membrane-bound forms with cholate (*24*). The final preparations thus obtained contained

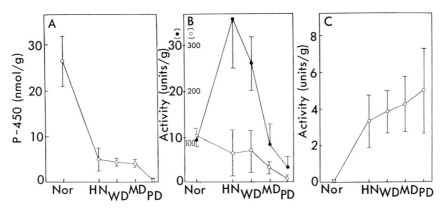

FIG. 3. Changes in the content of cytochrome P-450 and activities of UDP-GTs and γGTP during rat chemical hepatocarcinogenesis. A, P-450; B, UDP-GT; C, γGTP. Nor, normal liver; HN, hyperplastic nodules; WD, MD and PD, well-, moderately-, and poorly-differentiated hepatomas, respectively. B, ● o-GT; ○ p-GT.

TABLE III. A Comparison of Properties of o-GT and p-GT (14, 24, 25)

	Properties	o-GT	p-GT
1.	Developmental	Late fetal form	Neonatal form
2.	Induction		
	a) By (in short term)	3-MC, DEN, FAA, BHA	PB
	b) In carcinogenesis		
	i) Hyperplastic nodule	Much increased	Slightly increased
	ii) Hepatoma	Increased[a]	Decreased
3.	Physico-chemical		
	Molecular weight (SDS-PAGE)	54,000	54,000–58,000
	pI	6.2	6.6
4.	Catalytic		
	Effector		
	Triton X-100	Activated	Activated
	Na-cholate	Activated	Inhibited
	DEN	Activated	Inhibited
5.	Immunological		
	a) Double diffusion	Identical	
	b) Activity inhibition by IgG to o-GT	Much inhibited	Inhibited

[a] Increased in well-differentiated hepatomas, but decreased in poorly-differentiated ones.
BHA, butylated hydroxyanisole (an antioxidant).

two proteins on SDS-PAGE (24). These two proteins were separated by isoelectric focusing and were identified as o-GT and p-GT (24). A comparison of the properties of the two forms is summarized in Table III. They differed in molecular weight, pI, and kinetic properties. Though the two forms could not be distinguished by a double immunodiffusion method, they were slightly different in activity inhibition by the antibody against o-GT, and hyperplastic nodules were stained more densely than the non-nodular areas using this antibody (data not shown).

Deviation Patterns of Other Enzymes during Hepatocarcinogenesis

Three typical patterns of other marker enzymes we examined are shown in Fig. 3. In hyperplastic nodules and hepatomas isolated at 10 or more weeks after the removal of carcinogen(s) from the diet, cytochrome P-450, one of the activating enzymes, was markedly decreased. Accordingly this enzyme is considered to be one of the enzymes with decreased activity listed in Table I, whereas γGTP activity was markedly increased from hyperplastic nodules during hepatocarcinogenesis and was retained at high levels in hepatomas with apparently no relation to the differentiation of hepatoma. *o*-GT of UDP-GT was increased in hyperplastic nodules and in well-differentiated hepatomas but rapidly decreased with dedifferentiation of hepatoma, while *p*-GT gradually decreased.

Changes in preneoplastic marker enzyme activities examined during chemical hepatocarcinogenesis are summarized schematically in Fig. 4. At the initiation stage, both activating and detoxicating enzymes fluctuate but the responses are not specific for hepatocarcinogenesis. However, with the appearance of enzyme-altered foci and hyperplastic nodules, activating enzymes such as P-450 and other hepatic marker enzymes rapidly decrease, while detoxicating enzymes, especially some specific molecular forms such as *o*-GT of UDP-GT increase. The A-form of GST and epoxide hydrase (EH), which has been reported to be a preneoplastic antigen (5), markedly increase. However, they again decrease with dedifferentiation of the hepatoma. Thus, they can be considered as preneoplastic marker enzymes. γGTP also increases from hyperplastic nodules but is retained during dedifferentiation of hepatoma. The fetal isozymes of glycolysis such as hexokinase and pyruvate kinase are increased markedly only in poorly differentiated hepatomas (15).

It has not yet been clarified whether or not these marker enzymes are actually functioning in preneoplastic cells. However, these cells are known to be resistant to cytotoxic agents such as carcinogens (5), and so decreased activities of activating enzymes and increased activities of detoxicating enzymes may have some roles in the mechanism of resistance of these cells that may affect cell growth through selection.

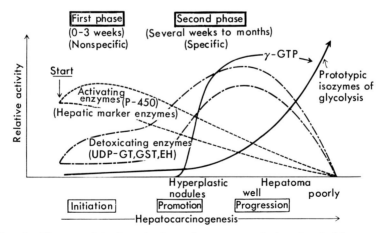

FIG. 4.   Changes of (pre)neoplastic marker enzymes during chemical hepatocarcinogenesis. Abbreviations used are described in Table I.

Acknowledgments

We thank Dr. Nobuyuki Ito and Dr. Hiroyuki Tsuda of Nagoya City University School of Medicine for their histological examination of tissues. We also thanks Dr. Masahiko Endo and Dr. Hajime Matsue of the First Department of Biochemistry of our medical school for analyses of sugars and amino acids of γGTPs.

This work was supported in part by Grants-in-Aid for Cancer Research from the Ministry of Education, Science and Culture of Japan.

REFERENCES

1. Berenblum, I. *Cancer Res.*, **14**, 471–477 (1954).
2. Bock, K. W., Josting, D., Lilienblum, W., and Pfeil, H. *Eur. J. Biochem.*, **98**, 19–26 (1979).
3. Chasseaud, L. F. *Adv. Cancer Res.*, **29**, 175–274 (1979).
4. Dutton, G. J. "Glucuronidation of Drugs and Other Compounds" (1980). CRC Press, Florida.
5. Farber, E. and Cameron, R. *Adv. Cancer Res.*, **31**, 125–226 (1980).
6. Ibsen, K. H. and Fishman, W. H. *Biochim. Biophys. Acta*, **560**, 243–280 (1979).
7. Inoue, M., Horiuchi, S., and Morino, Y. *Eur. J. Biochem.*, **78**, 609–615 (1977).
8. Iwama, K., Yasumoto, K., Fushiki, I., Takigawa, Y., and Mitsuda, H. *J. Biochem.*, **84**, 1237–1243 (1978).
9. Kitagawa, T., Imai, F., and Sato, K. *Gann*, **71**, 362–366 (1980).
10. Kitagawa, T., Watanabe, R., and Sugano, H. *Gann*, **71**, 536–542 (1980).
11. Kitahara, A., Satoh, K., and Sato, K. *Biochem. Biophys. Res. Commun.*, **112**, 20–28 (1983).
12. Meister, A. *Science*, **180**, 33–39 (1973).
13. Rao, M. S., Lalwani, N. D., Scarpelli, D. G., and Roddy, J. K. *Carcinogenesis*, **3**, 1231–1233 (1982).
14. Sato, K., Kitahara, A., Yin, Z., Ebina, T., Satoh, K., Hatayama, I., Nishimura, K., Yamazaki, T., Tsuda, H., Ito, N., and Dempo, K. *Ann. N.Y. Acad. Sci.*, in press.
15. Sato, K., Hatayama, I., Hoshino, K., Imai, F., Tsuchida, S., Sato, T., Nishimura, K., Tatematsu, M., and Ito, N. *Cancer Res.*, **41**, 4147–4153 (1981).
16. Sawabu, N., Toya, D., Ozaki, K., Wakabayashi, T. Nakagen, M., and Hattori, N. This volume, pp. 291–298.
17. Sawabu, N., Nakagen, M., Yoneda, M., Makino, H., Kameda, S., Kobayashi, K., Hattori, N., and Ishii, N. *Gann*, **69**, 601–605 (1978).
18. Solt, D. and Farber, E. *Nature*, **263**, 701–703 (1976).
19. Takahashi, S., Steinman, H. M., and Ball, D. *Biochim. Biophys. Acta*, **707**, 66–73 (1982).
20. Taniguchi, N., Saito, K., and Takakuwa, E. *Biochim. Biophys. Acta*, **391**, 265–271 (1975).
21. Tsuchida, S., Hoshino, K., Sato, T., Ito, N., and Sato, K. *Cancer Res.*, **39**, 4200–4205 (1979).
22. Tsuchida, S., Imai, F., and Sato, K. *J. Biochem.*, **89**, 775–782 (1981).
23. Tsuchida, S. and Sato, K. *Biochim. Biophys. Acta*, **756**, 341–348 (1983).
24. Yin, Z. *Hirosaki Med. J.*, **34**, 677–701 (1982) (in Japanese).
25. Yin, Z., Sato, K., Tsuda, H., and Ito, N. *Gann*, **73**, 239–248 (1982).
26. Yokosawa, N., Taniguchi, N., Tukada, Y., and Makita, A. *Oncodev. Biol. Med.*, **2**, 165–177 (1981).

II. MEMBRANE PHENOMENA
IN TUMOR CELLS

METASTATIC TUMOR CELL ATTACHMENT TO VASCULAR ENDOTHELIAL CELLS AND DESTRUCTION OF THEIR BASAL LAMINA-LIKE MATRIX

Tatsuro Irimura, Motowo Nakajima, and
Garth L. Nicolson

Department of Tumor Biology, The University of Texas System Cancer Center,
*M. D. Anderson Hospital and Tumor Institute**

Important steps in blood-borne tumor metastasis are the attachment of circulating malignant cells to the vascular endothelium and subsequent penetration of the endothelial cell layer and underlying basal lamina. Using cultured vascular endothelial cells we have found that metastatic cells attach more strongly and rapidly to the endothelial basal lamina-like matrix than to the apical surface of endothelial cells. This difference may be due, in part, to the exclusive presence of adhesive molecules such as fibronectin in the matrix. Tumor cell surface glycoproteins also appear to be involved, because blocking their appearance on metastatic cell surfaces with tunicamycin inhibits malignant cell binding to endothelial cells or their matrix and abolishes blood-borne implantation properties. During invasion metastatic cells degrade the basal lamina-like matrix using proteases and glycosidases. The release of [^{35}S] sulfate-labeled glycosaminoglycans from the endothelial matrix and degradation of a purified lung heparan sulfate substrate correlates with the metastatic properties of a series of malignant murine melanoma sublines. Analysis of the heparan sulfate degradation products indicates that one of these melanoma enzymes is capable of cleaving heparan sulfate at intrachain glucuronoside linkages producing its intermediate molecular weight fragment.

Of the important and life threatening properties of cancer cells, the most critical are their abilities to invade surrounding tissues and metastasize to distant organ sites. Metastasis accounts for the vast majority of cancer related deaths, and though primary cancer is often quite treatable by surgery alone or in combination with other therapeutic modalities, treatment of metastatic cancer has remained one of the most difficult tasks facing the clinical oncologist (*46, 65*).

In several species, including man, there are numerous examples of maligant tumors metastasizing to specific, distant secondary sites where the metastatic tumor colonies grow and ultimately kill their host (*46, 65*). Although most regional metastases can be explained strictly on anatomical or mechanical considerations such as efferent venous and lymphatic drainage or presence of large tumor cell emboli in these vessels (*65*), distant organ colonization often does not follow this pattern (*46*). This suggests that distant metastasis requires recognition of target organ cells or stroma by metastatic cells (*46*), or

* Houston, Texas 77030, U.S.A. (入村達郎, 中島元夫).

selective survival and/or growth at specific distant sites (25), or a combination of these (46).

The development of metastases is the result of a complex series of unique interactions between tumor and host tissues and cells. There are several properties of malignant cells that appear to be required for the successful completion of each step of the metastatic process, such as: invasion of surrounding normal tissues, penetration of blood and/or lymphatic vessels, dislodgement from the primary tumor mass, transport in lymph or blood to regional lymph nodes or distant capillaries, arrest and invasion at these sites, and survival and growth to form gross secondary lesions (15, 25, 46, 55, 65). In addition, the ability of malignant cells to escape from host defense mechanisms may be another important characteristic of metastatic cells (15, 46).

Malignant tumors are composed of heterogenous mixtures of cells possessing widely different metastatic potentials (14, 46, 49). Because of this heterogeneity cell sublines with unique metastatic properties can be obtained using selection techniques (46, 55). For example, Fidler (10) selected murine B16 melanoma cells for their increased abilities to colonize lung after intravenous inoculation, and after ten sequential selections obtained a subline (B16-F10) which possessed high lung colonization potential. Similar in vivo selection procedures have yielded B16 melanoma sublines with high ovary (B16-O13) (3) or brain (B16-B15b) (40) colonization potentials. Using in vitro selection procedures a highly metastatic subline possessing increased potential for tissue invasion (B16-BL6) has also been obtained (24, 57).

Malignant cell surface properties appear to be very important in at least certain events of metastasis such as blood-borne tumor cell implantation in the microcirculation. In support of this are experiments where the surface membranes of cells of low metastatic potential have been modified by fusion and incorporation of plasma membrane in the form of vesicles released spontaneously from cells of high metastatic potential. The vesicle-modified tumor cells transiently and specifically display enhance arrest and experimental metastasis formation compared to the unmodified tumor cells or cells modified by fusion with vesicles shed from low metastatic potential cells (56). In addition, there are numerous examples where cell surface differences in the display, dynamics, amounts, or structures of cell proteins/glycoproteins exist between tumor cell sublines selected in vivo or in vitro for altered metastatic properties (46).

During blood-borne metastasis the most important steps are probably the attachment of the circulating malignant cells to the vascular endothelium and their subsequent extravasation out of the blood vessel and invasion into surrounding tissues. The interactions between metastatic tumor cells and vascular endothelium have been extensively studied using cultured endothelial cell monolayers. These cell monolayers are well contact inhibited, and they synthesize an underlying basal lamina-like structure containing collagens, glycoproteins such as fibronectin and laminin, and proteoglycans (1, 38, 58). We have been particularly interested in the proteoglycans of the endothelial matrix, because proteoglycans and/or their sugar side chains (glycosaminoglycans) are important constituents of the endothelial basal lamina and are known to be uniquely distributed in various organs (9, 68). The mechanisms by which metastatic cells attach to vascular endothelial cells and their underlying matrix, as well as their abilities to invade and degrade these structures, may be important in determining preferences of distant metastasis.

Interactions of Blood-borne Metastatic Tumor Cells with Host Cells

Metastatic tumor cells in the circulation have the potential of forming distant metastases, but few cells survive to colonize organ sites. Fidler (*12*) has determined that fewer than 0.1 % of ^{125}IUDR-labeled B16 melanoma cells eventually survive to form experimental lung tumor colonies after their entry into the blood, indicating that metastasis is an inefficient process. Before lodgement at specific organ sites, blood-borne tumor cells interact with a wide variety of blood cells and blood components (*15, 46*). Some of these cellular interactions, such as those with natural killer (NK) cells, may be effective in eliminating malignant cells from the circulation (*22, 23*), while other interactions may actually increase the chance of arrest, survival and metastatic colonization. For example, homotypic interactions with other tumor cells (*44, 48*) heterotypic interactions with platelets (*18, 53*), lymphocytes (*11, 13*), or soluble blood components (*16*) can increase the chance of successful metastatic colonization. Since many tumor cells are thromboplastic, they can elicit fibrin formation during blood-borne transport or soon after their arrest in capillary beds (*4, 5, 71*). During blood-borne arrest fibrin clots can form around the embolus (*5*), and under certain conditions this can result in vessel wall damage and accumulation of neutrophils (*71*) or platelets (*26*). Various drugs which induce thrombocytopenia or reduce fibrin formation can decrease metastasis in many but not all malignant systems (*16, 19, 27, 66*). Finally, circulating tumor cells can interact with the vascular endothelium resulting in their attachment or implantation (next section).

After escape out of the circulatory compartment, metastatic tumor cells interact with parenchymal cells and the stroma of organs. These interactions have been estimated *in vitro* using various experimental approaches. By measuring the abilities of B16 cells to heterotypically adhere to suspended organ cells we have found that lung colonizing B16 cells adhere at faster rates to lung than to other organ cells (*47*), and using small pieces of organ tissue we have noted that different organ-selected melanoma lines display differing abilities to attach and invade tissues such as lung, ovary and heart (*46*). Other experiments on organ selective cell aggregation have been reported recently by Phondke *et al.* (*54*). Using leukemia cells that colonize spleen they found that the leukemia cells bind to spleen but not to isolated lung cells (*54*). Additionally, Schirrmacher *et al.* (*60*) have determined that liver colonizing mouse lymphoma cells adhere to hepatocytes in relation to their metastatic properties. The actual mechanisms of these cellular interactions are unknown, but, they can only be possible after the malignant cells have penetrated through the vascular endothelium and its underlying basal lamina.

There have been several studies on the interactions of metastatic tumor cells with culture substratum. Unfortunately, these studies probably bear little relationship to the important adhesive events that occur *in vivo* during metastasis, even in experiments where adhesive properties correlated well with metastasis formation. For example, adhesion of MCB-31 carcinoma cells to glass surfaces correlates inversely with metastatic potential (*6*), while B16 melanoma (*2*) or fibrosarcoma cells (*70*) resistant to removal from culture substratum by ethylenediamine tetraacetic acid (EDTA) or trypsin treatment are more metastatic when assayed *in vivo*. Such desparate results suggest wide differences in the properties of the experimental systems used to study metastasis. Although Varani *et al.* (*70*) have found a correlation between attachment to plastic surfaces or detachment from endothelial cell monolayers and metastasis, projecting such experimental results to the *in vivo* situation is not easily achieved.

Endothelial cells are the first cell type encountered at sites where tumor cells initiate distant blood-borne organ colonization. This type of interaction could well be specific, because endothelial cells from different locations appear to possess unique characteristics that may determine their tissue origin. This has been suggested by our experiments where brain colonizing B16 melanoma cells attach at higher rates to murine brain endothelial cells compared to murine lung endothelial cells (45). Each organ may therefore have its own recognition system based on unique vascular cell determinants.

Metastatic Tumor Cell Attachment to Endothelial Cells and Their Basal Lamina-like Matrix

Blood-borne tumor cells usually escape rapidly from the blood circulation after their implantation at distant sites. If they remain in the blood vessels, detachment and re-circulation can occur. During each passage through the circulatory system simple mechanical or shear forces and transcapillary distortions probably result in significant loss in cell viabilities (46, 59). It follows that stable attachment to the vascular endothelium and subsequent penetration of this structure should allow a greater chance for survival.

It has been shown that metastatic tumor cells possess greater affinities to basal lamina-like matrix made by endothelial cells than to the apical surface of the endothelial cells (37, 50). This may explain why metastatic tumor cells move from the lumen of the blood vessel to an extravascular position. After initial attachment at the apical endothelial cell surface, tumor cells appear to induce local endothelial cell retraction, and they then migrate to and spread on the underlying basal lamina (36, 45). Eventually they underlap

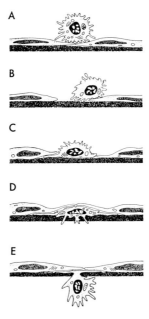

Fɪɢ. 1.   Schematic illustration of the sequence of events during blood-borne metastatic cell attachment and invasion of vascular endothelium and underlying basal lamina-like matrix. A, malignant cell attachment to endothelial cells; B, endothelial cell retraction; C, tumor cell migration and attachment to the underlying matrix; D, local destruction of the endothelial basal lamina-like matrix; E, invasion of the malignant cell into surrounding tissue (reproduced from Nicolson, Ref. 46).

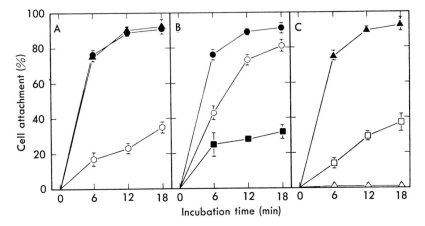

FIG. 2. Rates of attachment of ^{51}Cr-labeled B16-F10 melanoma cells to endothelial cell monolayers, extracellular matrix produced by endothelial cells or immobilized bovine serum fibronectin. A, adhesion of untreated B16-F10 cells to untreated endothelial cell monolayers (○), endothelial extracellular matrix (●), or immobilized fibronectin (▲). B, adhesion of B16-F10 melanoma cells to endothelial extracellular matrix (●) or matrix pretreated with 400 μg/ml purified anti-fibronectin antibody (○); adhesion of B16-F10 melanoma cells were pretreated with 0.5 μg/ml tunicamycin for 24 hr (■) to endothelial matrix. C, adhesion of B16-F10 cells to immobilized fibronectin (▲), or the immobilized fibronectin pretreated with 400 μg/ml anti-fibronectin (△); adhesion of B16-F10 melanoma cells pretreated with 0.5 μg/ml tunicamycin for 24 hr to immobilized matrix (□).

adjacent endothelial cells, solubilize local regions of the basal lamina and exit into the surrounding tissues (Fig. 1).

Components in the basal lamina that differ from the apical endothelial cell surface and are likely to be involved in metastatic cell adhesion are matrix glycoproteins, collagens and proteoglycans (reviewed in Ref. 46). For example, metastatic melanoma cells adhere with the same rapid kinetics to immobilized fibronectin, a prominent component of the endothelial basal lamina (1, 37), compared to the apical endothelial surface (37, 50). However, while adhesion to immobilized fibronectin is completely blocked by an affinity-purified antibody to fibronectin, adhesion to basal lamina-like matrix is only partially inhibited at high antibody concentrations (Fig. 2). These results suggest that metastatic tumor cells probably use a variety of adhesive mechanisms collectively to attach to endothelial basal lamina, and each class of adhesive interaction may act independently and play only a partial role in cell adhesion (50).

In other studies Murray *et al.* (41) noted that metastatic tumor cells attach to type IV collagen but not other collagen types in relation to their metastatic potentials. Recently, Terranova *et al.* (67) have found that laminin, another major glycoprotein component of endothelial matrix, plays an important role in adhesion of metastatic tumor cells to collagen. In their experiments laminin-dependent adhesion correlates with the metastatic capacities of the tumor lines that they used (67).

Tumor cell surface molecules have been implicated in metastatic cell attachment to endothelial basal lamina as well as to immobilized fibronectin, and these appear to be glycoproteins. Evidence for this comes from a series of experiments utilizing tunicamycin, an inhibitor of glycoprotein biosynthesis. Tunicamycin effectively blocks tumor cell-endothelial cell adhesion as well as tumor cell-fibronectin adhesion (Fig. 2). Tunicamycin treatment also modifies B16 cell surface glycoproteins, but not the major surface proteins detected by lactoperoxidase-catalyzed iodination. The effects are reversible within one day after drug removal from cultures of B16 melanoma cells. By examining the kinetics of loss of metastatic properties we could relate these biologic properties to the disappearance of a specific class of surface components (the sialogalactoproteins) on the B16 cells (29, 31). Treatment of B16 melanoma cells with this drug also prevented blood-borne arrest and experimental metastasis in syngeneic hosts (29, 31). Since modification of tumor cell glycoconjugates by enzymes can also result in loss of cell recognition and metastatic properties (21, 61), we attempted to purify the B16 cell surface sialogalactoproteins and examine the affinity of these glycoproteins to endothelial basal lamina (30). In contrast to intact B16 cells, isolated sialogalactoproteins only possess very low affinities to edothelial basal lamina-like matrix. This result suggests that B16 cellular adhesion to matrix results from multiple adhesive interactions and is not explainable by simple models based on a single molecular mechanism (50).

Degradation of Basal Lamina-like Endothelial Matrix by Metastatic Tumor Cells

The actual mechanisms of tumor cell extravasation through microvascular walls and basal lamina have been elusive. Mechanical disruption and alternatively enzymatic degradation have been postulated as important processes in basal lamina penetration by metastatic cells. As candidate enzymes, collagenase specific for type IV collagen and proteases capable of degrading matrix glycoprotein components are proposed as important (46). Mechanical disruption of basal lamina is postulated based strictly on morphological observations, although under the usual staining conditions extracellular matrix is not well visualized. In fact, according to the findings of Wight and Ross (74) the space beneath the endothelium appears to be filled with glycosaminoglycans. Moreover, Kanwar and Farquhar (33) have shown that a permeability barrier exists at the glomerular basement membrane, and the barrier can be destroyed by enzymatic or chemical degradation of heparan sulfate (HS). It is unlikely that simple mechanical disruption can explain the mechanism of extravasation, because metastatic tumor cells easily penetrate endothelial basal lamina-like matrix (41, 45) and intact blood vessel walls (24, 57) *in vitro* under conditions with minimal mechanical effects.

Enzymatic mechanisms of extravasation, and in particular, basal lamina destruction are probably more likely, because these do not require special circumstances such as excessive cell proliferation or increased tissue pressures (46). Liotta *et al.* (39) have shown that highly metastatic B16 cells possess higher collagenase activities, but only against type IV collagen. Several B16 sublines have been measured for collagenase activities against type I or II collagen; they are similar, indicating that these metastatic cells can degrade the major fibrous components of endothelial basal lamina. B16 melanoma cells also have several lysosomal proteases and glycosidases. Sloane *et al.* (62, 64) have reported that higher levels of lysosomal enzymes such as cathepsin B correlate with metastatic potential in the B16 system. This particular enzyme is a lysosomal cystein protease, and it may be involved in the activation of latent or procollagenase to collagenase. In addition, the production of prostaglandin D_2 inversibly correlates with metastatic potential (17) in this system, and the cellular release of the lysosomal enzymes may be controlled by such prostaglandins (63).

Metastatic tumor cells have the capacities to degrade the major components of the endothelial basal lamina-like matrix. When metastatic B16 cells are seeded onto metabolically-labeled, cell-free endothelial matrix, the [³H] leucine label is released into the media in the form of solubilized macromolecules that are 90–95% precipitable with 10% trichloroacetic acid (38, 45). Highly metastatic B16 sublines release [³H] leucine-labeled molecules from endothelial matrix at higher rates compared to B16 parental cells of lower metastatic potential (45). Using the endothelial cell matrix we have found that the predominant glycoprotein components solubilized by B16 melanoma cells are fibronectin and laminin. In the case of fibronectin, it appears in the media in a new form of slightly lower ($\sim$10,000) molecular weight (M_r). Analysis of endothelial matrix fibronectin by sodium dodecyl sulfate (SDS)-polyacrylamide gel electrophoresis indicates that the fibronectin subunits are approximately 230,000 in M_r (38). This suggests that the melanoma solubilized fibronectin is acted on by a tumor cell protease, or perhaps a glycosidase.

Metastatic cells also have enzymes capable of solubilizing basal lamina proteoglycans. Kramer *et al.* (38) have measured the abilities of B16 melanoma cells to solubilize [³⁵S] sulfated proteoglycans from endothelial matrix, and they find that the glycosaminoglycan HS is degraded from a molecule of approximately 25,000–30,000 M_r to a fragment approximately one-third the original size (38). These fragments are >95% HS and appear only when the B16 melanoma cells are incubated with matrix. It is not a normal endothelial cell degradation product of the matrix. The composition of this fragment indicates that B16 melanoma cells possess an endoglycosidase activity against the HS glycosaminoglycan that cleaves these molecules at intrachain sites. Subsequently, we have determined that the highly metastatic sublines of B16 melanoma release sulfated glycosaminoglycan

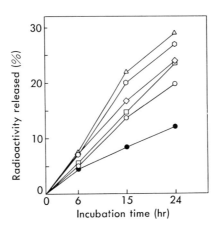

FIG. 3.   Solubilization of sulfated glycosaminoglycans from subendothelial matrix by B16 melanoma metastatic variants. Endothelial cell cultures were labeled metabolically with sodium [³⁵S]sulfate (25 μCi/ml) in sulfate-depleted medium plus 10% fetal bovine serum for one week, and subendothelial matrix was prepared according to Kramer *et al.* (37). B16 melanoma cells were grown, harvested and 2 ml of cell suspension plated on matrix in 35 mm culture dish at a concentration of 1.5× 10⁵ cells/ml. At various times during the incubation at 37° aliquots of the media were removed and centrifuged at 40,000×g for 30 min. The radioactivity in the supernatants were determined by liquid scintillation counting. ● control; △ B15b, ◯ BL6; ◇ O13; □ F10; ○ F1.

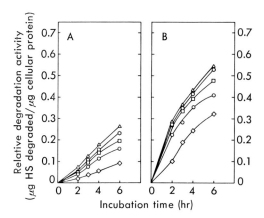

Fig. 4. Time course of HS degradation by cell homogenates of B16 melanoma cells. Fifty μg of purified bovine lung HS was incubated with each B16 cell homogenate (30 μg protein) or boiled cell homogenate in 70 μl of 0.1 M sodium phosphate, 0.2% Triton X-100, 0.15 M sodium chloride, pH 6.0 at 37° for various times. After incubation, the mixtures were centrifuged to remove debris, and 2 μl of the supernatants were applied to 6% polyacrylamide gels in 50 mM 1,3-diaminopropane-acetate buffer, pH 9.0. Electrophoresis was performed at 120 V for 60 min at 4°. Electrophoresed gels were fixed and then stained with 0.1% toluidine blue in 1% acetic acid, destained and scanned at 525 nm to quantitate the glycosaminoglycans. The relative degradation activities were calculated from the decrease in total area of the HS peak (A) or the decrease in area of the high molecular weight half of the HS peak (B). Results are expressed as μg HS degraded/μg cellular protein. Each symbol represents the average of quadruplicate samples (S.D.<10% of data). △ B15b; ○ BL6; □ F10; ○ F1; ◇ O13.

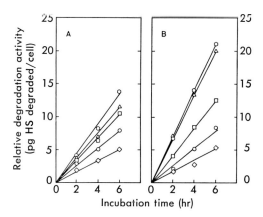

Fig. 5. Time course of HS degradation by intact, viable B16 melanoma cells. B16 cells (1×10^5) were incubated with 50 μg purified bovine lung HS for various times in 200 μl medium containing 20 mM Tricine (pH 7.3) at 37°. Upon incubation with B16 cells the relative degradation activities were calculated from the decrease in total area of the HS peak (A) or the decrease in area of the high molecular weight half of the HS peak (B). Results are expressed as pg HS degraded/cell. Each symbol represents the average of quadruplicate samples (S.D.<10% of data). ○ BL6; △ B15b; □ F10; ○ F1; ◇ O13.

fragments from endothelial matrix at higher rates than B16 sublines of low metastatic and invasive potentials (Fig. 3) (*43*).

We have also examined five B16 sublines for their abilities to degrade purified lung HS *in vitro*. In this assay we measured the appearance of HS degradation products using polyacrylamide gel electrophoresis in 1,3-diaminopropane-acetate buffer according to Dietrich *et al*. (*7, 8*).The rates of total HS degradation by the B16 variant sublines and the rates of appearance of HS degradation products of decreased molecular weights indicated that high molecular weight HS is degraded to a few large fragments rather than monosaccharides. This suggests that B16 melanoma cells have an endoglycosidase capable of acting on HS. When various B16 sublines were compared for their HS degrading activities using either or their cell-free homogenates (Fig. 4) or, intact cells (Fig. 5),

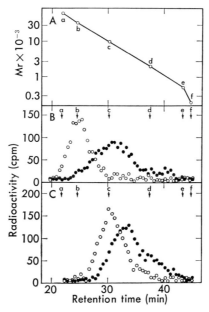

FIG. 6. High-performance liquid chromatographic analysis of HS and its fragments produced by B16 melanoma cell heparanases. A, logarithmic plot of the retention times of standard glycans separated on two sequential 0.7×75 cm columns of Fractogel-TSK (Toyopearl) HW-55(S). Elution was performed with 0.2 M NaCl at a flow rate of 1.0 ml/min at 55°. Standard glycans used are: a, chondroitin 6-sulfate from shark cartilage ($M_r \sim 60,000$); b, HS from bovine lung ($M_r \sim 34,000$); c, heparin from porcine mucosal tissue ($M_r \sim 11,000$); d, monosialosyl-biantennary complex-type glycopeptide from porcine thyroglobulin; e, tri-N-acetylchitotriose; f, N-acetylglucosamine. B, elution profiles of ³H-labeled bovine lung HS (○) and its degradation fragments produced by heparanase derived from B16-F10 melanoma cells (●). Incubations were performed in a solution containing 60 μg cellular protein with 2,000 cpm HS in the presence of 20 mM D-saccharic acid 1,4-lactone at 37° for 3 hr with occasional mixing. The reaction was stopped by chilling and the addition of one-tenth volume of cold 50% trichloroacetic acid. After centrifugation at $9,000 \times g$ the supernatant was delivered directly into the injection port. Fractions corresponding to 30 sec were collected and counted; a–f indicate the eluting positions of the standard glycans. C, elution profiles of cellular HS produced by PYS-2 embryonic carcinoma (○) and its degradation products by B16-BL6 melanoma cell heparanase (●). Experimental conditions were the same in B except that the incubation time was 1.5 hr

we found that the sublines with the highest lung colonization potentials such as B16-BL6 and B16-F10 have the highest lung HS degradation activities while the sublines with the lowest lung colonization potentials such as B16-O13 and B16-F1 have the lowest activities. These results indicate that HS degradative activity correlates with the lung colonization abilities of murine B16 melanoma sublines.

We have recently developed an analytical system to determine the size distribution of a variety of glycosaminoglycans and their fragments using high performance liquid chromatography (32). Using this system, we have found that lung HS and also HS from various other sources are degraded into large molecular weight fragments by melanoma cell-derived glycosidases. The average size of the fragments produced appear to be specific for each of the HS substrates. For example, ^{3}H-labeled bovine lung HS (M_r of about 34,000) is cleaved into molecules of M_r about 10,000 and lower, while [^{35}S]-labeled HS synthesized by PYS-2 embryonic carcinoma cells ($M_r \sim 11,000$) is clipped into fragments of average $M_r \sim 6,000$ (Fig. 6). This result was more easily seen when the incubation is performed in the presence of D-saccharic acid 1,4-lactone, an inhibitor of exo-β-glucuronidase. Our results indicate that metastatic melanoma cells have an endoglycosidase which recognizes a sequence which occurs periodically in the HS chains. While heparin is a poor substrate, it inhibits HS degradation. This suggests the possibility that an enzymatic mechanism may also be involved in modifying blood-borne metastasis by heparin or other sulfated glycans (20, 69).

In order to determine more precisely the enzymatic activity involved in B16 melanoma glycosidase cleavage of HS, the HS fragments derived from bovine lung HS previously reduced with NaBH$_4$ at the reducing terminal have been isolated and labeled at their newly formed reducing terminal ends with NaB[^{3}H]$_4$. After acid hydrolysis or nitrous acid deamination followed by mild acid hydrolysis, the labeled reducing terminal sugar(s) are analyzed by descending paper chromatography and high voltage paper electrophoresis. More than 90% of reducing terminal sugar of HS fragments have been identified as glucuronic acid, indicating that the B16 heparanase is an endoglucuronidase (42).

Similar HS degrading endoglycosidases have been described in various tissues such as skin fibroblasts (35), rat liver cells (28), human platelets (73), and placenta (34); but their physiological function remains unknown. Ögren and Lindahl (51) have reported that murine mastocytoma cells contain a heparin-specific endoglucuronidase that is capable of converting macromolecular heparin to physiologically active, intermediate molecular weight fragments, and Oosta et al. (52) have recently purified an endoglycosidase specific for HS from normal human platelets. Although normal cells also possess endoglycosidases similar to metastatic tumor cells, it remains to be determined if there are regulatory or structural differences between the heparanases of tumor and nontumor cells. Nonetheless, the degradation of endothelial matrix glycosaminoglycans by tumor cell heparanases may explain, in part, the specific extravasation seen in distant metastasis of some tumors.

Acknowledgment

These studies were supported by National Institutes of Health grant RO1-28867 and RO1-CA28844 from the National Cancer Institute (to G. L. Nicolson) and institutional grant IN-121B (to T. Irimura) from the American Cancer Society.

REFERENCES

1. Birdwell, C. R., Gospodarowicz, D., and Nicolson, G. L. *Proc. Natl. Acad. Sci. U.S.*, **75**, 3273–3277 (1978).
2. Briles, E. B. and Kornfeld, S. *J. Natl. Cancer Inst.*, **60**, 1217–1222 (1976).
3. Brunson, K. W. and Nicolson, G. L. *J. Supramol. Struct.*, **11**, 517–528 (1979).
4. Chew, E. C. and Wallace, A. C. *Cancer Res.*, **36**, 1904–1909 (1976).
5. Chew, E. C., Josephson, R. L., and Wallace, A. C. *In* "Fundamental Aspects of Metastasis," ed. L. Weiss, pp. 121–150 (1976). North Holland Publishing, Amsterdam.
6. Cottler-Fox, M., Ryd, W., Hagmar, B., and Fox, C. H. *Int. J. Cancer*, **26**, 689–694 (1980).
7. Dietrich, C. P. and Dietrich, S.M.C. *Anal. Biochem.*, **70**, 645–647 (1976).
8. Dietrich, C. P. and Nader, H. B. *Biochim. Biophys. Acta*, **343**, 34–44 (1974).
9. Dietrich, C. P., Sampaio, L. O., and Toledo, O.M.S. *Biochem. Biophys. Res. Commun.*, **71**, 1–10 (1976).
10. Fidler, I. J. *Nature New Biol.*, **242**, 148–149 (1973).
11. Fidler, I. J. *Cancer Res.*, **35**, 218–224 (1975).
12. Fidler, I. J. *In* "Fundamental Aspects of Metastasis," ed. L. Weiss, pp. 275–289 (1976). North Holland Publishing, Amsterdam.
13. Fidler, I. J. and Bucana, C. *Cancer Res.*, **37**, 3945–3951 (1977).
14. Fidler, I. J. and Kripke, M. L. *Science*, **197**, 893–895 (1977).
15. Fidler, I. J. and Nicolson, G. L. *Cancer Biol. Rev.*, **2**, 174–234 (1981).
16. Fisher, B. and Fisher, E. R. *Surgery*, **50**, 240–247 (1961).
17. Fitzpatrick, F. A. and Stingfellow, D. A. *Proc. Natl. Acad. Sci. U.S.*, **76**, 1765–1769 (1979).
18. Gasic, G. J., Gasic, T. B., Galanti, N., Johnson, T., and Murphy, S. *Int. J. Cancer*, **11**, 704–718 (1973).
19. Gestpart, H. *J. Med.*, **8**, 103–121 (1977).
20. Hagmar, B. *Acta Pathol. Microbiol. Scand.*, *Sect. A*, **80**, 357–366 (1972).
21. Hagmar, B. and Norrby, K. *Int. J. Cancer*, **11**, 663–675 (1973).
22. Hanna, N. *Cancer Res.*, **42**, 1337–1342 (1982).
23. Hanna, N. and Fidler, I. J. *J. Natl. Cancer Inst.*, **65**, 801–809 (1980).
24. Hart, I. R. *Am. J. Pathol.*, **97**, 587–600 (1979).
25. Hart, I. R. *Cancer Metastasis Rev.*, **1**, 5–16 (1982).
26. Hilgard, P. *Br. J. Cancer*, **28**, 429–435 (1973).
27. Honn, K. V., Cifone, B., and Skoff, A. *Science*, **212**, 1270–1272 (1980).
28. Höök, M., Wasteson, Å., and Oldberg, Å. *Biochem. Biophys. Res. Commun.*, **67**, 1422–1428 (1975).
29. Irimura, T. and Nicolson, G. L. *J. Supramol. Struct. Cell. Biochem.*, **17**, 325–336 (1981).
30. Irimura, T. and Nicolson, G. L. *J. Cell Biol.*, **91**, 119a (1981).
31. Irimura, T., Gonzalez, R., and Nicolson, G. L. *Cancer Res.*, **41**, 3411–3418 (1981).
32. Irimura, T., Nakajima, M., Di Ferrante, N., and Nicolson, G. L. *Anal. Biochem.*, **130**, 461–468 (1983).
33. Kanwar, Y. S. and Farquhar, M. G. *Proc. Natl. Acad. Sci. U.S.*, **76**, 1303–1307 (1979).
34. Klein, U. and von Figura, K. *Biochem. Biophys. Res. Commun.*, **73**, 569–576 (1976).
35. Klein, U., Kresse, H., and von Figura, K. *Biochem. Biophys. Res. Commun.*, **69**, 158–166 (1976).
36. Kramer, R. H. and Nicolson, G. L. *Proc. Natl. Acad. Sci. U.S.*, **76**, 5704–5708 (1979).
37. Kramer, R. H., Gonzalez, R., and Nicolson, G. L. *Int. J. Cancer*, **26**, 639–645 (1980).
38. Kramer, R. H., Vogel, K. G., and Nicolson, G. L. *J. Biol. Chem.*, **257**, 2678–2686 (1982).
39. Liotta, L. A., Tryggvason, K., Garbisa, S., Hart, I. R., Foltz, C. M., and Shafie, S. *Nature*, **284**, 67–68 (1980).
40. Miner, K. M., Kawaguchi, T., Uba, G., and Nicolson, G. L. *Cancer Res.*, **42**, 4631–

    4638 (1982).

41. Murray, J. C., Liotta, L. A., Rennard, S. I., and Martin, G. *Cancer Res.*, **40**, 347–351 (1980).

42. Nakajima, M., Irimura, T., Di Ferrante, N., and Nicolson, G. L. *J. Cell Biol.* 95, 135a (1982).

43. Nakajima, M., Irimura, T., Di Ferrante, D., Di Ferrante, N., and Nicolson, G. L. *Science*, **220**, 611–613 (1983).

44. Nicolson, G. L. *Am. Zool.*, **18**, 71–80 (1978).

45. Nicolson, G. L. *J. Histochem. Cytochem.*, **30**, 214–220 (1982).

46. Nicolson, G. L. *Biochim. Biophys. Acta*, **695**, 113–176 (1982).

47. Nicolson, G. L. and Winkelhake, J. L. *Nature*, **255**, 230–232 (1975).

48. Nicolson, G. L., Winkelhake, J. L., and Nussey, A. *In* "Fundamental Aspects of Metastasis," ed. L. Weiss, pp. 291–303 (1976). North Holland Publishing, Amsterdam.

49. Nicolson, G. L., Brunson, K. W., and Fidler, I. J. *Cancer Res.*, **30**, 4105–4111 (1978).

50. Nicolson, G. L., Irimura, T., Gonzalez, R., and Rouslahti, E. *Exp. Cell Res.*, **134**, 461–465 (1981).

51. Ögren, S. and Lindahl, U. *J. Biol. Chem.*, **250**, 2690–2697 (1975).

52. Oosta, G. M., Favreau, L. V., Beeler, D. L., and Rosenberg, R. D. *J. Biol. Chem.*, **257**, 11249–11255 (1982).

53. Pearlstein, E., Salk, P. L., Yogeeswaran, G., and Karpatkin, S. *Proc. Natl. Acad. Sci. U.S.*, **77**, 4336–4339 (1980).

54. Phondke, G. P., Madyastha, K. R., Madyastha, P. R., and Barth, R. F. *J. Natl. Cancer Inst.*, **66**, 643–647 (1981).

55. Poste, G. and Fidler, I. J. *Nature*, **283**, 139–146 (1980).

56. Poste, G. and Nicolson, G. L. *Proc. Natl. Acad. Sci. U.S.*, **77**, 399–403 (1980).

57. Poste, G., Doll, J., Hart, I. R., and Fidler, I. J. *Cancer Res.*, **40**, 1636–1644 (1980).

58. Sage, H., Crouch, E., and Bornstein, P. *Biochemistry*, **18**, 5433–5442 (1980).

59. Sato, H., Khato, J., Sato, T., and Suzuki, M. *GANN Monogr. Cancer Res.*, **20**, 3–13 (1977).

60. Schirrmacher, V., Cheinsong-Popov, R., and Arnheiter, H. *J. Exp. Med.*, **151**, 984–989 (1981).

61. Sinha, B. K. and Goldenberg, G. J. *Cancer*, **34**, 1956–1961 (1974).

62. Sloane, B. F., Dunn, J. R., and Honn, K. V. *Science*, **212**, 1151–1153 (1981).

63. Sloane, B. F., Makim, S., Dunn, J. R., Lacoste, R., Theodorou, M., Battista, J., Alex, R., and Honn, K. V. *In* "Prostaglandins and Cancer," ed. T. Powels, R. S. Bockman, K. V. Honn, and P. Ramwell, pp. 789–792 (1981). Alan R. Liss, New York.

64. Sloane, B. F., Honn, K. V., Slader, J. G., Turner, W. A., Kimpson, J. J., and Taylor, J. D. *Cancer Res.*, **42**, 980–986 (1982).

65. Sugarbaker, E. V. *Cancer Biol. Rev.*, **2**, 235–278 (1981).

66. Tanaka, K., Kohga, S. Kinjo, M., and Kodama, Y. *GANN Monogr. Cancer Res.*, **20**, 97–119 (1977).

67. Terranova, V. P., Liotta, L. A., Russo, R., and Martin, G. *Cancer Res.*, **42**, 2265–2269 (1982).

68. Toledo, O. M. and Dietrich, C. P. *Biochim. Biophys. Acta*, **498**, 114–122 (1977).

69. Tsubura, E., Yamashita, T., Kobayashi, M., Higuchi, Y., and Isobe, J. *GANN Monogr. Cancer Res.*, **20**, 147–161 (1977).

70. Varani, J., Orr, W., and Ward P. A. *J. Natl. Cancer Inst.*, **64**, 1173–1178 (1980).

71. Warren, B. A. *J. Med.*, **4**, 150–177 (1973).

72. Wasteson, Å., Höök, M., and Westermark, B. *FEBS Lett.*, **64**, 218–221 (1976).

73. Wasteson, Å., Glimelius, B., Bush, C., Westermark, B., Heldin, C-H., and Norling, B. *Thromb. Res.*, **11**, 309–311 (1977).

74. Wight, T. N. and Ross, R. *J. Cell Biol.*, **67**, 660–674 (1975).

GANN Monograph on Cancer Research 29, 1983

SHEDDING FROM CANCER CELLS AND ITS IMPORTANCE IN DETERMINING THE PATHOPHYSIOLOGY OF CANCER

Debra D. POUTSIAKA and Paul H. BLACK

*Hubert H. Humphrey Cancer Research Center and Department of Microbiology, Boston University School of Medicine**

Shedding, the release of components or structures of the plasma membrane, is an important part of membrane turnover. It is not comparable to secretion, the exocytosis of soluble cellular products within vesicles. Shedding is a characteristic of activated cells; thus, it is observed in normal growing cells or normal cells activated by stimuli such as mitogens. Examples are the shedding of plasminogen activator from macrophages and the shedding of membrane enclosed discs from photoreceptor cells. Cancer cells, which exist in an abnormally activated state, exhibit increased shedding. The shedding of plasminogen activator from malignant or transformed cells is a model of shedding by cancer cells. The increased shedding exhibited by cancer cells is likely to be responsible for several characteristics of cancer. These include invasion, metastasis, evasion of the immune system and aberrations in the clotting system. The inhibition of shedding, which is seen after *in vitro* treatment of transformed cells with interferon, may be exploited as a possible therapeutic approach to cancer.

The plasma membrane of mammalian cells is more than a partition between the cytoplasm and its constituents and the extracellular environment. It is a dynamic component of the cell which is intimately involved in cellular functions. An important aspect of the dynamics of the plasma membrane is its turnover. One mechanism by which membranes turn over is shedding, the release of constituents of the plasma membrane in soluble or particulate form, into the extracellular fluid or culture medium (see Ref. *4* for review). Shedding is distinguished from secretion (Table I), which is the release through exocytosis of soluble cellular products packaged within vesicles. An example of secretions is the release of digestive enzymes by exocytosis of zymogen granules from acinar cells in the pancreas. There are severl characterisitics of shedding:
1) Material which is shed is derived from the cell surface. 2) Material which is shed is made by the cell. 3) Shedding is an active metabolic process which is characteristic of viable cells and therefore is not the result of cell lysis. 4) Shedding follows first order kinetics, indicating that molecules are shed in a manner not influenced by the length of tenure of a particular molecule in the membrane. 5) Shedding is a property of activated cells.

Cellular activation can result from a number of stimuli such as the addition of serum to quiescent, serum-deprived cultures, exposure of cells to mitogens such as the tumor promoter, phorbol myristate acetate (PMA), or the lectin, concanavalin A, or, in the

---

* Boston, Massachusetts 02118, U.S.A.

TABLE I. General Comparison of Secretion and Shedding

	Secretion	Shedding
Cell surface association of released product	No	Yes (peripheral and/or integral)
Intracellular existence of released product	Contained in soluble form within vesicle or granule	Membrane associated
External surface labeling of product prior to release	Not labeled	Labeled
Release of product by exocytosis	Yes	No
Energy requirement for release	Yes	Yes
Coupling of protein synthesis with release	No	Yes
Lag period from stimulation to release	Short	Long
Augmented by cell activation, cell proliferation, mitogenesis, or transformation	Not necessarily	Yes

case of the immune system, from exposure to antigen. Malignantly transformed cells may be viewed as being perpetually activated and are distinguished from normal cells in that cancer cells lack the mechanisms which limit cell activation. During activation there is an increase in synthesis of various proteins already being made. New proteins may also be synthesized during activation. If destined to become integral membrane proteins, they are inserted into the membrane of the endoplasmic reticulum and reach the cell surface through the process of membrane flow. The biosynthesis of peripheral membrane proteins, the means by which they are placed on the cell surface, and the nature of the attachment between peripheral membrane proteins and the plasma membrane are unclear. Either integral membrane proteins or peripheral membrane proteins may be shed, in a linear, soluble form or on a vesicle which has been released from the plasma membrane.

In large part, the mechanism of shedding remains unknown. Molecules shed in linear form may be released by a proteolytic event or through other unknown mechainsms. The shedding of vesicles may occur *via* a mechanism similar to the budding and shedding of enveloped viruses, that is through a process of membrane fusion with subsequent release of a vesicle.

Shedding is a characteristic of many diverse cell types, either normal or malignant. Normal cells exhibit shedding under various circumstances. For instance, granulosa cells shed plasminogen activator (PA) as ovulation approaches. Trophoblast cultures release PA at a time corresponding to the invasion of the uterine wall. Murine spleen cells shed immune response-associated (Ia) antigens and histocompatibility antigens in culture (18). Since the shedding of various cell products from normal cells is important in cell function, it appears that under certain circumstances, shedding may contribute to disease states. For instance, the failure of pigmented epithelial cells in the eye to phagocytose shed discs from photoreceptor cells may be important in the pathogenesis of certain retinal dystrophies. In another example, it has been proposed that there may be a link between the shedding of PA by macrophages treated with the tumor promoter, PMA, and tumor production after PMA treatment (25).

The following paper will be confined to a discussion of shedding from cancer cells. The shedding of PA from simian virus 40 (SV40)-transformed Swiss 3T3 cells as a model of shedding from cancer cells will be discussed in detail. Finally, the influence of shedding on the expression of the malignant phenotype will be examined.

The Release of PA as a Model System for Shedding from Cancer Cells

Although it had been known since 1925 that cancer cells could lyse a fibrin clot (20), the features of the fibrinolytic system in transformed cells have been delineated only recently by Reich and his group. Their early studies and other studies revealed that cells transformed by a variety of viruses and chemicals, as well as cells from spontaneously arising cancer, contained and released into the medium a serine protease, PA, which was not present in untransformed cells. This protease converts the serum zymogen plasminogen to plasmin, which hydrolyzed fibrin (65).

Early studies of the fibrinolytic activity of untransformed cells emphasized the low or background levels of PA when cells were assayed soon after plating (65). Subsequently, Chou *et al.* in our laboratory found that the fibrinolytic activity of untransformed mouse cells varies greatly during the cell growth curve (9). An increse in cell-associated activity, with a considerable increase in released PA, occurs in actively growing untransformed mouse cells. However, the release of PA decreases when the cells become confluent, indicating a density-dependent control of release. In contrast, transformed cells, which continue to grow, continue to release PA (9, 10). Cell lysate activities remain at approximately the same level (10) or increase for a period of time (36) in confluent, untransformed mouse cells. In subsequent studies of cells from a number of other species, cell-associated and released PA were also shown to increase as the cells grew prior to confluency. Evidence was presented that this was due to increased synthesis of PA rather than to changes in cellular inhibitor levels or to adsorption of released molecules to the cell (49). These studies indicate that an increase in synthesis and release of PA occurs in growing normal cells and that release decreases upon cell confluence. These findings, together with the turnover studies presented, further indicate that shedding is associated with cell growth.

The plasma membrane association of PA has been found in a number of cell types from different species. The increase in PA activity in cell homogenates, which occurs after addition of the detergent Triton X-100 but not after treatments that would normally solubilize the contents of vesicles, suggests that the enzyme is not contained within a vesicle, but rather exists in a membrane-bound form (28). In addition, PA has been shown to be associated with plasma membrane-enriched fractions of virus-transformed cells from a number of species (11). The requirement for detergent treatment to solubilize the enzyme suggests that it may be an integral membrane protein, but this is not known for certain (28). All available evidence, however, indicates the plasma membrane association of PA; its release, therefore, is likely to be by shedding rather than by secretion.

When the intracellular distribution of PA activity in growing and non-growing mouse cells is compared, approximately 70% of PA activity is found to be associated with the plasma membrane-enriched fraction of the growing cells, whereas only 20–25% of PA activity is associated with a similar fraction in the nongrowing cells; in nongrowing cells, the remainder of the activity is associated with a heavier membrane fraction, presumably the rough endoplasmic reticulum (RER) (28). This suggests that PA molecules move from heavy RER to lighter (plasma membrane-enriched) fractions during growth. Such movement of PA is associated with its shedding, since there is a correlation between shedding of PA and its predominantly plasma membrane location (28).

Molecular weight determinations of partially purified PA from normal and transformed cells have revealed some differences between species (see Ref. *48* for review). In general, there is a major component of approximately 50,000 daltons (d) and two minor components of approximately 75,000 d and 35,000 d; all have PA activity. Both the 50,000 d and 35,000 d, but not the 75,000 d, species of human PA cross-react with an antiserum prepared against human urokinase, suggesting that the lower-molecular-weight forms of PA are related (*67*). Whether the 75,000 d form represents a separate gene product is not known. In quiescent mosue cells, the predominant form of PA is a 75,000 d species that is associated with a heavy membrane fraction (as determined by sucrose gradients). In growing and transformed mouse cells, however, nearly all the PA activity is present as the 50,000 d form that is associated with a plasma membrane-enriched fraction (*29, 31*). Following stimulation of quiescent cells with PMA, calcium, or serum, there is an induction of the 50,000 d species, an increase in plasma membrane-associated activity, and release of PA (*29, 31*). This indicates that with activation and movement of PA to the plasma mambrane, the 50,000 d species of PA is generated, but whether a precursor-product relationship exists between the 75,000 d and 50,000 d species of PA is not known.

From these studies, one may conclude that cell surface proteolytic activity increases with growth and that proteolytic activity from growing cells may be shed into the medium; such activity is diminished or absent from nongrowing cells. Growing cells, then, resemble cancer cells in having increased surface proteolytic activity that may be shed.

Influence of Shedding on the Phenotype of Cancer Cells

1. Shedding and tumor immunity

A number of mechanisms by which animal tumor cells escape host immune destruction have been described (see Ref. *30* for review). Tumor antigens may be masked or covered by another molecule. Another escape mechanism is antigenic modulation, which may result when tumor cells are exposed to antibody specific for cell surface antigens (*43*). The antibody causes a redistribution (patching, capping, then endocytosis with or without shedding) and eventual elimination of the tumor antigen from the cell surface; reappearance of antigen does not occur in the presence of antibody, and the cell effectively escapes from the cytotoxic effect of complement in this *in vitro* model (*56*). Aside from masking or modulation of tumor antigen, a change in or, more rarely, loss of tumor antigen may occur in certain tumors. The former may result from immunoselective pressures that tend to select for cells with "weaker" tumor antigens, whereas a loss of tumor antigen(s) may occur in rapidly growing tumors (*3*) or after prolonged cultivation of certain tumors as organ cultures *in vitro* (*45*). Although the mechanism of such change in or loss of antigenicity is not known, shedding is one mechanism whereby cell surface tumor antigens are lost. Shedding may play a key role in tumor escape not only by eliminating tumor antigen, but also by the capacity of the shed product to generate other blocking factor(s).

Much evidence indicates that at least a portion of the host antitumor response is mediated by effector T cells with specific receptors for the tumor antigen and that engagement of the receptor by cellular tumor antigen is necessary for killing (*33*). Lymphocytes from tumor-bearing animals or humans often kill cells from their respective tumors *in vitro* (*23*). Sera from tumor-bearing animals block the killing of tumor cells by autologous lymphocytes *in vitro* in an immunologically specific manner; this has been thought to represent the *in vitro* correlate of tumor enhancement (*26*). Most evidence indicates that blocking activity in serum is related either directly to free circulating tumor antigen and/or antigen-antibody complexes or indirectly to suppressor factor(s).

Blocking of cellular immune reactions mediated by lymphocytes from humans and animals bearing tumors and autologous tumor cells *in vitro* has been achieved in many instances by tumor antigen alone; this suggests that tumor antigen may be the active blocking factor (see Ref. *47* for review). Blocking by antigen is of the central type, which occurs at the level of the effector lymphocyte after its interaction with tumor antigen. Blocking centrally by tumor antigen is generally specific and is dependent on the amount of antigen present in the blocking serum (*5*). The tumor antigen in serum originates by shedding from the surface of tumor cells (*4*).

Immune complexes can also block *in vitro*. The incidence of immune complexes in cancer sera is fairly high, ranging from 50–80%, depending on the type of assay employed (*63*). Immune complexes in cancer sera may be composed of cell surface material of varying antigenic specificity, *e.g.*, tumor antigen (*37*), fetal antigen (*13*), or viral antigen (*44*). Such antigens, having evoked a humoral immune response in the tumor-bearing hosts, are likely to combine with antibody in the circulation subsequent to their shedding from the tumor cell surface (*63*). Immune complexes may also be formed by stripping of cell surface antigen with specific antibody (*42*).

Although immune complexes can act as blocking factors, it is not clear whether blocking occurs centrally or at the target cell level. Binding of immune complexes to the crystallizable fragment (Fc) receptor of tumor cells (*62*) or to tumor antigen (*35*), may occur. Immune complexes may also facilitate binding of antigen to the effector T lymphocyte by antibody-mediate cross-linking processes, resulting in specific blockade and low zone tolerance (*15*). Whether immune complexes act centrally or peripherally may depend on whether they occur in antigen or antibody excess, respectively (*63*). There is also evidence that immune complexes can bind to the Fc receptor of the killer (K) cell and block antibody dependent cell-mediated cytotoxicity (ADCC) (*60*). Immune complex binding to macrophages *via* the Fc receptors has also been demonstrated (*51*).

The presence of blocking factors in serum is related to the size of the tumor and the extent of metastases (*63*). With a number of human and animal tumors, blocking factors are present with growing tumors (*2, 66*) and not in hosts with regressed tumors; cell-mediated immune reactivity against autochthonous tumor cells is present in both, however. Moreover, the most rapidly growing tumors in certain experimental animal systems (*i.e.*, those accompanied by metastases) are associated with the largest amount of blocking factor(s); and elevation of blocking factor(s), especially tumor antigen, frequently precedes metastases (*32*). A number of such metastasizing and nonmetastasizing tumors have been studied; the former shed cell surface components more rapidly and to a greater extent, have less glycocalyx, and are less immunogenic than their nonmetastasizing counterparts (*14, 32*). In addition, a greater lability of cell surface molecules is found in metastasizing tumors than in nonmetastasizing tumors (*i.e.*, antigenic modulation occurred much more readily in the former than in the latter tumors) (*14*).

Excision of tumor has generally been accompanied by a loss of blocking factors (*57*) and may occur within 24 hr with certain experimental animal tumors (*55*). Furthermore, treatment of patients with chemotherapy has resulted in a loss of serum blocking activity, whereas recurrence of disease may be accompanied by an increase in blocking activity (8).

There is evidence that host suppressor cells, which are found in the spleens or thymuses of tumor-bearing animals, or specific soluble products, which may be shed from and can substitute for suppressor cells (64), play a role in promoting tumor growth by decreasing the effective host antitumor immune response (see Ref. 7 for review). Suppressor cells are a subset of T cells, but non-T cells which nonspecifically suppress a wide spectrum of immunological functions may also be present in tumor-bearing animals and humans.

Certain studies suggest that suppressor cells are evoked in response to antigenic stimulation. With respect to tumor antigen, immunization may stimulate a host immune response against a transplanted tumor; however, a paradoxical effect may result and growth of a transplanted tumor may be enhanced. Suppressor cells specific for the tumor have been demonstrated in such instances (17, 27). Such a sequence of events apparently occurs during the growth of a transplanted tumor (38). There is evidence that tumor antigens enhance tumor growth *in vivo* by interacting with a radiosensitive population of T cells; suppressor cells are generally sensitive to sublethal doses of X-irradiation (27). The induction of such suppressor activity by large amounts of free tumor antigen in tumor-bearing animals is presumably responsible for the depressed tumor-specific immunity and results in what might be viewed as a state of immunological tolerance (17).

Although the aforementioned studies suggest that tumor antigen evokes suppressor activity, it is not always clear from these studies whether the specific immunosuppressive effect is due to tumor antigen or to suppressor factor (17). In this connection, a tumor-specific blocking factor (a glycoprotein of molecular weight approximately 56,000 d) has been purified from the serum of mice bearing a methylcholanthrene-induced fibrosarcoma (purification utilzed affinity chromatographic techniques and an antiserum raised against tumor cells) (41). Such a factor could represent either tumor antigen or a suppressor molecule. The role of tumor antigen in inducing suppression is further suggested by the relationship that exists between the presence of tumor and suppressor factors, both specific and nonspecific. Thus, a parallelism of tumor growth and the presence of specific suppressor cells has been observed (46). Moreover, spleen cells from animals with progressively growing tumors contained suppressor cells for lymphocyte mitogenesis and the mixed lymphocyte reaction, whereas spleen cells from regressor animals did not (22). In addition, excision of tumor results in loss of a factor that inhibited the response of spleen cells to phytohemagglutinin (PHA) (21).

In summary, both specific and nonspecific immunosuppressive factors are present in cancer patients. The relationship between shedding of tumor antigens and malignancy suggests that shedding is an essential element in the abrogation of the immune response in cancer and that one approach to reduction of suppressor activity might involve attempts to reduce shedding.

2. *Derangements of the clotting system in cancer*

The hemostatic mechanism in cancer seems to be poised between hyperactivity of the coagulation system (with widespread fibrin deposition and thrombosis) and excessive stimulation of the fibrinolytic system (this occurs with disseminated intravascular coagulation (DIC)). Examples of the former are the high incidence of thrombosis in autopsied cancer cases (*52*) and the thromboses that occur with occult tumors of pancreas, lung, stomach, and other neoplasms. Pathologic activation of both the coagulation and fibrinolytic systems, however, results in thrombolytic and hemorrhagic events (DIC). In this syndrome, consumption of platelets, fibrinogen, and other factors occurs during coagulation, while hydrolysis of fibrinogen/fibrin with generation of split products results from the fibrinolytic activity. Much evidence indicates that the consumptive process is initiated by the release of thromboplastin-like material into the circulation, with resulting coagulation; the fibrinolytic activity is thought to be induced secondarily (*58*).

Tissue factor (TF), also known as thromboplastin, is a glycoprotein which can bind to clotting factor VII and generate an enzyme which can activate factor X. A number of reactions then ensue, culminating in the formation of a fibrin clot. TF is thought to be sequestered on the surface of a number of cell types (including fibroblasts (*39, 69, 70*), endothelial, and smooth muscle cells) and may also be associated with subendothelial structures such as collagen and basement membrane (*40*). It is the "procoagulant activity," described in cultures of fibroblast cells (*69*), that was later identified as TF (*55*). Early studies indicate that TF activity of human fibroblasts in culture increased with time, and it was thought that attachment and spreading triggered the synthesis of TF. However, total cellular and surface activities have been found to be highest in growing fibroblast and endothelial cells, whereas confluent cells have little or no surface activity; the appearance of TF activity requires RNA and protein synthesis (*40, 69*).

One may interpret these findings in light of the model presented in this review: cell growth evokes new TF synthesis, transport, and insertion into the cell membrane. The cryptic nature of TF in confluent cells indicates that either little TF is present on the cell surface or that it is masked; the former is likely to be the case if TF resembles PA in its metabolism. This, of course, would be desired especially in endothelial cells. If total and cell surface TF activity are increased in growing cells, the same situation might be expected to occur in cancer cells. Indeed, tumor cells are particularly rich in thromboplastic activity (*53*). Recent evidence also indicates that TF is shed from tumor cells *in vitro* (*16*), and it is likely that such shedding from tumor cells occurs *in vivo*. Such release of TF is presumably responsible for activation of the extrinsic pathway of clotting and may occur both locally and systemically in cancer.

3.   *Invasion and metastasis*

The ability of cells to invade normal tissues and metastasize to distant sites characterizes them as malignant cells. If one hopes to interrupt this process, the mechanisms underlying these events must be known. For invasion, and/or metastasis to occur, cells must separate from the primary tumor mass. In addition, during the process of metastasis, cells must enter vascular channels, be disseminated throughout the body, become arrested, penetrate the endothelium, move out of the vascular space, and infiltrate and grow in the extravascular space.

The mechanism(s) whereby cells separate from the primary tumor mass is not understood. Increased tumor tissue pressure, the loss of certain cell-to-cell junctions, the known motility of cancer cells, a decrease in cell surace and/or released proteolytic activity may all be factors (*61*). The loss of adhesive forces between cancer cells, which facilitates separation, has been known for some time (*12*). Such loss presumably results from some change in the physicochemical bonds on the surface of adjacent cells or between the cell and intercellular matrix. The decrease or absence of adhesion proteins such as fibronectin or a fibronectin-glycosaminoglycan (*e.g.*, heparan sulfate) complex (*50*) would influence such interactions and is likely to be an important factor in the loss of adhesion.

More insight into the mechanism of separation can be gained by considering the properties of peripheral tumor cells, which separate, infiltrate, and may metastasize. This area of a tumor is usually well vascularized and the cells have a high rate of DNA synthesis compared to the more hypoxic core (*61*). It is known that in culture an increased growth rate of both normal and cancer cells is associated with cell detachment from a solid surface; furthermore, cells in mitosis round up and partially detach from the monolayer. It is also known that the most actively dividing tumors (and also the most anaplastic) have the greatest tendency to infiltrate and metastasize (*68*).

The aforementioned evidence suggests that actively growing cells are associated with separation and metastasis. The shedding of cell surface molecules, particularly the adhesion proteins and glycoproteins, which occurs during activation and cell cycle traverse, is likely to be involved in separation. Whether cell surface proteases, either directly or indirectly, affect the separation process is uncertain.

The possible involvement of proteolytic enzymes elaborated by tumor cells (particularly collagenase) in modifying surrounding normal tissues to facilitate invasion and metastasis has received much attention (see Ref. *59* for review). A number of studies indicate a relationship between malignancy and collagenase activity (*1, 24*). Moreover, metastatic cells may also have high proteolytic activity. These results, together with reports of the selection of supermetastatic sublines from tumors (*19*), indicate that cells in the tumor population are heterogeneous and that cells that have exposed or are releasing proteases may more successfully infiltrate and metastasize (*6*); metabolically active cells at the periphery of tumors are more likely to exhibit these characteristics.

Throughout the cascade of events that occur during metastasis, there is continuous selection: certain cells separate, infiltrate, and enter the vascular space; only a fraction of circulating cells successfully adhere and penetrate; and only a proportion acquire a vascular supply and stroma and successfully grow. One may hypothesize that dividing and shedding tumor cells are involved in separation, infiltration, and metastasis. Such cells are relatively devoid of adhesion proteins and contain and shed surface proteases. Such proteases, either alone or together with others activated either on the cell surface or in the immediate tumor vicinity, may induce the tissue hydrolysis necessary for invasion and metastasis. Surface and/or released TF activity is likely to promote fibrin formation associated with both the primary tumor and the tumor emboli.

CONCLUSIONS

The release of cellular constituents by the process of shedding has been discussed in this paper. It is distinguished from secretion, the release of cellular products *via* exocytosis. Shedding is an important aspect of normal cell physiology as it is involved in membrane turnover and the release of cellular products necessary for cellular function. Shedding is a characteristic of cell activation and, as such, is subject to the controls of cell activation operative in normal cells. However, in cancer cells, there is a defect in the control of cell activation. Consequently, a control of shedding by malignant cells may be lacking. Unregulated shedding of various tumor cell products may account for some of the properties of malignant cells. They include invasion, metastasis, evasion of the immune system and induction of irregularities in the clotting pathway. Interferon treatment has been shown to inhibit the shedding of PA from SV40-transformed 3T3 cells (54) and has increased the presence of surface antigens on lymphoid cell lines (34). It is possible that the effect on shedding of interferon may contribute to its antitumor effect. In this regard, the imposition of control on shedding by malignant cells may constitute a means of therapy for cancer in the future.

REFERENCES

1. Abramson, M., Huang, C.-C., Schilling, R. W., and Salome, R. G. *Ann. Otol.*, **84**, 158–163 (1975).
2. Bennett, B. T., Debelak-Fehir, K. M., and Epstein, R. B. *Cancer Res.*, **35**, 2942–2947 (1975).
3. Biddison, W. E. and Palmer, J. C. *Proc. Natl. Acad. Sci. U.S.*, **74**, 329–333 (1977).
4. Black, P. H. *Adv. Cancer Res.*, **23**, 75–199 (1980).
5. Bonavida, B. *J. Immunol.*, **112**, 926–934 (1974).
6. Bosmann, H. B., Bieber, G. F., Brown, A. E., Case, K. R., Gersten, D. M., Kimmerer, T. W., and Lione, A. *Nature*, **246**, 487–489 (1973).
7. Broder, S. and Waldmann, T. A. *N. Engl. J. Med.*, **299**, 1281–1284 and 1335–1341 (1978).
8. Brown, C. A., Hall, C. L., Long, J. C., Carey, K., Weitzman, S. A., and Aisenberg, A. C. *Am. J. Med.*, **64**, 289–294 (1978).
9. Chou, I.-N., Black, P. H., and Roblin, R. O. *Nature*, **250**, 739–741 (1974).
10. Chou, I.-N., O'Donnell, S. P., Black, P. H., and Roblin, R. O. *J. Cell. Physiol.*, **91**, 31–37 (1977).
11. Christman, J. K., Acs, G., Silagi, S., and Silverstein, S. C. *In* "Proteases and Biological Control," ed. E. Reich, D. Rifkin, and E. Shaw, pp. 827–839 (1975). Cold Spring Harbor Laboratory, Cold Spring Harbor.
12. Coman, D. R. *Cancer Res.*, **4**, 625–629 (1944).
13. Costanza, M. E., Pinn, V., Schwartz, R. S., and Nathanson, L. *N. Engl. J. Med.*, **289**, 520–522 (1973).
14. Davey, G. C., Currie, G. A., and Alexander, P. *Br. J. Cancer*, **33**, 9–14 (1976).
15. Diener, E. and Feldman, M. *Transplant. Rev.*, **8**, 76–103 (1972).
16. Dvorak, H. F., Orenstein, N. S., Carvalho, A. C., Churchill, W. H., Dvorak, A. M., Galli, S. J., Feder, J., Bitzer, A. M., Rypysc, J., and Giovinco, P. *J. Immunol.*, **122**, 166–174 (1979).
17. Embleton, M. J. *Int. J. Cancer*, **18**, 622–629 (1976).
18. Emerson, S. G. and Cone, R. E. *J. Immunol.*, **127**, 482–486 (1981).
19. Fidler, I. J. and Kripke, M. L. *Science*, **197**, 893–895 (1977).
20. Fischer, A. *Arch. Mikrosk. Anat. Entwicklungsmech.*, **104**, 210–261 (1925).
21. Gillette, R. W. and Boone, C. W. *Cancer Res.*, **35**, 3774–3779 (1975).
22. Glaser, M., Kirchner, H., and Herberman, R. B. *Int. J. Cancer* **16**, 384–393 (1975).
23. Golub, S. H. *In* "Cancer 4. Biology of Tumors: Surfaces, Immunology, Comparative Pathology," ed. F. F. Becker, pp. 259–300 (1975). Plenum Press, New York.
24. Hashimoto, K., Yamanishi, Y., Maeyens, E., Dabbous, M. K., and Kanzaki, T. *Cancer Res.*, **33**, 2790–2801 (1973).
25. Hamilton, J. A. *Cancer Res.*, **40**, 2273–2280 (1980).
26. Hellstrom, K. E. and Hellstrom, I. *Annu. Rev. Microbiol.*, **24**, 373–398 (1970).
27. Hellstrom, K. E. and Hellstrom, I. *Proc. Natl. Acad. Sci. U.S.*, **75**, 436–440 (1978).
28. Jaken, S. and Black, P. H. *Proc. Natl. Acad. Sci. U.S.*, **76**, 246–250 (1979).

29. Jaken, S. and Black, P. H. *J. Cell Biol.*, **90**, 721–726 (1981).
30. Klein, G. *In* "The Harvey Lectures," Ser. 69, pp. 71–102 (1975). Academic Press, New York.
31. Jaken, S. and Black, P. H. *J. Cell Biol.*, **90**, 727–731 (1981).
32. Jamasbi, R. J., Nettesheim, P., and Kennel, S. J. *Int. J. Cancer*, **21**, 387–394 (1978).
33. Kuppers, R. C. and Henney, C. S. *J. Immunol.*, **118**, 71–76 (1977).
34. Lindahl, P., Gresser, I., Lear, P., and Tovey, M. *Proc. Natl. Acad. Sci. U.S.*, **73**, 1284–1287 (1976).
35. Long, J. C., Hall, C. L., Brown, C. A., Stamatos, C., Weitzman, S. A., and Carey, K. N. *Engl. J. Med.*, **297**, 295–299 (1977).
36. Loskutoff, D. J. and Paul, D. *J. Cell. Physiol.*, **97**, 9–16 (1978).
37. Loughbridge, L. W. and Lewis, M. G. *Lancet*, **i**, 256–258 (1971).
38. Manor, Y., Treves, A. J., Cohen, I. R., and Feldman, M. *Transplantation*, **22**, 360–366 (1976).
39. Maynard, J. R., Heckman, C. A., Pitlick, F. A., and Nemerson, Y. *J. Clin. Invest.*, **55**, 814–824 (1975).
40. Maynard, J. R., Freyer, B. E., Stemerman, M. B., and Pitlick, F. A. *Blood*, **50**, 387–396 (1977).
41. Nepom, J. T., Hellstrom, I., and Hellstrom, K. E. *Proc. Natl. Acad. Sci. U.S.*, **74**, 4605–4609 (1977).
42. Nordquist, R. E., Anglin, J. H., and Lerner, M. P. *Science*, **197**, 366–367 (1977).
43. Old, L. J., Stockert, E., Boipe, E. A., and Kim, J. H. *J. Exp. Med.*, **127**, 523–539 (1968).
44. Oldstone, M.B.A., Theofilopoulos, A. N., Gunven, P., and Klein, G. *Intervirology*, **4**, 292–302 (1974).
45. Parks, R. C. *J. Natl. Cancer Inst.*, **54**, 1473–1474 (1975).
46. Poupon, M.-F., Kolb, J.-P., and Lespinats, G. *J. Natl. Cnacer Inst.*, **57**, 1241–1247 (1976).
47. Price, M. R., and Baldwin, R. W. *In* "Dynamic Aspects of Cell Surface Organization," ed. G. Poste and G. L. Nicolson, pp. 423–471 (1977). Elsevier-North Holland, New York.
48. Roblin, R. O., Chou, I.-N., and Black, P. H. *Adv. Cancer Res.*, **22**, 203–260 (1975).
49. Rohrlich, S. T. and Rifkin, D. B. *J. Cell Biol.*, **75**, 31–42 (1977).
50. Rollins, B. J. and Culp, L. A. *Biochemistry*, **18**, 141–148 (1979).
51. Ryan, J. L., Arbeit, R. D., Dickler, H. B., and Henkart, P. A. *J. Exp. Med.*, **142**, 814–826 (1975).
52. Sack, G. H., Jr., Levin, J., and Bell, W. R. *Medicine*, **56**, 1–37 (1977).
53. Sakuragawa, N., Takahashi, K., Hoshiyama, M., Jimbo, C., Ashizawa, K., Matsuoka, M., and Ohnishi, Y. *Thromb. Res.*, **10**, 457–463 (1977).
54. Schroder, E. W., Chou I.-N., Jaken, S., and Black, P. H. *Nature*, **276**, 828–829 (1978).
55. Siekevitz, P. *J. Theor. Biol.*, **37**, 321–334 (1972).
56. Stackpole, C. W., Jacobson, J. B., and Lardis, M. P. *J. Exp. Med.*, **140**, 939–953 (1974).
57. Steele, G., Jr., Sjogren, H. O., Rosengren, J. E., Lindstrom, C., Larsson, A., and Leandoer, L. *J. Natl. Cancer Inst.*, **54**, 959–966 (1975).
58. Straub, P. W., Riedler, G., and Frick, P. G. *J. Clin. Pathol.*, **20**, 152–157 (1967).
59. Strauch, L. *In* "Tissue Interactions in Carcinogenesis," ed. D. Tarin, pp. 399–434 (1972). Academic Press, London.
60. Sugamura, K. and Smith, J. B. *Cell. Immunol.*, **30**, 353–357 (1977).
61. Sugarbaker, E. V. and Ketcham, A. S. *Sem. Oncol.*, **4**, 19–32 (1977).
62. Targowski, S. P., Abeyounis, C. J., and Milgrom, F. *Proc. Soc. Exp. Biol. Med.*, **154**, 365–367 (1977).
63. Theofilopoulos, A. N., Andrews, B. S., Urist, M. M., Morton, D. L., and Dixon, R. J. *J. Immunol.*, **119**, 657–663 (1977).

64. Treves, A. J., Cohen, I. R., and Feldman, M. *J. Natl. Cancer Inst.*, **57**, 409–414 (1976).
65. Unkeless, J. C., Tobia, A., Ossowski, L., Quigley, J. P., Rifkin, D. B., and Reich, E. *J. Exp. Med.*, **137**, 85–111 (1973).
66. Urovitz, E. P., Czitrom, A. A., Langer, F., Gross, A. E., and Pritzker, K.P.H. *J. Bone Joint Surg.*, **58** A, 308–311 (1976).
67. Vetterlein, D., Young, P. L., Bell, R. E., and Roblin, R. *J. Biol. Chem.*, **254**, 575–578 (1979).
68. Weiss, L. *Sem. Oncol.* **4**, 5–17 (1977).
69. Zacharski, L. R. and McIntyre, O. R. *Nature*, **232**, 338–339 (1971).
70. Zacharski, L. R. and McIntyre, O. R. *Proc. Soc. Exp. Biol. Med.*, **139**, 713–715 (1972).

GANN Monograph on Cancer Research 29, 1983

TURNOVER OF PLASMA MEMBRANE GLYCOPROTEINS FROM LIVER AND HEPATOMA

Werner Reutter and Rudolf Tauber

Institut für Molekularbiologie und Biochemie, Freie Universität Berlin

1. Based on the findings of increased protein-bound fucose and an enhancement in the fucoprotein pattern in plasma membranes of Morris hepatoma 7777, measurements on the biosynthesis and degradation of membrane fucoproteins have been performed.

2. With respect to turnover, it could be shown that in hepatoma the regulation of degradation of overall membrane glycoproteins is different from that of normal or regenerating liver.

3. Using isolated membrane glycoproteins of liver, an intramolecular heterogeneity of glycoprotein degradation can be revealed. The terminal carbohydrates, especially fucose, are turning over at the highest rate.

4. Three possible mechanisms of the involvement of this new membrane glycoprotein characteristic in biological functions are presented.

The most susceptible alterations of cancer cells are observed in the nucleus and in the plasma membrane. The former sets the pace for carcinogenesis and the latter is highly correlated to metastasis (7). Their interdependence is still unknown. Research on membrane alterations revealed that after oncoviral transformation both the glycoproteins and the glycolipids of plasma membranes are significantly altered (see also the contributions of Warren, Kobata, or Davidson (4, 12, 18) in this volume). In our studies membrane glycoproteins of a solid growing tumor (Morris hepatoma) has been compared with normal liver and in some cases with regenerating liver (as a fast growing/ but controlled differentiating liver tissue). Advantages of this system have been outlined previously (10).

Large Fucosylglycoprotein in Plasma Membrane

The present studies have been prompted by two observations. Firstly, the concentration of protein-bound L-fucose in hepatoma plasma membranes is more than four times that of liver (Table I). Secondly, the pattern of fucopolypeptides of plasma membranes of Morris hepatoma 7777 is significantly different from that of normal liver (Fig. 1 and Ref. *17*): in hepatoma, many glycoproteins exhibit an increased fucose labelling. In the high molecular range, a 190 kilodaltons (kD)-glycoprotein (Mr. 190,000) is labelled with L-fucose forty times (in dpm/mg protein) more than the average hepatoma plasma membrane. Neither finding (Table I and Fig. 1) was seen in regenerating liver. This increase of fucosylpolypeptides of apparently high molecular weight seems, therefore, to be a characteristic feature of malignant hepatic tissue. The high-molecular weight fucoproteins may be correlated to the occurrence of the "early eluting" glycopeptides in virus-trans-

---

* D-1000 Berlin 33, West Germany.

TABLE I.   Content of Protein-bound Carbohydrates in the Plasma Membranes
of Hepatoma and Host Liver

Sugar	Content (nmol/mg protein)	
	Morris hepatoma 7777	Host liver
L-Fucose	26.1±3.7	6.1±1.7
N-acetylneuraminic acid	60.7±8.7	50.1±8.7
Galactose	100.3±9.1	81.4±8.4
Mannose	44.6±4.2	35.2±2.5
N-acetyl-glucosamine	127.4±32.9	95.8±8.8
N-acetyl-galactosamine	78.4±12.9	49.8±6.6

Adapted to Ref. 17.

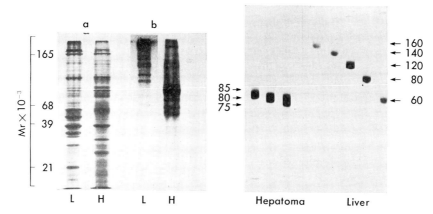

FIG. 1 (left).   Fucosylated plasma membrane glycoproteins from liver and Morris
hepatoma 7777. Buffalo rats bearing hepatoma were labeled in vivo with 100 μCi
L-[14C]-fucose per 100 g body weight. Plasma membranes from host liver (L) and
hepatoma (H) were isolated 1 hr after injection of the label, followed by separation
on a 10% SDS-polyacrylamide slab gel and fluorographed. The position of molecular weight (×10⁻³) standards is indicated. a, Coomassie staining; b, fluorogra-
phic pattern. For further details see Refs. 15 and 17.

FIG. 2 (right).   Glycoproteins isolated from the plasma membrane of liver and
Morris hepatoma 7777. The purified glycoproteins (16) were separated by SDS-
polyacrylamide gel electrophoresis and stained with Coomassie blue. Adapted to
Ref. 16.

formed cells as originally found by the groups of Robbins (19), Warren (3), and Emmelot (6).

These findings suggested experiments to elaborate possible mechanisms responsible
for these specific alterations of the fucoprotein pattern in hepatoma plasma membranes.

Metabolism of Fucoproteins

Since alterations either of biosynthesis or degradation of fucoproteins may be responsible for this disturbance, the following measurements have been performed.

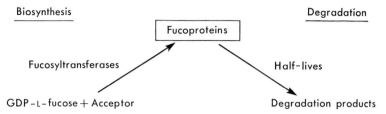

With respect to biosynthesis, it could be shown that in Morris hepatomas the concentration of guanosine-5′-diphosphate (GDP)-L-fucose is increased two-fold (from 6 to 12 nmol/g wet weight) (10, 17). No alterations were found in regenerating liver. Also the concentration of the protein acceptors available for fucosylation is two to three times higher in hepatoma, but not in regenerating liver. Furthermore, the activities of α_2- and α_3-fucosyltransferases are elevated in hepatoma tissue (2). These enzyme activities are also increased in regenerating liver, indicating characteristics of rapidly growing tissue but not of malignancy (C. H. Bauer, unpublished results).

The degradation of fucoproteins was studied in the plasma membranes of liver and hepatoma, since no data are available on the possible role of glycoprotein catabolism for the altered pattern of membrane glycoproteins in malignant cells (11). Three main characteristics of glycoprotein breakdown were found in the plasma membranes: during enhanced growth of regenerating liver the overall half-life of plasma membrane glycoproteins is increased (13, 14). This down-regulation of plasma membrane breakdown may be interpreted as part of the restoration process after resection of two-thirds of the liver. By contrast, in Morris hepatoma the rate of degradation of plasma membrane glycoproteins is evidently not regulated by the same mechanism as in the regenerating liver. Depending on the time after transplantation and the type of tumor, protein half-lives in hepatoma were increased or decreased or were in the same range as in liver plasma

TABLE II. Rate Constants of Degradation and Half-lives of Plasma Membrane Proteins in Hepatoma

Tissue	Days after inocula-tion	Plasma membrane		Soluble fraction		Total cell protein	
		K_d	$T_{1/2}$	K_d	$T_{1/2}$	K_d	$T_{1/2}$
Hepatoma 7777	13	0.44±0.01	1.6	—		0.38±0.01	1.8
Host liver		0.52±0.02	1.3	—		0.29±0.02	2.3
Hepatoma 7777	26	0.53±0.02	1.3	0.52±0.01	1.3	0.39±0.03	1.7
Host liver		0.52±0.04	1.3	0.24±0.02	2.8	0.27±0.01	2.5
Hepatoma 3924A	15	0.44±0.02	1.6	—		0.19±0.04	3.6
Host liver		0.62±0.02	1.1	—		0.40±0.02	1.7
Hepatoma 3924A	28	0.25±0.07	2.7	0.26±0.05	2.7	0.28±0.02	2.5
Host liver		0.54±0.04	1.3	0.46±0.1	1.5	0.38±0.05	1.8
Hepatoma 9121	20	0.67±0.01	1.0	0.52±0.01	1.3	0.57±0.01	1.2
Host liver		0.53±0.05	1.3	0.36±0.01	1.9	0.39±0.01	1.8
Hepatoma 9121	27	0.31±0.01	2.2	—		0.20±0.02	3.5
Host liver		0.53±0.01	1.3	—		0.29±0.02	2.4

Plasma membranes, a soluble fraction and total cell homogenates of Morris hepatoma were prepared at various times after *in vivo* labelling with sodium [^{14}C] carbonate.

Rate constant (per day) of degradation K_d and half-lives $T_{1/2}$ (days) were calculated from the decay of specific radioactivity assuming first order kinetics. Means±S.E.M. From Ref. *14*.

membranes (Table II). This dysregulation of membrane glycoprotein degradation may also contribute to alteration of the fucopolypeptide pattern observed in hepatoma plasmamembrane. Whether the dysregulation of membrane glycoprotein degradation or the dysregulation of acceptor protein biosynthesis is mainly responsible for the described alteration of hepatoma plasma membrane pattern cannot be decided on the basis of overall measurements. This unsatisfactory situation prompted studies on isolated membrane glycoproteins.

Molecular Species of Plasma Membrane Fucoproteins

The aim of our research project is to compare biosynthesis and degradation of single defined glycoproteins isolated from the plasma membrane of liver with antigenically identical glycoprotein (identical in its protein part) isolated from the hepatoma plasma membrane. First, experiments were done studying the degradation of defined plasma membrane glycoproteins isolated from normal liver. With respect to the observed alterations of fucoproteins in hepatoma, we intended to isolate plasma membrane glycoproteins with a high content of fucose. Since we had no hint of any enzymatic activity of those fucoproteins, glycoprotein fractions were enriched and selected for their incorporation of radioactivity after *in vivo* labelling with ³H-fucose. After appropriate solubilization, lectin affinity chromatography and sodium dodecylsulfate (SDS) gel electrophoresis a fucose-enriched glycoprotein could be isolated from rat liver plasma membrane with an apparent molecular weight of 110 kD (*8*). Further experiments established that it is the monomer of the dipeptidylpeptidase IV (DPP IV) which has an apparent molecular weight of 220 kD (*9*). In the last two years the isolation and partial characterization was made of five further membrane glycoproteins with apparent molecular weights of 160 kD (GP 1), 140 kD (GP 2), 120 kD (GP 3), 80 kD (GP 4), and 60 kD (GP 5) and, further, three glycoproteins from hepatoma plasma membranes (Fig. 2). The methodologic difference between the isolation of DPP IV and that of the latter glycoproteins was mainly in the extraction step. All of these isolated glycoproteins are characterized by a high content of protein-bound fucose, especially GP2 (*16*).

Half-lives of Fucoproteins

The degradation of the isolated plasma membrane glycoproteins was measured *in vivo* in pulse-chase experiments (Table III). Comparing the half-lives of the carbohy-

TABLE III. Half-lives of Carbohydrate and Protein Moieties
of the Glycoproteins from Normal Rat Liver

Precursor	Half-life (hr)					
	GP 60	GP 80	DPP IV[a]	GP 120	GP 140	GP 160
[³H] leucine	62	85	60	88	78	52
[¹⁴C] mannose	58	38	56	51	66	26
[¹⁴C] fucose	21	17	12	21	16	16
N-[³H] acetyl-mannosamine	33	31	30	27	29	26

For methods see Table II and Refs. *8* and *16*.
[a] DPP IV is a monomer with a molecular weight of 110,000.

drate and protein moieties of these glycoproteins a general characteristic of membrane glycoprotein breakdown was apparent: in each of the glycoproteins investigated the half-life of the carbohydrate portion was found to be significantly shorter than that of the protein backbone. Moreover, within the carbohydrate moiety two domains could be distinguished with respect to splitting off carbohydrates. The domain of terminal sugars is characterized by a very rapid turnover (mobile region). In DPP IV the half-life of protein-bound fucose is at least one fifth of the protein moiety. Surprisingly, in DPP IV and the other glycoproteins investigated the half-life of N-acetylneuraminic acid is significantly longer than that of the other terminal carbohydrate, fucose. Therefore, it is assumed that the core fucose-α 1, 6-linked to the innermost N-acetylglucosamine is turning over faster than any other terminal carbohydrate. Secondly, the domain of the core sugars of the oligosaccharide moiety is degraded with half-lives corresponding to that of the protein moiety (immobile region). This is mostly expressed in DPP IV and GP 5, where the core sugar mannose had the same half-life as did the protein backbone. In GP 4, GP 3, and GP 2 mannose half-lives were somewhat shorter than that of the polypeptide, but were significantly longer compared to the terminal sugars. The results obtained in GP 1, where mannose is turning over as fast as N-acetylneuraminic acid, point to individual differences in the breakdown of the core region of the carbohydrate moiety. This intramolecular heterogeneity seems to be a general characteristic of membrane glycoproteins in liver (8, 16). The observed short half-lives of terminal carbohydrates compared to the core sugars and protein backbone show that they are rapidly split off from the glycoproteins. At present the site and the mechanism of this deglycosylation is unknown. Moreover, since so far no accumulation of deglycosylated glycoproteins has been observed in the plasma membrane, a reglycosylation of the glycoproteins is assumed. Therefore, the aim of current studies is to localize the site and the mechanisms of a de- and reglycosylation of the isolated membrane glycoproteins.

Perspectives

The following working hypotheses should be tested experimentally.

1. Both de- and reglycosylation are taking place in endomembranes. Deglycosylation may be performed by neutral glycosidases of the endoplasmic reticulum or acid glycosidases of lysosomes (limited hydrolysis only), followed by reglycosylation in the Golgi complex and reinsertion into the plasma membrane. This possibility may be working during receptor recycling (Fig. 3). The trigger for interiorization of a receptor glycoprotein might be the recognition and fixation of a receptor-specific extracellular ligand. This complex is interiorized, *e.g.*, *via* endocytosis. The ligand and the fixing terminal carbohydrates are split off. Whereas the ligand has now to find its intracellular target (*e.g.*, the nucleus or lysosomes), the deglycosylated glycoprotein receptor is reglycosylated within the Golgi complex and is reinserted into the plasma membrane *via* membrane flow. A candidate for a similar mechanism may be the asialoglycoprotein receptor (1). This rather economic view of receptor recycling implies the existence of an only partially glycosylated receptor glycoprotein in the cytosol, which is the subject of the current research.

2. De- and reglycosylation take place at the level of plasma membranes by transglycosylation. Sugar transfer may occur (Fig. 4A) from one glycoprotein to another within the same membrane or (B) from one glycoprotein to another in the plasma membranes

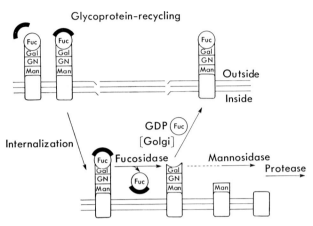

FIG. 3. Hypothetical model of intramolecular heterogeneity and receptor recycling. ⌒ means extracellular ligand. GN, N-acetylglucosamine. The fucose in this model can also be the core-fucose, linked to the innermost N-acetylglucosamine.

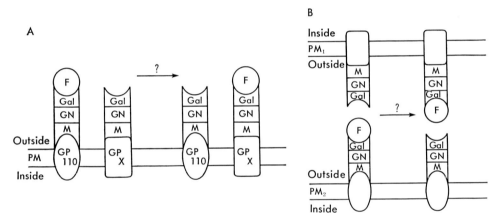

FIG. 4A. Hypothetical model of intramolecular heterogeneity and transglycosylation within the same membrane. GP 110 and GP X are two different membrane glycoproteins.

FIG. 4B. Hypothetical model of intramolecular heterogeneity and transglycosylation between two different cells. PM$_1$ and PM$_2$ indicate plasma membranes of these two cells. M, mannose.

of two neighboring cells. A hint of the existence of the latter possibility may be given by previous findings of Yogees-Waran *et al.* (*20*) showing the transfer of labelled carbohydrates to glycolipids attached to glass beads when in contact with the cell surface of NIL or BHK cells. With respect to cell-cell interaction transglycosylation would be of a simple kind of mediating intercellular communication. It may be assumed that its disturbance in the hepatoma is responsible for the alterations of the fucoprotein pattern in the plasma membrane.

    3. Deglycosylation may occur in the plasma membrane followed by glycosylation in the Golgi complex and reinsertion into the plasma membrane. Based on the findings of Ashwell (*1*) which demonstrated that some serum glycoproteins are recognized taken up and degraded by liver cells, and based on the report of partial reglycosylation of

serum glycoproteins by Debanne and Regoeczi (5), deglycosylated membrane glycoproteins may be similarily internalized and reglycosylated. Provided clusters of such
glycoproteins existed in defined membrane regions, endocytosis and membrane recycling
could be induced by such a mechanism.

REFERENCES

1. Ashwell, G. and Harford, J. *Annu. Rev. Biochem.*, **51**, 531–554 (1982).
2. Bauer, C. H., Vischer, P., Grünholz, H.-J., and Reutter, W. *Cancer Res.*, **37**, 1513–1518 (1977).
3. Buck, C. A., Fuhrer, J. P., Soslaw, G., and Warren, L. *J. Biol. Chem.*, **249**, 1541–1550 (1973).
4. Davidson, E. A., Bhavanandan, V. P., Barsoum, A. L., Hatae, Y., and Hatae, T. This volume, pp. 139–147.
5. Debanne, M. T. and Regoeczi, E. *J. Biol. Chem.*, **256**, 11266–11272 (1981).
6. Emmelot, P., van Beek, W. P., and Smets, L. A. *In* "Membrane Alterations as Basis of Liver Injury," ed. H. P. Popper, L. Bianchi, and W. Reutter, pp. 179–195 (1977). MTP Press, Lancaster.
7. Finne, J., Tao, T. W., and Burger, M. M. *Cancer Res.*, **40**, 2580–2587 (1980).
8. Kreisel, W., Volk, B. A., Büchsel, R., and Reutter, W. *Proc. Natl. Acad. Sci. U.S.*, **77**, 1828–1831 (1980).
9. Kreisel, W., Heussner, R., Volk, B., Büchsel, R., Reutter, W., and Gerok, W. *FEBS Lett.*, **147**, 85–88 (1982).
10. Reutter, W. and Bauer, C. *In* "Morris Hepatomas: Mechanisms of Regulation," ed. H. P. Morris and W. E. Criss, pp. 405–437 (1978). Plenum Press, New York.
11. Reutter, W., Tauber, R., Vischer, P., Grünholz, H.-J., and Bauer, C. H. *In* "Protein Turnover and Lysosome Function," ed. H. L. Segal and D. Doyle, pp. 779–790 (1978). Academic Press, New York.
12. Takasaki, S., Yamashita, K., and Kobata, A. This volume, pp. 129–137.
13. Tauber, R. and Reutter, W. *FEBS Lett.*, **87**, 135–140 (1978).
14. Tauber, R. and Reutter, W. *Eur. J. Biochem.*, **83**, 37–45 (1978).
15. Tauber, R. and Reutter, W. *Eur. J. Cell Biol.*, **26**, 35–43 (1981).
16. Tauber, R., Park, Ch.-S. and Reutter, W. *Proc. Natl. Acad. Sci. U.S.*, in press.
17. Vischer, P. and Reutter, W. *Eur. J. Biochem.*, **84**, 363–368 (1978).
18. Warren, L. and Cossu, G. This volume, pp. 107–112.
19. Wu, H. C., Meezan, E., Black, P. H., and Robbins, P. W. *Biochemistry*, **8**, 2509–2514 (1969).
20. Yogeeswaran, G., Laine, R. A., and Hakomori, S. *Biochem. Biophys. Res. Commun.*, **59**, 591–599 (1974).

III. DIFFERENTIATION OF TUMOR CELLS AND CELL SURFACE CHANGES

MEMBRANE GALACTOSYL SITES: ROLE IN LYMPHOCYTE PROLIFERATION AND DIFFERENTIATION

Abraham Novogrodsky[*1] and Kurt H. Stenzel[*2]

*The Rogoff-Wellcome Medical Research Institute, Beilinson Medical Center, Tel Aviv University Sackler School of Medicine[*1] and The Rogosin Kidney Center, Departments of Biochemistry and Medicine, Cornell University Medical College[*2]*

The lymphocyte membrane serves to transmit external signals that induce lymphocyte proliferation and differentiation. Most of the agents that induce polyclonal proliferation of T-cells interact with cell-surface saccharide moieties. These mitogens include lectins and the oxidizing agents; sodium periodate and galactose oxidase (GO). The target sites for the mitogenic action of periodate and GO are surface membrane sialyl and galactosyl residues, respectively, that yield on oxidation an aldehyde moiety that is involved in the triggering process. Galactosyl residues exposed after neuraminidase (NA) treatment serve as the target site(s) for the mitogenic action of GO and the galactosyl binding lectins; soybean agglutinin, peanut agglutinin (PNA), and hepatic binding protein. Aldehyde-induced blastogenesis could be associated with the formation of a cross-linked structure on the aldehyde-modified cell itself or between adjacent cells. Proliferation of peripheral blood mononuclear cells (PBL) can be stimulated by irradiated autologous PBL that have been treated with NA and GO (NAGO). NAGO-treated macrophages are the most potent stimulatory cells followed in order of stimulatory potency by B and finally T-cells. T-cells are the responding cells. Lymphoblastoid cell lines treated with NAGO, were stimulatory. B-cell lines were more potent than T-cell lines and the membrane fractions from NAGO-treated B-cell lines retained stimulatory activity. Chemical and enzymic modifications of the cell surface of malignant cells and lymphocytes may provide a useful tool in modulating the immune response to tumor cells. Membrane-galactosyl sites also serve as differentiation markers of lymphoid cells and other cell types. Murine lymphocytes could be fractionated according to their interaction with PNA. PNA[+] cells are immature cells that fail to respond to phytohemagglutinin (PHA) in the absence or presence of interleukin 1 (IL-1). PNA[-] cells are more mature cells that respond to PHA and can produce interleukin 2 (IL-2). 12-O-tetradecanoylphorbol-13-acetate (TPA) mimics the effect of IL-1 on mouse thymocytes. Both IL-1 and TPA stimulate IL-2 production by PHA-treated PNA[-] cells. IL-2 stimulates both PHA-treated PNA[+] and PNA[-] cells. Chemical agents that are known to induce cell differentiation markedly inhibit thymocyte mitogenesis *via* inhibition of IL-2 production.

[*1] Petah-Tikva, Israel.
[*2] New York, N.Y. 10021, U.S.A.

These agents also markedly inhibit proliferation of human leukemia *in vitro*, and may offer additional therapeutic agents for malignant disease.

DNA replication, cell-cell interactions and the invasiveness of cells are controlled by biochemical events occurring at the level of the cell membrane. Thus, many studies in recent years have focused on alterations in the membrane of cancer cells. Immunological mechanisms, including affector and effector reactions, are also mediated by membrane interactions. The lymphocyte provides a most useful cell for the study of membrane structure and function that is related to the control of cell proliferation and differentiation. We will discuss in this paper the role of membrane galactosyl sites in lymphocyte proliferation and differentiation.

Nature of Lymphocyte Mitogenic Site

The lymphocyte membrane serves to transmit external signals that induce lymphocyte proliferation. The signals that interact with the cell membrane and trigger proliferation may be either immunologically specific and induce a monoclonal proliferation, or may be immunologically non-specific and induce polyclonal proliferation. Most T-cell mitogens, agents that induce polyclonal proliferation of T-cells, interact with cell-surface polysaccharide moieties. These mitogens include certain lectins and the oxidizing agents, sodium periodate (IO_4^-) and galactose oxidase (GO). We discovered that mitogenic properties of the latter agents several years ago (15–17), and since then they have been studied in several laboratories. The initial step in the triggering of lymphocyte activation is mitogen binding to, or alteration of, cell surface structures. The nature of this interaction is central to understanding the mechanisms responsible for lymphocyte activation.

Lymphocytes from many species, such as human, rat, mouse, rabbit, and guinea pig, are stimulated by IO_4^- (1, 7, 15, 16, 25, 27). Treatment of lymphocytes with neuraminidase (NA) markedly reduces their response to IO_4^- (16). Mitogenesis induced by IO_4^- is also decreased when the treated lymphocytes are reacted with aldehyde blocking agents, such as borohydride or NH_2OH (16, 37). These findings led to the conclusion that the target site for IO_4^- action is a surface membrane sialyl residue, yielding on oxidation an aldehyde moiety, that is involved in the triggering process. This conclusion is further supported by the studies of Van Lenten and Ashwell (36) who showed that IO_4^-, under mild conditions, selectively oxidezes sialyl residues in sialo-glycoproteins, to yield a seven carbon sialic acid analogue containing an aldehyde moiety. Liao *et al.* (11) have also shown that the main targets of IO_4^- oxidation of human erythrocytes are sialic acid moieties of surface membrane sialoglycoproteins. More recently, Presant and Parker (28) and Durand *et al.* (5) have provided direct evidence that aldehyde is generated on sialyl moieties following treatment of lymphocytes with IO_4^-.

The observation that IO_4^- triggers lymphocyte activation *via* the formation of aldehyde moieties on the cell surface, prompted us to search for an enzymic modification of the cells that could mimic the IO_4^- effect. Sialic acid in glycoproteins always occupies a non-reducing terminal position, and is glycosidically linked either to D-galactose or N-acetylgalactosamine (32). Studies on plasma glycoproteins have shown that galactosyl residues exposed by the action of NA could be oxidized at the carbon six position to yield 6-aldehyde analogues (13). We found that treatment of lymphocytes with GO

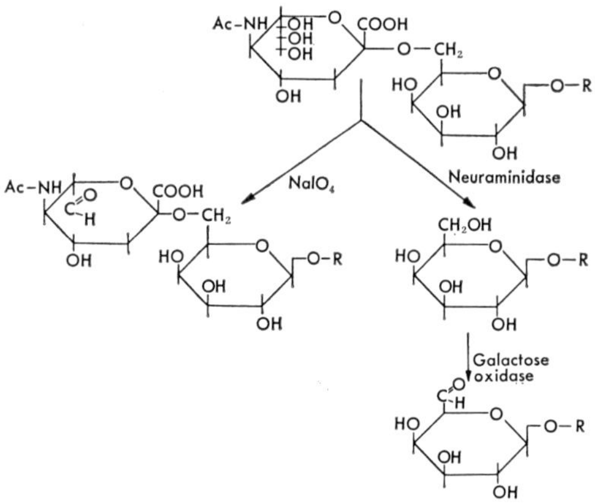

Fig. 1. Generation of aldehyde moieties on cell surface sialyl and NA-exposed galactosyl residues.

after incubation with NA induces extensive blastogenesis (17). Blastogenesis induced by the sequential treatment of cells with NA and GO (NAGO) is similar to that induced by IO_4^- in that it also was decreased upon reacting treated cells with reagents that interact and block aldehyde groups (4, 16, 17, 24, 37). The latter treatments do not affect transformation of cells induced by concanavalina A (Con A) (16). These findings led us to conclude that galactosyl residues on the cell membrane, exposed by the action of NA, are oxidized by GO and that the aldehyde moieties formed are involved in the induction of blastogenesis (Fig. 1).

In evaluating possible mechanisms responsible for aldehyde induced lymphocyte proliferation, we considered the possibility that the surface aldehyde interacts with functional groups on the cell surface to form a cross-linked structure. Cross-linking of cell surface sites has been implicated as playing a major role in lymphocyte activation by lectins. We designed the following experiment to examine this possibility. Biotin was conjugated to cells by sequential treatment of the cells with periodate, biotin hydrazide and borohydride. Cells treated in this way do not undergo blastogenesis since the aldehyde groups are effectively blocked. We then asked the question—would binding of avidin to the biotin-conjugated cells result in a proliferative response? The results indicated that avidin treatment of biotin-conjugated cells induced marked blastogenesis (14). Using similar experimental procedures, we have conjugated dinitrophenyl (DNP) moieties to lymphocytes, and measured the mitogenic properties of antibodies directed against the DNP group. The results indicate that the antibody, as well as its divalent fragment (F_{ab}) both induced a proliferative response in DNP-conjugated lymphocytes. In contrast, univalent antibodies failed to stimulate these cells (29).

The role of galactosyl sites in the triggering of lymphocyte activation was demonstrated directly by reacting galactosyl binding lectins with cells with exposed galactosyl sites. The galactosyl sites in human lymphocytes are partially exposed, whereas in mouse lymphocytes, these binding sites are completely masked by sialyl moieties that can be exposed by NA treatment. The galactosyl-membrane sites are heterogeneous. For instance, untreated human lymphocytes failed to respond to the galactosyl binding lectin, peanut agglutinin (PNA), whereas they undergo a partial response to another galactosyl binding lectin, soybean agglutinin. Following treatment with NA, lymphocytes undergo extensive mitogenesis in response to these lectins (*18, 19*). It is of interest to note that the mammalian lectin, hepatic binding protein, is also mitogenic for NA-treated lymphocytes. Sequential treatment of lymphocytes with NA and β-galactosidase, renders them unresponsive to the mitogenic effect of GO and the galactosyl binding lectins (*20*).

Cells treated with NAGO and rendered incapable of division by irradiation, were found to be mitogenic for untreated lymphocytes. The nature of the stimulatory cells and responding cells are different. T-cells are the responding cells whereas there is a hierarchy of stimulatory potency among peripheral blood mononuclear cells. Macrophages are the most potent stimulating cells followed by B and T cells. We investigated the stimulatory properties of a variety of human B and T lymphoblastoid cell lines following NAGO treatment. Among the lines we tested, we also noted a hierarchy in stimulatory potential. For instance, B lymphoblastoid lines were the most potent, whereas several T lines, MOLT 4 and 8402, were weak stimulatory cells. Another T-lymphoblastoid line, however, CEM, induced marked proliferation in responding cell populations. We are currently studying structural and functional requirements for stimulatory activity of these lymphoblastoid cells. These studies should provide information on mechanisms of stimulation of the immune system by malignant cells. From a practical standpoint, we are attempting to amplify the stimulatory potency of cells. This will be accomplished by chemical and enzymic methods as well as by introducing stimulatory components by fusion techniques. Cell membranes isolated from lymphoblastoid cell lines that are stimulatory following NAGO treatment, retain their stimulatory capacity. This finding provides the basis for further purification and identification of the stimulatory moieties involved in indirect stimulation by the cell lines.

Galactosyl Sites as Differentiation Markers

Galactosyl sites have been implicated as differentiation markers for malignant cells. Springer (*33*) has reported an increased binding of anti-T panagglutinin to mammary cancer cells as compared to cells from benign breast tumors. This agglutinin recognizes saccharide sites that are also recognized by PNA. Mouse thymocytes have been found to consist of at least two populations of cells. The major population contains undifferentiated cells that possess exposed sites for PNA. A minor population of cells among murine thymocytes lacks exposed sites for PNA, and consists of more differentiated cells. These two populations of thymocytes can be separated by agglutination techniques based on these properties (*31*). We have investigated the properties of these two populations in terms of their ability to respond to mitogens. Unfractionated mouse thymocytes do not respond to the mitogenic lectin, phytohemagglutinin (PHA), alone, but do proliferate when a macrophage-produced lymphocyte activating factor, or interleukin 1 (IL-1) is added to the PHA-treated cells. We have found that the tumor promoter, 12-O-tetradecanoylphorbol-13-acetate (TPA), mimics the effect of this physiologic lymphocyte growth factor (*30*). That is, while not mitogenic itself for mouse thymocytes, TPA induces extensive proliferation when added to PHA-treated thymocytes. Analysis of the isolated subpopulations of mouse thymocytes, namely the PNA+ and PNA− cells, yielded unexpected results. The major population, the PNA+ cells, failed to respond to PHA and TPA, or to PHA and IL-1. The population of PNA− cells, that accounts for a very small percent of the total cells in unfractionated thymocyte popula-

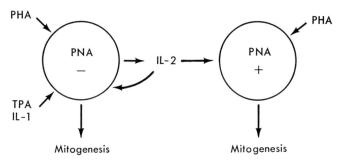

F<small>IG</small>. 2.   The co-mitogenic effect of TPA and IL-1 on murine thymocytes.

tions, responded in a manner similar to the responses seen in unfractionated cells. That is, extensive proliferation was induced by PHA and TPA and by PHA and IL-1. A clue to the solution of this apparent paradox was the finding that the T cell growth factor, interleukin 2 (IL-2), induced proliferation in both populations of thymocytes following exposure to PHA. This finding suggested that the PNA⁻ subpopulation was induced to produce IL-2 by PHA and TPA or PHA and IL-1. The mitogenic lymphokine, IL-2, then induced proliferation in both of the PHA-treated thymocyte subpopulations. We addressed this problem directly by measuring IL-2 production by PNA⁻ cells. The supernatant of PNA⁻ cells treated with either PHA and TPA or PHA and IL-1 induced proliferation in PHA treated PNA⁺ cells. We also quantitated IL-2 production by PNA⁻ cells with the use of a long-term mouse cytotoxic T lymphocyte line. PNA⁺ cells did not produce IL-2. Thus, activation of unfractionated thymocytes by PHA and TPA or by PHA and IL-1, depends on cell cooperativity, in which a minor population of cells produces a growth factor which activates the bulk of the cells in the unfractionated thymocyte preparations (Fig. 2).

Effects of Differentiating Agents on Lymphocyte Proliferation

A variety of agents, such as polar organic solvents, short chain fatty acids, purine derivatives, bisacetamides, and hemin, have been found to induce cell differentiation in murine erythroleukemia cells and several other cell lines. We found that there is a direct parallelism between the ability of a compound to induce cell differentiation on one hand, and to inhibit lymphocyte proliferation on the other hand (Table I) (*21, 34*). Human lymphocytes undergo mitogenesis in response to TPA alone. This stimulation was inhibited by the differentiating agents to a greater extent than were lymphocyte responses to mitogenic lectins or oxidizing agents. However, at high concentrations of the differentiating agents, these latter responses were also impaired. We recently found that murine thymocyte responses to PHA and TPA or to PHA and IL-1, are also exquisitely sensitive to the inhibitory effects of the differentiating agents (*22*). We asked the question—at what point in the activation process of mouse thymocytes outlined above (Fig. 2) did the differentiating agents act to inhibit proliferation? We found that thymocyte responses induced by IL-2 were resistant to inhibition by the differentiating agents (Fig. 3). This suggested that the site of inhibition was on the production of IL-2, stimulated by PHA and TPA or by PHA and IL-1, rather than on the response to IL-2. This was verified by demonstrating that the production of IL-2 was inhibited by the differentiating agents.

A. NOVOGRODSKY AND K. H. STENZEL

TABLE I. Inhibition of Lymphocyte Mitogenesis by Cellular Differentiating Agents

Compound tested	Concentration range (mM) resulting in 50% inhibition of ^{3}H-thymidine incorporation		Concentration (mM) reported to induce maximum erythroid differentiation in FL cells
	PMA-induced responses	PHA-induced responses	
1. Polar organic solvents			
DMSO	60	>210	70–300
Dimethylformamide	75	120	60–150
N,N-dimethylacetamide	5–10	25	20–30
Dimethylurea	20	50	40–50
Tetramethylurea	5	15	10–20
2. Short chain fatty acids			
Propionic acid	1–1.5	10	2
n-Butyric acid	0.1–0.4	1.4	1–2
n-Valeric acid	1.6	>4.0	2
Caproic acid	10	>10	Inactive
3. Butyric acid analogues			
Isobutyric acid	4–5	>10	30
β-OH-butyric acid	>10	>10	Inactive
γ-OH-butyric acid	>10	>10	
α-Amino-butyric acid	>10	>10	
β-Amino-butyric acid	>10	>10	
γ-Amino-butyric acid	>10	>10	Inactive
4. Purine analogues			
Hypoxanthine	1–2	>5.0	3.7
1-Methyl hypoxanthine	0.5–1.0	3–5.0	3.3
Xanthine	>5.0	>5.0	Inactive
Allantoin	>5.0	>5.0	Inactive
5. Hexamethylene bisacetamide	2	4	2–4
6. Hemin	0.05	0.1	0.1

PMA, phorbol myristate acetate.

The mechanism by which the differentiating agents inhibit IL-2 production is unknown. One group of the differentiating agents, the polar organic solvents, are known to be scavengers of activated oxygen radicals. We postulated that a free radical mediated mechanism might be involved in the propagation of the mitogenic signal (22). Consistent with this notion was the finding that additional free radical scavengers, such as benzoate, thiourea, and tryptophan, that are not known to induce cellular differentiation, share with the differentiating agents the property of inhibition of TPA-induced responses.

·OH could be generated by several cellular mechanisms. TPA activates membrane-bound NAD(P)H oxidase in neutrophils and results in the generation of free radicals (35). Free radicals are also generated by peroxidases involved in the lipoxygenase and cyclooxygenase pathways of arachidonic acid metabolism (6). Mitogens are known to enhance the release of arachidonic acid (26), the initial substrate for these pathways and inhibition of the lipoxygenase pathway inhibits lectin-induced lymphocyte proliferation (10). In addition, various intracellular oxidases are capable of generating free radicals.

What cellular biochemical events could be mediated by free radicals? An attractive possibility is the activation of guanylate cyclase by ·OH. Goldberg and his colleagues (9) and others (12) have shown that guanylate cyclase is subject to modulation by oxidative-reductive mechanisms and, in point of fact, is activated by ·OH. A possible role

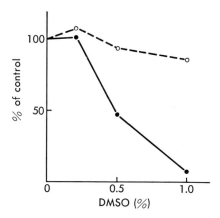

FIG. 3.   Effect of DMSO on proliferative responses of PHA-treated PNA⁻ murine thymocytes induced by IL-2 (○) and TPA (●).

for cGMP in mediating the mitogenic signal has previously been postulated (8), and the mitogenic lectin PHA has been reported to increase guanylate cyclase activity (3). We found that TPA stimulation increased guanylate cyclase activity in most experiments, a finding also recently reported by Coffey and Hadden (2). In addition, we found that the TPA-dependent increase in guanylate cyclase was inhibited in three of six experiments by the ·OH scavenger Me₂SO. Clearly, more studies are required to determine the relationship between ·OH scavenging and guanylate cyclase activity in PBM.

·OH could also inactivate enzymes and thus result in alterations of metabolic pathways. For instance, ·OH has been shown to inactivate cyclooxygenase and peroxidases involved in arachidonic acid metabolism (6).

Effect of Differentiating Agents on Poorly Differentiated Cells

The anti-proliferative effect of the differentiating agents for TPA-driven mitogenic responses prompted us to examine the effect of the differentiating agents on proliferation of cells from patients with leukemia (23). Butyric acid, dimethylsulfoxide (DMSO), dimethylacetamide, and dimethylformamide, all potent differentiating agents, inhibited thymidine incorporation in these cells. Propionic, isobutyric, and β-hydroxybutyric acids, on the other hand, compounds that have little differentiating effect, did not significantly affect the proliferative responses of the leukemic patients' cells. Most of the patients studied had either acute myelocytic or acute lymphocytic leukemia. Decreased thymidine uptake following incubation of leukemic cells from several of the patients with the differentiating agents was associated with cell damage. This damage was manifested initially by vacuolization of the cytoplasm and nucleus, followed by disintegration of the cells. The cytotoxic effect of the differentiating agents on leukemic cells is in marked contrast to their effect on normal cells. Incubation of normal cells with these agents for the same duration, at the maximal concentrations used, either with or without mitogenic stimulation, did not affect cell viability. The potency of the organic compounds to inhibit thymidine incorporation and to induce morphologic changes in leukemic cells, closely paralleled both their potency to induce differentiation in murine erythroleukemia cells and to inhibit mitogen-induced lymphocyte responses. The anti-proliferative properties of butyrate, its ability to induce differentiation in different cell types *in-vitro* and our

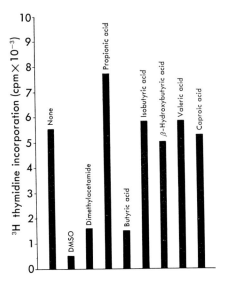

FIG. 4.   Effect of differentiating agents on proliferation of leukemic cells from a patient with acute myelocytic leukemia. The concentration of DMSO was 120 mM, dimethylacetamide 10 mM, and the fatty acids 1 mM.

finding of its selective cytotoxic effect on human leukemic cells, prompted us to determine possible *in-vivo* anti-leukemic effects of butyrate in a patient with acute myelogenous leukemia. This patient was in relapse and resistant to conventional therapy after repeated bouts of remissions and relapses. Butyrate (1 mM) treatment of the patient's cells *in vitro* induced cytotoxic changes concomitant with a decrease in thymidine incorporation (Fig. 4). Intravenous administration of butyrate resulted in remarkable changes in the leukemic peripheral blood cells. The number of myeloblasts gradually decreased and by the 15th day following initiation of intravenous butyrate, they were no longer detectable in the peripheral blood. This reduction in myeloblasts was followed by the appearance of mature myeloid cells, the most prominent being giant granulocytes, along with an increase in monocytes. Bone marrow myeloblasts decreases from 70–80% prior to butyrate treatment to approximately 20%. The patient again relapsed several weeks following discontinuation of butyrate.

The mechanism of the effect of differentiating agents on the leukemic cells could be related to the induction of differentiation in these cells or to the direct anti-proliferative effect. Nevertheless, the use of chemical differentiating agents may provide a new modality for the therapy of leukemia.

CONCLUSIONS

Membrane galactosyl sites on PNA[+] thymocytes appears to be one of several differentiation markers. It is certainly difficult to relate all the differences in functional properties between PNA[−] and PNA[+] cells to this particular structure. However, since the galactosyl site is a mitogenic site, it is tempting to speculate that this site might provide for mitogenic signals for these undifferentiated, rapidly dividing cells. This signal could be provided by an endogenous galactosyl binding lectin. Murine thymocytes provide a useful experimental system for investigating lymphocyte proliferation, differentiation, and the complex interrelationships between these two phenomena.

Acknowledgment

This work was supported in part by a grant from The National Science Foundation (Grant No. PCM 8208933).

REFERENCES

1. Biniaminov, M., Ramot, B., and Novogrodsky, A. *Clin. Exp. Immunol.*, **16**, 235–242 (1974).
2. Coffey, R. G. and Hadden, J. W. *Biochem. Biophys. Res. Commun.*, **101**, 584–590 (1981).
3. Coffey, R. G., Hadden, E. M., and Hadden, J. W. *J. Biol. Chem.*, **256**, 4418–4424 (1981).
4. Dixon, J.F.P., O'Brien, R. L., and Parker, J. W. *Exp. Cell Res.*, **96**, 383–387 (1975).
5. Durand, G., Guenounou, M., Feger, J., and Agenfray, J. *Biochem. Biophys. Res. Commun.*, **83**, 114–123 (1978).
6. Egan, R. W., Gale, P. H., and Kuchl, R. H., Jr. *J. Biol. Chem.*, **254**, 3295–3302 (1979).
7. Greineder, D. K. and Rosenthal, A. L. *J. Immunol.*, **115**, 932–938 (1975).
8. Hadden, J. W., Hadden, E. M., Haddox, M. K., and Goldberg, N. D. *Proc. Natl. Acad. Sci. U.S.*, **69**, 3024–3027 (1972).
9. Haddox, M. D., Stephenson, J. H., Moser, M. E., and Goldberg, N. D. *J. Biol. Chem.*, **253**, 3143–3152 (1978).
10. Kelly, J. P., Johnson, M. C., and Parker, C. W. *J. Immunol.*, **122**, 1563–1571 (1979).
11. Liao, T., Gallop, P. M., and Blumenfeld, O. O. *J. Biol. Chem.*, **248**, 8247–8253 (1973).
12. Mittel, C. K. and Murad, F. *Proc. Natl. Acad. Sci. U.S.*, **74**, 4360–4364 (1977).
13. Morell, A. G., Vanden Hamer, C.J.A., Scheinberg, I. H., and Ashwell, G. *J. Biol. Chem.*, **241**, 3745–3749 (1966).
14. Novogrodsky, A. *In* "Biogenesis and Turnover of Membrane Macromolecules," ed. J. S. Cook, pp. 221–233 (1976). Raven Press, New York.
15. Novogrodsky, A. and Katchalski, E. *FEBS Lett.*, **12**, 297–300 (1971).
16. Novogrodsky, A. and Katchalski, E. *Proc. Natl. Acad. Sci. U.S.*, **69**, 3207–3210 (1972).
17. Novogrodsky, A. and Katchalski, E. *Proc. Natl. Acad. Sci. U.S.*, **70**, 1824–1827 (1973).
18. Novogrodsky, A. and Katchalski, E. *Proc. Natl. Acad. Sci. U.S.*, **70**, 2515–2518 (1973).
19. Novogrodsky, A., Lotan, R., Ravid, A., and Sharon, N. *J. Immunol.*, **115**, 1243–1248 (1975).
20. Novogrodsky, A. and Ashwell, G. *Proc. Natl. Acad. Sci. U.S.*, **74**, 676–678 (1977).
21. Novogrodsky, A., Rubin, A. L., and Stenzel, K. H. *J. Immunol.*, **124**, 1892–1897 (1980).
22. Novogrodsky, A., Ravid, A., Rubin, A. L., and Stenzel, K. H. *Proc. Natl. Acad. Sci. U.S.*, **79**, 1171–1174 (1982).
23. Novogrodsky, A., Dvir, A., Ravid, A., Schkolnik, T., Stenzel, K. H., Rubin, A. L., and Zaizov, R. *Cancer*, in press.
24. O'Brien, R. L., Parker, J. W., Paolilli, P., and Steiner, J. *J. Immunol.*, **112**, 1884–1890 (1979).
25. Ono, M. and Hozumi, M. *Biochem. Biophys. Res. Commun.*, **53**, 342–349 (1973).
26. Parker, C. W., Kelly, J. P., Falkenheinn, S. F., and Huber, M. G. *J. Exp. Med.*, **149**, 1487–1503 (1979).
27. Parker, J. W., O'Brien, R. L., Lukes, R. J., and Steiner, J. *Lancet*, i, 103–104 (1972).
28. Presant, C. A. and Parker, S. *J. Biol. Chem.*, **251**, 1864–1870 (1976).
29. Ravid, A., Novogrodsky, A., and Wilchek, M. *Eur. J. Immunol.*, **8**, 289–294 (1978).
30. Ravid, A., Rubin, A. L., Stenzel, K. H., and Novogrodsky, A. Submitted for publication.

31. Reisner, Y., Linker-Israeli, M., and Sharon, N. *Cell. Immunol.*, **25**, 129–134 (1976).
32. Spiro, R. G. *Annu. Rev. Biochem.*, **39**, 599–638 (1970).
33. Springer, G. S., Besai, P. R., Yang, H. J., and Murthy, V. N. *Clin. Immunol. Immunopathol.*, **7**, 426–441 (1977).
34. Stenzel, K. H., Schwartz, R., Rubin, A. L., and Novogrodsky, A. *Nature*, **285**, 106–108 (1980).
35. Suzuki, Y. and Lehrer, R. I. *J. Clin. Invest.*, **66**, 1409–1418 (1980).
36. Van Lenten, L. and Ashwell, G. *J. Biol. Chem.*, **246**, 1889–1894 (1971).
37. Zatz, M. M., Goldstein, A. L., Blumenfeld, O. O., and White, A. *Nature*, **240**, 252–255 (1972).

ASSOCIATION OF MEMBRANE PHOSPHOLIPID METABOLISM WITH DIFFERENTIATION OF MOUSE MYELOID LEUKEMIA CELLS

Motoo Hozumi, Yoshio Honma,
and Takashi Kasukabe

Department of Chemotherapy, Saitama Cancer Center Research Institute*

Mouse myeloid leukemia M1 cells could be induced by various substances to differentiate into macrophages and granulocytes. When M1 cells were cultured with an inducer, the ratio of phosphatidylethanolamine to phosphatidylcholine increased during their differentiation reaching nearly that of normal mouse macrophages. During differentiation the incorporation of methyl groups into phosphatidylethanolamine in M1 cells was decreased, while the incorporation of choline into phosphatidylcholine was slightly increased, suggesting that decrease of cellular phospholipid methylation is partly due to decrease of methyltransferase activity.

Culture of M1 cells with the choline analogues N-monomethylethanolamine and N, N'-dimethylethanolamine resulted in accumulation of phosphatidyl-N-monomethylethanolamine and phosphatidyl-N, N'-dimethylethanolamine, respectively, in the cell membrane. This change on treatment with choline analogues was associated with morphological and functional differentiation of the M1 cells into macrophages and granulocytes. These results suggest that phospholipid metabolism is involved in the mechanism of differentiation of M1 cells.

The mouse myeloid leukemia cell line M1, established from a spontaneous myeloid leukemia in an SL mouse, can be induced by various substances, including dexamethasone, lipopolysaccharide and protein factors, to differentiate into macrophages and granulocytes (*11, 12, 14, 17*). In differentiating M1 cells, expression of differentiation-associated properties, such as Fc and C3 receptors on the cell surface, phagocytosis, migrating activity, adhesion to the substratum, agglutinability by some lectins and secretion of lysozyme, may result from changes in structure of the cell membrane during differentiation of the cells. We found that a glycoprotein with a molecular weight of 180,000 (p180) was induced in the cell surface of differentiated M1 cells by the protein inducers, dexamethasone, dibutyryl cyclic AMP, and prostaglandin E1 (*19, 20*). p180 was suggested to be involved in the mechanisms of cell-substrate adhesion and increase in agglutination by concanavalin A during differentiation of M1 cells.

We also examined the changes in phospholipid composition of M1 cells during their differentiation into macrophages and granulocytes, and found that both phospholipid methylation and the content of phosphatidylcholine in membrane phospholipids decreased during differentiation of M1 cells (*7, 8*). O-alkyllysophospholipids, which may cause serious disturbance of phospholipid metabolism, were also found to induce dif-

---

* Ina-machi, Kitaadachi-gun, Saitama 362, Japan (穂積本男, 本間良夫, 粕壁　隆).

ferentiation of M1 cells (9). Consistent with our findings, Masuda et al. (16) reported that the percentage of phosphatidylcholine in total phospholipids decreased during differentiation of M1 cells, although Saito et al. (18) could not detect any change of phospholipid composition in lipopolysaccharide-treated M1 cells.

Based on these findings that changes in phospholipid metabolism are involved in the mechanism of differentiation of M1 cells, we modified the membrane phospholipids of M1 cells by adding choline analogues to the culutre medium and examined the effect of this modification on differentiation of the cells. We found that accumulation of methylated phospholipids in the cell membrane was associated with morphological and functional differentiation of the M1 cells into macrophages and granulocytes (10). This paper reports differentiation-associated changes in the phospholipid composition of M1 cells and induction of differentiation of the M1 cells by choline analogues.

Changes in Phospholipid Composition in Differentiating M1 Cells

We examined changes in phospholipid composition in differentiated M1 cells treated with inducers such as dexamethasone, lipopolysaccharide, and protein inducer, which was prepared from the ascitic fluid of rats with hepatoma AH-130 as reported previously (6, 13). M1 cells treated with these inducers differentiated into forms that are functionally and morphologically similar to macrophages and granulocytes (7). Although there was no difference in the phospholipid compositions of sensitive and resistant M1 cells, the percentage of phosphatidylcholine was less in differentiated M1 cells than in untreated M1 cells, while the percentage of phosphatidylethanolamine was greater in the differentiated M1 cells (Table I). Changes in the percentages of other phospholipids, such as lysophosphatidylcholine and sphingomyelin during differentiation were slight. On the other hand, the phospholipid composition of the differentiated M1 cells was similar to that of a macrophage-like cell line (Mm-1) developed spontaneously from M1 cells or normal mouse peritoneal macrophages (7). Moreover, no difference was observed between the phospholipid compositions of non-confluent and confluent M1 cells.

The ratio of phosphatidylethanolamine to phosphatidylcholine increased markedly during differentiation of M1 cells induced by various inducers, such as dexamethasone,

TABLE I. Changes in Ratio of Phosphatidylethanolamine (PE) to Phosphatidylcholine (PC) in Differentiating M1 Cells

Experiment	Cells	Treatment	Ratio $\left(\dfrac{PE}{PC}\right)$
1	M1	None	0.31
		Dexamethasone $(5 \times 10^{-7}$ M$)$[a]	0.52
		Lipopolysaccharide $(0.5 \ \mu g/ml)$[b]	0.54
		Protein inducer $(5\%, \ v/v)$[c]	0.54
2	M1	None	0.32
		Dexamethasone $(5 \times 10^{-7}$ M$)$	0.51
	Mm-1	None	0.64
	Normal		
	Macrophages	None	0.67

[a-c] M1 cells were incubated with various inducers for 4 days.

lipopolysaccharide and protein inducer and reached nearly that of Mm-1 cells or normal macrophages (Table I). Although growth of M1 cells was inhibited by treatment with the inducers, it is unlikely that the changes in phospholipid composition were due to inhibition of cell growth because 5-fluorodeoxyuridine inhibited growth of M1 cells but did not induce differentiation of the cells, and the phospholipid composition of cells treated by 5-fluorodeoxyuridine was similar to that of untreated cells (7). Furthermore, the phospholipid composition of exponentially growing Mm-1 cells was similar to that of normal macrophages or differentiated M1 cells (7).

We then examined incorporation of ^{32}P into different phospholipids of M1 cells (7). Most of the radioactivity was found in the fractions containing phosphatidylethanolamine, phosphatidylcholine, and phosphatidylinositol. Phosphatidylinositol synthesis of the cells was markedly inhibited by treatment with dexamethasone, probably mainly owing to inhibition of cell growth since phosphatidylinositol synthesis was correlated with cell growth (1, 2). Although inhibition of incorporation of ^{32}P into phosphatidylethanolamine was only 10%, that of incorporation of ^{32}P into phosphatidylcholine was 39%. These results suggest that phosphatidylethanolamine synthesis is specifically maintained during differentiation of M1 cells and that these changes in phospholipid metabolism are closely associated with cell differentiation.

Decrease in Phospholipid Methylation in Differentiating M1 Cells

From the finding that the ratio of phosphatidylethanolamine to phosphatidylcholine increased during differentiation of M1 cells, reaching nearly that of normal macrophages, we examined the change in phosphatidylcholine synthesis in differentiating M1 cells.

Phosphatidylcholine is synthesized *via* two pathways, the stepwise addition of three methyl groups from S-adenosyl-L-methionine to the amino group of phosphatidylethanolamine, and the enzymatic coupling of cytidine diphosphate (CDP) choline to a 1,2-diacylglycerol. We examined the synthesis of phosphatidylcholine *via* the two pathways in M1 cells by treatment of the cells with L-[methyl-^{3}H]methionine and with [^{14}C] choline (8).

When M1 cells were induced to differentiate into macrophages and granulocytes by dexamethasone, lipopolysaccharide or protein inducer, methylation of cellular phospholipids decreased markedly (Table II). In contrast, treatment with an inducer produced a slight, but significant, increase in the incorporation of [^{14}C]choline into the phospholipid fraction of the cells. Therefore, decrease of phospholipid methylation during dif-

TABLE II. Decrease in Phospholipid Methylation in M1 Cells Treated with Various Inducers of Cell Differentiation

Inducer[a]	Concentration	Relative extent of incorporation of [^{3}H] methyl into phospholipids[b]
None		100
Dexamethasone	4×10^{-7} M	65.5
Lipopolysaccharide	0.5 μg/ml	60.7
Protein inducer	5%, v/v	61.8

[a] M1 cells were treated with various inducers for 30 hr.

[b] L-[Methyl-^{3}H] methionine was used as a donor of methylation. Incorporation of [^{3}H]-methyl group into untreated 10^7 M1 cells was 45.5 pmol/hr.

ferentiation of M1 cells was unlikely to be due to general inhibition of phospholipid synthesis.

Next we tested whether the decrease of cellular phospholipid methylation was due to accelerated degradation of these phospholipids in the newly synthesized membrane (8). M1 cells were prelabeled for 80 min at 37° with 0.1 μM L-[methyl-³H]methionine, and then washed extensively and resuspended in culture medium containing 0.1 mM unlabeled methionine and incubated for various periods. Measurement of the total amount of phospholipid-associated radioactivity remaining in the cells showed that no significant loss of cellular radioactivity of labeled phospholipid occurred in either untreated cells or differentiated M1 cells induced with dexamethasone. On the other hand, the phospholipid methyltransferase activity in isolated membranes decreased during differentiation of M1 cells. Therefore, the decrease of cellular phospholipid methylation may be partly due to decrease of phospholipid methyltransferase activity, but could not be explained by increased degradation of preformed methylated phospholipids.

The ratio of phosphatidylcholine to phosphatidylethanolamine decreased during differentiation of M1 cells and this decrease was detectable only 3 days later (7), while the decrease of stepwise methylation of phosphatidylethanolamine was detectable within 20 hr. This change in phospholipid composition might be indirectly involved in the decrease of phospholipid methylation, since the transmethylation pathway is minor compared with the CDP-choline pathway for phosphatidylcholine synthesis (21). The relation between the change in phospholipid composition and the decrease of phospholipid methylation remains to be elucidated.

Induction of Differentiation of M1 Cells by Choline Analogues

It has been reported that the compositions of membrane phosphlipids of various mammalian cultured cells are modified by addition of choline analogues to the culture medium (3–5, 15). Therefore, we modified the membrane phospholipids of M1 cells by adding choline analogues to the culture medium and examined the effect of this modification on differentiation of the cells (10).

The changes in phospholipid composition of the M1 cell membranes with this addition to the medium are summarized in Table III. Although choline caused no change in phospholipid composition, N-monomethylethanolamine (ME), and N,N-dimethyletha-

TABLE III.   Effects of Choline Analogues on Phospholipid Composition and Differentiation-associated Properties of M1 Cells

Choline analogue[a]	Concentration (μg/ml)	Phospholipid composition (%)				Differentiation	
		PE	PME	PDME	PC	Lysozyme activity[b] (U/10⁷ cells)	Phagocytic cells (%)
None		16.5	<0.5	<0.5	54.9	<0.8	1.5
ME	100	11.0	31.4	1.2	36.5	14.3	15.2
DME	100	14.5	<0.5	45.1	17.4	5.7	8.1
Choline	100	17.8	<0.5	<0.5	57.3	<0.8	1.2
Ethanolamine	10	20.7	<0.5	<0.5	48.0	<0.8	2.6

[a] M1 cells were grown for 5 days in medium with choline or one of its analogues.
[b] One unit of activity is defined as the amount equivalent to that of 1 μg of egg white lysozyme.

TABLE IV. Induction of Differentiation of Ml Cells by Treatment
with ME and/or Dexamethasone

Treatment[a]	Morphological changes (%)			Lysozyme activity (U/10^7 cells)
	Myeloblasts	Cells in intermediate stages of differentiation	Mature granulocytes and macrophages	
None	97.5	2.5	0	0.8
ME (150 μg/ml)	56.5	37.5	6.0	12.3
Dexamethasone (10^{-8} M)	93.0	7.0	0	8.3
Dexamethasone (10^{-8} M) +ME (150 μg/ml)	20.5	58.5	21.0	42.7

[a] Ml cells were cultured for 5 days in the presence of ME with or without a suboptimal concentration of dexamethasone.

nolamine (DME) increased the corresponding phospholipids, phosphatidyl-N-monomethylethanolamine (PME), and phosphatidyl-N,N'-dimethylethanolamine (PDME), respectively, with concomitant decrease of phosphatidylethanolamine and phosphatidylcholine. Ethanolamine at a concentration of 10 μg/ml caused a slight increase of phosphatidylethanolamine in membrane phospholipids. A higher concentration of ethanolamine (20 μg/ml) could not be used because it was too toxic to M1 cells.

When M1 cells were cultured with choline or ethanolamine, differentiation-associated properties, such as lysozyme activity and phagocytic activity, were not induced but these properties were significantly induced by ME and DME, the former being more effective (Table III). ME significantly inhibited cell growth but induced differentiation without any apparent cytotoxic effects; it was not cytotoxic to the cells even at high concentration (200 μg/ml).

Finally, we examined the effect of ME on the morphology of M1 cells (10). ME induced M1 cells to differentiate morphologically into mature granulocytes and macrophages. It also had a synergistic effect on differentiation with a suboptimal concentration of dexamethasone, another inducer of differentiation of M1 cells (Table IV).

The present results suggest that changes in phospholipid metabolism are closely associated with differentiation of M1 cells and that modification of membrane phospholipid by choline analogues causes induction of differentiation of the cells.

Acknowledgment

This work was partly supported by Grants-in-Aid from the Ministry of Education, Science, and Culture of Japan.

REFERENCES

1. Ciechanover, A. and Hershko, A. *Biochem. Biophys. Res. Commun.*, **73**, 85–91 (1976).
2. Cunningham, D. D. *J. Biol. Chem.*, **247**, 2463–2470 (1972).
3. Engelhard, V. H., Esko, J. D., Storm, D. R., and Glaser, M. *Proc. Natl. Acad. Sci. U.S.*, **73**, 4482–4486 (1976).
4. Finkel, R. S. and Volpe, J. J. *Biochim. Biphys. Acta*, **572**, 461–471 (1979).
5. Glaser, M., Ferguson, K. A., and Vagelos, P. R. *Proc. Natl. Acad. Sci. U.S.*, **71**, 4072–4076 (1974).
6. Honma, Y., Kasukabe, T., and Hozumi, M. *Cancer Res.*, **39**, 2190–2194 (1979).

7. Honma, Y., Kasukabe, T., and Hozumi, M. *Biochem. Biophys. Res. Commun.*, **93**, 927–933 (1980).

8. Honma, Y., Kasukabe, T., and Hozumi, M. *Biochim. Biophys. Acta*, **664**, 441–444 (1981).

9. Honma, Y., Kasukabe, T., Hozumi, M., Tsushima, S., and Nomura, H. *Cancer Res.*, **41**, 3211–3216 (1981).

10. Honma, Y., Kasukabe, T., and Hozumi, M. *Biochim. Biophys. Acta*, **721**, 83–86 (1982).

11. Hozumi, M. *Cancer Biol. Rev.*, **3**, 153–211 (1982).

12. Hozumi, M. *Adv. Cancer Res.*, **38**, 121–169 (1983).

13. Hozumi, M., Honma, Y., Okabe, J., Tomida, M., Kasukabe, T., Takenaga, K., and Sugiyama, K. *In* "Oncogenic Viruses and Host Cell Genes," ed. Y. Ikawa and T. Odaka, pp. 341–353 (1979). Academic Press, New York.

14. Ichikawa, Y. *J. Cell. Physiol.*, **74**, 223–234 (1969).

15. Maeda, M., Tanaka, Y., and Akamatsu, Y. *Biochem. Biophys. Res. Commun.*, **96**, 876–881 (1980).

16. Masuda, T., Kannagi, R., Kyoizumi, S., Kino, M., and Saito, K. *Proc. Japan. Cancer Assoc.*, **39**, 159 (1980).

17. Sachs, L. *Nature*, **274**, 535–539 (1978).

18. Saito, M., Nojiri, H., and Yamada, M. *Biochem. Biophys. Res. Commun.*, **97**, 452–462 (1980).

19. Sugiyama, K., Tomida, M., and Hozumi, M. *Biochim. Biophys. Acta*, **587**, 169–179 (1979).

20. Sugiyama, K., Tomida, M., Honma, Y., and Hozumi, M. *Cancer Res.*, **40**, 3387–3391 (1980).

21. Vance, D. E. and Kruijff, B. *Nature*, **288**, 277–278 (1980).

GANN Monograph on Cancer Research 29, 1983

ALTERATIONS OF GLYCOLIPID COMPOSITION AND METABOLISM DURING THE DIFFERENTIATION OF MOUSE MYELOID LEUKEMIA CELLS (M1)

Takao Taki[*1], Mitsuhiro Kawamoto,[*1] Hiroyuki Seto,[*1] Nobuhiro Noro,[*2] Tohru Masuda,[*2] Reiji Kannagi,[*2,*3] and Makoto Matsumoto[*1]

*Department of Biochemistry, Shizuoka College of Pharmacy[*1], Institute for Immunology, Faculty of Medicine, Kyoto University,[*2] and Division of Biochemical Oncology, Fred Hutchinson Cancer Research Center, University of Washington[*3]*

Differentiation-associated changes of glycolipid composition and metabolism were investigated using a mouse myeloid leukemia cell line (M1) which can be differentiated into macrophage type (M1[+]) cells. Gangliotriaosylceramide (GA_2) and gangliotetraosylceramide (GA_1) were found to be major glycolipid components in M1 and Mm1 (a subclone of M1) cells. As a result of the differentiation of M1 cells into M1[+] cells, globotriaosylceramide (CTH) which was newly synthesized became a major glycolipid in the differentiated cells. Metabolic study confirmed that the biosynthetic pathway, glucosylceramide (CMH) → lactosylceramide (CDH) → GA_2 → GA_1 → monosialoganglioside (GM_{1b}), was a main route in M1 as well as Mm1 cells. In M1[+] cells, activity of a galactosyltransferase catalyzing the formation of CTH from CDH increased about 10-fold over that in M1 cells. The appearance of CTH in the differentiated M1[+] cells could be attributed to the induction of the galactosyltransferase. Both CTH as a surface marker and galactosyltransferase as an enzyme marker are proposed to be valuable differentiation markers in M1 cells.

Glycosphingolipids are known to be membrane components of mammalian cells. A glycolipid is composed of a ceramide moiety embedded in the lipid bilayer of the membrane and a carbohydrate moiety exposed to the outer environment of the cell. The oligosaccharide moiety of glycolipids has been demonstrated to be involved in many biological functions such as antigens and receptors of bacterial toxins (7, 17, 27), hormones and of virus (5, 9, 19, 26). Besides these functional roles, glycolipids have been reported as surface markers of some cells (12, 29) and tumor-associated antigens (20).

As for the study in the alteration of glycolipid composition and metabolism accompanying tumorigenesis of cells, a number of papers have been published (4, 5). The observations made so far can be summarized as follows: 1, incomplete synthesis of glycolipids; 2, accumulation of precursor lipids; 3, appearance of unusual glycolipids and metabolism. On the other hand, very limited information is available from studies on

---

[*1] Oshika 2-2-1, Shizuoka 422, Japan (滝　孝雄, 河本光宏, 瀬戸博幸, 松本　亮).

[*2] Yoshidakonoe-cho, Kyoto 606, Japan (野呂信弘, 増田　徹, 神奈木玲児).

[*3] Seattle, Washington 98104, U.S.A.

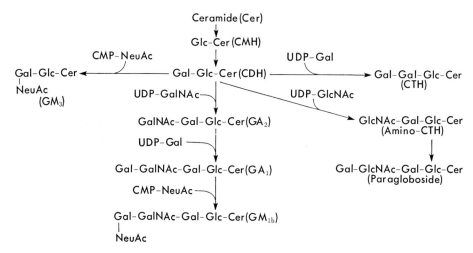

FIG. 1.   Glycolipids and synthetic routes examined in the present study.

the relationship of glycolipid metabolism and differentiation (*1, 2*). With an ideal cell line for the study of differentiation, research on the changes of glycolipid composition during differentiation would seem to be useful in elucidating the role of glycolipid in cell function. If a special glycolipid is induced during differentiation, the glycolipid might be associated with a new function.

The mouse myeloid leukemia cell line (M1) was established from an SL-strain mouse by Ichikawa in 1969 (*10*). M1 cells can be differentiated into macrophage type cells (M1$^+$) by incubation with the culture supernatant of mouse embryonic fibroblast, continued medium (CM). The differentiated cell, M1$^+$, acquires adhesiveness and phagocytic activity in association with the expression of Fc receptor (FcR), but loses leukemogenicity *in vivo* and proliferative activity *in vitro* (*10, 11, 28*). Moreover, it has been noted that M1$^+$ cells exhibit accessory cell (A cell) activities for lymphocytes in immune response, with the concomitant appearance of Ia antigen in the membrane. In contrast, Mm1 (a subclone of M1) cells subcloned from M1 cells, lack the A cell activities and Ia antigen in spite of the presence of both FcR and phagocytic activities (*14, 16*).

In this study, M1, Mm1, and M1$^+$ cells were studied for differentiation-associated changes of glycolipid composition and metabolism. Glycolipids including abbreviations and their synthetic pathways investigated in the present sutdy are shown in Fig. 1.

Glycolipid Composition of M1, Mm1, and M1$^+$ Cells

In M1 cells, neutral glycolipids corresponding to glucosylceramide (CMH), lactosylceramide (CDH), gangliotriaosylceramide (GA$_2$), and gangliotetraosylceramide (GA$_1$) were detected (Fig. 2). In Mm1 cells, GA$_2$ as well as GA$_1$ were found to be major glycolipids. After differentiation of M1 into M1$^+$ cells, a dramatic change in glycolipid composition was observed; asialogangliosides in M1 cells decreased and became minor components in M1$^+$ cells, while a glycolipid moving slightly faster than GA$_2$ appeared and became a major glycolipid in M1$^+$ cells. This observation indicates that functional differentiation of the cells was accompanied by changes in glycolipid composition, which should influence membrane properties.

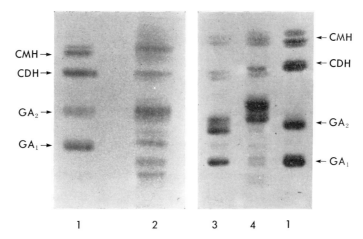

Fɪɢ. 2.   Thin layer chromatography of glycolipids from M1, Mm1, and M1⁺ cells. Lane 1, CMH, CDH, GA₂, and GA₁ from top to bottom; Lane 2, glycolipids from M1 cells; Lane 3, glycolipids from Mm1 cells; Lane 4, glycolipids from M1⁺ cells. Glycolipids were separated using a solvent mixture of $CHCl_3$: CH_3OH: H_2O (60: 35: 8, v/v/v).

In order to clarify what kind of structural change had occurred, major glycolipids in these cells were purified and subjected to glycosidase treatment (6, 15, 22) and methylation analysis (3). The structural analysis showed that the major glycolipid in M1 and Mm1 cells was GalNAc(β1–4)Gal(β1–4)Glc-Cer (GA₂) and the major glycolipid in M1⁺ was Gal(α1–4)Gal(β1–4)Glc-Cer (globotriaosylceramide (CTH)). The change of glycolipid composition observed during differentiation suggests that induction of glycosyltransferases might occur, especially those acting upon CDH.

Change of Glycolipid Metabolism

The glycosyltransferase activities shown in Fig. 1 were investigated with respect to the differentiation of M1 to M1⁺ cells. The cells used for enzyme sources were harvested at 0 hr, 12 hr, 24 hr, and 44 hr after the addition of CM. These cells were also used for the assay of FcR as a marker of the degree of differentiation. When the process of differentiation of M1 to M1⁺ cells was examined in terms of the appearance of FcR which can be detected by EA-rosette formation (18), the formation increased proportionally with incubation time, reaching about 90% of the cells after 44 hr.

1.   N-acetylgalactosaminyltransferase

N-acetylgalactosaminyltransferase which acts on CDH is a key enzyme for the synthesis of monosialoganglioside (GM₁ᵦ), through asialogangliosides. When M1 cells were assayed for the N-acetylgalactosaminyltransferase activity during differentiation, the enzyme activity level was almost unchanged for 2 days. On the other hand, enzyme activity of M1 cells was 5-times more active than that of M1 cells, and exhibited the highest level of all the glycosyltransferase activities examined.

2.   Galactosyltransferase

Two galactosyltransferase activities for the synthesis of GA₁ from GA₂ and of CTH

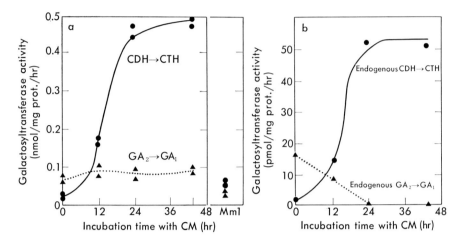

FIG. 3a.   Change of galactosyltransferase activities towards exogenous CDH and GA₂ during the differentiation of M1 to M1⁺ cells. ● galactosyltransferase for CTH synthesis; ▲ galactosyltransferase for GA_1 synthesis. The enzyme activity in Mm1 cells are shown in the right side of the figure.

FIG. 3b.   Change of galactosyltransferase activities towards endogenous acceptor lipids during the differentiation of M1 to M1⁺ cells. ● galactosyltransferase for CTH synthesis; ▲ galactosyltransferase for GA_1 synthesis.

from CDH were assayed. Since GA_1 was markedly reduced in M1⁺ cells, the synthetic activity of GA_1 was expected to decrease during differentiation. However, no significant change of this enzyme activity was observed as shown in Fig. 3a, when GA_2 was an exogenous acceptor lipid. This fact suggests two possibilities for the decrease of GA_1 in M1⁺ cells: one is that GA_1 could be hydrolyzed as soon as the lipid was synthesized by induced glycosidases. The second is that the microenvironment surrounding endogenous GA_2 in the cells changes, hindering the interaction between galactosyltransferase and acceptor lipid resulting in an inhibition in synthesis of GA_1. In order to examine the second possibility, galactosyltransferase activity was determined without adding GA_2 exogenously. Figure 3b shows that the galactosyltransferase activity towards endogenous GA_2 was decreasing in accordance with differentiation of M1 to M1⁺ cells. The results shown in Fig. 3b may best be explained by alternative mentioned above. However, the changes seen in Fig. 3b may not be sufficient to explain the decrease of GA_1 in M1⁺ cells, and the first possibility cannot be ruled out, because hydrolytic enzyme was induced during differentiation (13).

The other galactosyltransferase responsible for synthesis CTH from CDH increased about 10-fold over that in M1 cells, during differentiation (Fig. 3a). A similar increase was observed in the experiment without any addition of exogenous acceptor glycolipid (Fig. 3b). The appearance of CTH in M1⁺ cells could be attributed to a great increase of galactosyltransferase activity.

In Mm1 cells, the galactosyltransferase activity for GA_1 synthesis was comparable to that in M1 cells. The galactosyltransferase activity for CTH synthesis was quite low.

3.   Sialyltransferases

Two sialyltransferase activities for synthesis of GM_{1b} from GA_1 and of GM_3 from CDH were assayed. The sialyltransferase for GM_{1b} synthesis was detected in M1 cells, and the activity did not change during differentiation (Fig. 4). The other sialyltransferase for GM_3 synthesis was detected only in Mm1 cells and seemed to be very characteristic for Mm1 cells.

4. N-acetylglucosaminyltransferase

In M1[+] and Mm1 cells paragloboside was detected. Paragloboside can be synthesized from amino-CTH by a galactosyltransferase. Accordingly, the synthesis of amino-CTH was assayed. The enzyme was detectable in these cells, increasing 3-fold over that in M1 cells during differentiation (Fig. 5). The enzyme activity in M1[+] cells was almost comparable to that in Mm1 cells. Since amino-CTH was detected neither in M1[+] nor in Mm1 cells, the synthesized amino-CTH seemed to be rapidly converted to paragloboside by a galactosyltransferase.

The results of the present study is summarized in Fig. 6. M1 cells showed all enzyme activities which are required to form GM_{1b} through asialogangliosides. The presence of asialogangliosides was demonstrated here, and the presence of GM_{1b} was reported previously (21). These results suggest that the biosynthetic pathway depicted in Fig. 6 is a major metabolic route in M1 cells. The same metabolic pathway also found in Mm1 cells. During differentiation CTH and the galactosyltransferase responsible for its synthesis were induced. Since CTH was undetectable in M1 cells, it was assumed to be a very useful surface differentiation marker. In fact, M1[+] cells were found to be stained by an immunofluorescence technique using a monoclonal antibody against CTH (data will be reported elsewhere). The appearance of CTH in M1[+] cells may be intimately correlated with the function of the cells. M1[+] cells acquire A cell activities in the immune response in parallel with the loss of proliferative or leukemogenic activities. Such

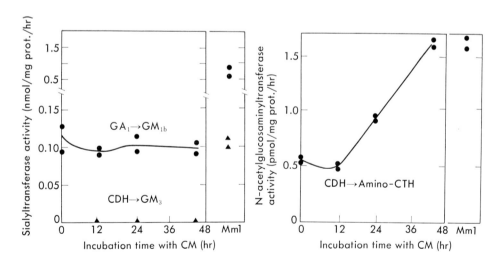

FIG. 4. (left) Change of sialyltransferase activities for GM_{1b} and GM_3 synthesis during the differentiation of M1 to M1[+] cells. ● sialyltransferase for GM_{1b} synthesis; ▲ sialyltransferase for GM_3 synthesis. The enzyme activities in Mm1 cells are shown in the right side of the figure.

FIG. 5. (right) Change of N-acetylglucosaminyltransferase activity for amino-CTH synthesis during the differentiation of M1 to M1[+] cells. ● N-acetylglucosaminyltransferase. The enzyme activity in Mm1 cells is shown in the right side of the figure.

90 T. TAKI ET AL.

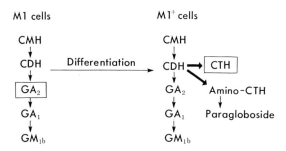

Fig. 6. Change of glycolipid metabolism of M1 cells during differentiation. □ a major glycolipid; ➡ increase of enzyme activity.

properties in M1+ cells are never seen in Mm1 cells which are able to proliferate *in vitro* as well as *in vivo* (5, 9, 19, 28, 29). Thus, CTH may be involved in the mechanism of either a cell activity or the cessation of growth of tumor cells.

The enzyme activities necessary for GM_3 synthesis in Mm1 cells are also very interesting. Mm1 cells have far greater adhesiveness to substrate than do M1+ cells. These facts may be correlated with those of our previous study on the glycolipid composition and metabolism of two types of rat ascites hepatoma cells (23, 24). The free type of rat ascites hepatoma cells contained asialogangliosides and GM_{1b} as glycolipid components, while the island type of hepatoma cells contained GM_3 as ganglioside but no GM_{1b} (8). When these tumor cells were cultured in butyrate-containing medium, an increase of GM_3 synthesis in the island type of tumor cells was observed prior to morphological differentiation and adhesion of cells to substrate. But GM_3 synthesis could not be induced in the free type hepatoma cells even if the butyrate concentration was increased (25). The appearance of GM_3 synthesis in Mm1 cells would seem to resemble the situation of the island type cells cultured in butyrate-containing medium. Synthesis of GM_3 would appear to be closely associated with cell adhesiveness.

From the present study, three kinds of cells—tumor cells, differentiated cells, and proliferative functional cells—were shown to be distinguishable by the glycosyltransferase which acted upon CDH. The glycosyltransferases can modify the cell membrane and its function.

Acknowledgments
We thank Professor S. Hakomori, Fred Hutchinson Cancer Research Institute, Washington, U.S.A., for the methylation analysis and valuable discussion and Mr. B. Levery for technical assistance with GC-MS. This work was supported in part by a grant from the Ministry of Education, Science and Culture of Japan.

REFERENCES

1. Fishman, P. H. and Henneberry, R. C. *In* "Cell Surface Glycolipid," ACS Symposium Series, ed. M. J. Comstock, pp. 223–240 (1980). American Chemical Society, Washington, D. C.
2. Glickman, R. M. and Bouhours, J. F. *Biochim. Biophys. Acta*, **424**, 17–26 (1975).
3. Hakomori, S. *J. Biochem.*, **55**, 205–208 (1964).
4. Hakomori, S. *Biochim. Biophys. Acta*, **417**, 55–89 (1975).
5. Hakomori, S. *Annu. Rev. Biochem.*, **50**, 733–764 (1981).

6. Hakomori, S., Siddiqui, B., Li, Y.-T., Li, S.-C., and Hellerqvist, C. G. *J. Biol. Chem.*, **246**, 2271–2277 (1971).

7. Higashi, H., Naiki, M., Matsuo, S., and Okouchi, K. *Biochem. Biophys. Res. Commun.*, **79**, 388–395 (1977).

8. Hirabayashi, Y., Taki, T., and Matsumoto, M. *FEBS Lett.*, **100**, 253–257 (1979).

9. Holmgren, J., Svennerholm, L., Elwing, H., Fredman, P., and Strannegård, O. *Proc. Natl. Acad. Sci. U.S.*, **77**, 1947–1950 (1980).

10. Ichikawa, Y. *J. Cell Physiol.*, **74**, 223–234 (1969).

11. Ichikawa, Y. *J. Cell Physiol.*, **76**, 175–184 (1970).

12. Kasai, M., Iwamori, M., Nagai, Y., Okumura, K., and Tada, T. *Eur. J. Immunol.*, **10**, 175–180 (1980).

13. Kasukabe, T., Honma, Y., and Hozumi, M. *Gann*, **68**, 765–773 (1977).

14. Kyoizumi, S., Noro, N., Teshigawara, K., Sakaguchi, S., and Masuda, T. *J. Immunol.*, **128**, 2586–2594 (1982).

15. Li, S.-C., Mazzota, N. Y., Chien, C. F., and Li, Y.-T. *J. Biol. Chem.*, **250**, 6786–6791 (1975).

16. Maeda, M. and Ichikawa, Y. *Gann*, **64**, 265–271 (1973).

17. McKibbin, J. M. *J. Lipid Res.*, **19**, 131–147 (1978).

18. Miyama, M., Kuribayashi, K., Yodoi, J., Takabayashi, A., and Masuda, T. *Cell Immunol.*, **35**, 253–265 (1978).

19. Mullin, B. R., Fishman, P. H., Lee, G., Aloj, S. M., Ledley, F. D., Winand, R. J., Kohn, L. D., and Brady, R. O. *Proc. Natl. Acad. Sci. U.S.*, **73**, 842–846 (1976).

20. Rosenfelder, G., Young, W. W., Jr., and Hakomori, S.-I. *Cancer Res.*, **37**, 1333–1339 (1977).

21. Saito, M., Nojiri, H., and Yamada, M. *Biochem. Biophys. Res. Commun.*, **97**, 452–462 (1980).

22. Svennerholm, L., Månsson, J.-E., and Li, Y.-T. *J. Biol. Chem.*, **248**, 740–742 (1973).

23. Taki, T., Hirabayashi, Y., Suzuki, Y., Matsumoto, M., and Kojima, K. *J. Biochem.*, **83**, 1517–1520 (1978).

24. Taki, T., Hirabayashi, Y., Ishiwata, Y., Matsumoto, M., and Kojima, K. *Biochim. Biophys. Acta*, **572**, 113–120 (1979).

25. Taki, T., Hirabayashi, Y., Kondo, R., Matsumoto, M., and Kojima, K. *J. Biochem.*, **86**, 1395–1402 (1979).

26. Van Heyningen, W. E. *Nature*, **249**, 415–417 (1974).

27. Yamakawa, T. and Nagai, Y. *Trends Biochem. Sci.*, **3**, 128–131 (1978).

28. Yodoi, J., Masuda, T., Miyama, M., Maeda, M., and Ichikawa, Y. *Cell Immunol.*, **39**, 5–17 (1978).

29. Young, W. W., Jr., Hakomori, S., Durdik, J. M., and Henney, C. S. *J. Immunol.*, **124**, 199–201 (1980).

MEMBRANE-ASSOCIATED GLYCOENZYMES AND GLYCOPROTEINS OF HUMAN RECTAL CANCER CELLS: THE EFFECT OF THREE DIFFERENTIATING AGENTS

Young S. KIM, Akira MORITA, and Steven H. ITZKOWITZ

Gastrointestinal Research Laboratory (151M2), Veterans Administration Medical Center[1] *and Department of Medicine, the University of California*[2]

Disordered cellular differentiation, as a consequence of aberrant programming of normal gene function, may result in neoplastic growth. Efforts to investigate the relationship between cellular differentiation and neoplasia have employed various differentiating agents that can alter the phenotypic expression of certain cancer cells.

A poorly-differentiated human rectal carcinoma cell line, HRT-18, was subjected to treatment with each of three putative differentiating agents (sodium butyrate, dimethylsulfoxide (DMSO), and retinoic acid) and the cells were analyzed for *in vitro* growth properties, tumorigenicity, cell morphology, cell surface membrane-associated glycoenzymes and proteins, and enzymes involved in glycoprotein synthesis and degradation. All three agents reversibly caused a marked increase in doubling times, a decrease in saturation densities, and reduced colony-forming efficiency in soft agar. Butyrate was remarkable for causing an increase in alkaline phosphatase, sucrase, and γ-glutamyltranspeptidase activities, carcinoembryonic antigen content, glycosyltransferase and nucleotide pyrophosphatase activities. Aminooligopeptidase, K^+-stimulated phosphatase and glycosidase activities were unchanged or decreased, demonstrating a selective rather than a general increase in gene expression. DMSO and retinoic acid induced less dramatic changes in the above parameters. The butyrate-induced changes resulted in phenotypic expression more consistent with normal colonic cells. A cell surface glycoprotein with 60,000 molecular weight (M.W.) appeared in butyrate-treated cells and may possibly be involved in the mechanism by which butyrate causes colon cancer cells to assume a more normal phenotype. Differentiating agents serve as useful tools for studying differentiation-associated changes and for elucidating the molecular events involved in tumorigenicity.

Although the precise relationship between cellular differentiation and neoplasia is not clear, it is now well known that neoplasia is the result of disordered cellular differentiation, resulting from an aberrant programming of normal gene function (*15, 21*). This view is supported by the findings that histological composition of some tumors changes to a more normal differentiated type (*3*), that many tumor cells produce gene products

---

[1] San Francisco, California 94121, U.S.A.
[2] San Francisco, California 94143, U.S.A.

often associated with their fetal counterpart (1, 6) and that teratocarcinoma cells contribute cells to many normal tissues and organs of the developing chimeric mouse when injected into the mouse blastocyst (17).

Many structurally unrelated chemicals have been reported to induce biochemical, functional, and morphological differentiation in some normal and cancer cells such as erythroleukemia, neuroblastoma, teratocarcinoma, and HeLa cells (5, 11, 13, 23). These include polar organic compounds, bisacetamides, short-chain fatty acids, purine and purine analogues, antimetabolites, and vitamin A. It would appear that different inducers of differentiation may not act by the same mechanisms and may induce different phenotypic expression. Available data obtained from studies on erythroleukemic cells (ELC) suggest that there are stages in the process of differentiation prior to the accumulation of hemoglobin or expression of other morphological and biochemical features of differentiation at which ELC become irreversibly committed to continue the developmental process in the absence of inducer (22).

These stages in the induction of ELC differentiation can be broadly divided into "early" and "late" events. "Early events" are those which occur in cultured cells prior to commitment in the presence of inducer and are reversible upon removal of the inducer. "Late events" are those which occur with or after commitment. Cells which become committed lose the capacity for unlimited cell proliferation, initiate their terminal cell divisions, and accumulate hemoglobin and red cell specific membrane antigens (22).

In induction studies, specific markers have been developed for the specific stages of development and differentiation of particular cell types. However, at the present time, very little is known about the specific developmental patterns of gene products of many cell types of solid tumors including colonic mucosal cells.

Effect of Butyrate, Dimethylsulfoxide (DMSO), and Retinoic Acid on Growth Properties of HRT-18 Cells

To gain some insight into the molecular mechanisms of cellular differentiation and tumorigenesis of colonic mucosal cells we examined the effects of three putative differentiating agents (sodium butyrate, DMSO, and retinoic acid) on a poorly-differentiated human rectal carcinoma cell line, HRT-18 provided by Dr. Tompkins (27). The cellular properties examined included *in vitro* growth properties, *in vitro* tumorigenicity, cellular morphology, cell surface membrane associated glycoenzymes, enzymes involved in glycoprotein synthesis and degradation and cell surface proteins (30).

When the growth curves of HRT-18 cells in the presence and absence of sodium butyrate, DMSO, and retinoic acid were examined, sodium butyrate caused a marked reduction in the growth rates of these cells at 2 mM, and complete inhibition of growth at 5 mM. At 2 mM, sodium butyrate had little effect on the viability of the cells as assessed by trypan blue exclusion, but at 5 mM dye uptake began to occur on the fourth day. Normal growth rate was restored upon removal of butyrate indicating reversibility of the effect. Treatment with 2% DMSO caused reduction in the growth rates similar to that observed with 2 mM butyrate. Retinoic acid at 3.3×10^{-5} M caused less inhibition of the growth rate than was observed with the other two agents. The growth rate was restored to normal upon removal of DMSO or retinoic acid and cells remained viable with both DMSO or retinoic acid.

The *in vitro* growth properties of treated cells are summarized in Table I. The

TABLE I. Growth Properties of a Human Rectal Adenocarcinoma Cell Line (HRT-18)

Conditions[a]	Doubling time (hr)	Saturation density ($\times 10^{-5}$ cells)	Colony-forming efficiency in soft agar (%)
Control	22	50.0	89
Sodium butyrate	77	12.4	0
DMSO	67	8.8	0
Retinoic acid	39	42.0	38

[a] Final concentrations in the media were: sodium butyrate, 2 mM; DMSO, 2%; retinoic acid, 3.3×10^{-5} M. (see Ref. 30)

doubling times of cells in the inducer-containing media were all considerably longer than those of untreated cells. The saturation densities of inducer-treated cells were reduced markedly after butyrate and DMSO treatment while retinoic acid-treated cells showed only a slight reduction in saturation density. Both sodium butyrate-treated cells and DMSO-treated cells did not form colonies in soft agar while retinoic acid treatment resulted in the formation of about one-half as many colonies as the control cells. Thus all three agents had marked effects on various growth properties of HRT-18 cells including prolongation of doubling time, decrease in saturation density and *in vitro* tumorigenicity as tested by growth in soft agar. These results suggest that the three inducers reversibly caused these tumor cells to acquire *in vitro* properties that are considered to be consistent with normal cell growth.

Morphological examination carried out at the light microscopic level showed that after four days butyrate-treated cells were spread out with a polygonal epithelioid configuration and had a marked increase in the number and the length of processes projecting from the expanded cytoplasm. DMSO- or retinoic acid-treated cells displayed a less pronounced increase in the length of membranous processes and showed no change in the cell size.

Effect of Butyrate, DMSO, and Retinoic Acid on the Activities of Membrane-associated Glycoenzymes

When the effect of differentiating agents on the activities of five plasma membrane-associated glycoenzymes were examined the following results were obtained (Table II). Butyrate caused a 10-fold increase in alkaline phosphatase activity, 3-fold increase in γ-glutamyltranspeptidase activity and 2-fold increase in sucrase activity but had no effect on aminopeptidase activity. K$^+$-stimulated phosphatase activity was reduced to about one-half of that in the untreated cells. DMSO caused no change in the enzyme activities except for alkaline phosphatase and K$^+$-stimulated phosphatase which were decreased. Retinoic acid caused a decrease in the activities of alkaline phosphatase and γ-glutamyltranspeptidase activity, while the activities of the other three enzymes remained unchanged.

In the small intestine, alkaline phosphatase, γ-glutamyltranspeptidase, sucrase, and aminooligopeptidases are associated with the apical microvillus membrane, while K$^+$-stimulated phosphatase is localized to the basolateral membrane of mucosal cells. Furthermore, the activities of these enzymes are higher in the more-differentiated villus cells than in the less-differentiated crypt cells. Although comparable data are not avail-

TABLE II. Effects on Membrane-associated Enzyme Activities of HRT-18 Cells

	Enzyme activities[a] (nmol/min/mg protein)				
	Alkaline phosphatase	γ-Glutamyl transpeptidase	Sucrase	Aminopeptidase	K[+]-stimulated phosphatase
Control	5.3 ± 0.6[b]	15.3 ± 4.7	4.4 ± 0.8	5.1 ± 1.3	2.2 ± 0.6
Sodium butyrate	55.5 ± 1.7	47.7 ± 6.5	9.6 ± 1.4	3.1 ± 0.6	1.2 ± 0.5
DMSO	1.7 ± 1.2	16.4 ± 7.3	4.2 ± 1.1	5.6 ± 1.9	2.1 ± 0.3
Retinoic acid	0.4 ± 0.2	7.4 ± 5.4	3.6 ± 0.9	5.6 ± 3.8	1.8 ± 0.1

[a] Final concentrations in the media were: sodium butyrate, 2 mM; DMSO, 2%; retinoic acid, 3.3×10^{-5} M.

[b] Mean $\pm$ S.D. of 4 experiments. (see Ref. *30*)

able for the colon, the alkaline phosphatase activity has been reported to be lower in colon cancer tissues than in normal colonic tissues by several investigators. Therefore the observed increase in the activities of alkaline phosphatase, γ-glutamyltranspeptidase, and sucrase in the butyrate-treated HRT-18 cells may reflect a more-differentiated phenotype when compared to untreated cancer cells. In the butyrate-treated cells the concomitant decrease in the activities of two other plasma membrane-associated enzymes, K[+]-stimulated phosphatase and aminooligopeptidases, indicates that there is not a generalized increase in gene expression with butyrate treatment in HRT-18 cells. Since alkaline phosphatase activity showed the most marked increase after butyrate treatment, we studied the induction of this enzyme in HRT-18 cells in detail.

Induction of Membrane-associated Alkaline Phosphatase of HRT-18 Cells by Sodium Butyrate

The effect of various concentrations of sodium butyrate on the specific activity of alkaline phosphatase in HRT-18 cells showed that increasing concentrations of sodium butyrate caused an increase in alkaline phosphatase activity in HRT-18 cells (*19*). The increase in the specific enzyme activity was maximum at 3 mM. However treatment of cells with sodium butyrate at concentrations above 2 mM caused some cellular uptake of trypan blue. Therefore, treatment of the cells with butyrate was performed at a concentration of 2 mM in subsequent experiments.

As shown in Fig. 1, specific activity of alkaline phosphatase per mg of cellular protein reached a maximal 73-fold increase compared to controls on day 4 and subsequently decreased with longer cell culture. When sodium butyrate was removed from the culture medium on day 4, the enzyme activity decreased significantly indicating that the effect of butyrate on alkaline phosphatase was reversible. A similar pattern was observed for enzyme activity expressed per cells but peak activity occurred on day 6.

A kinetic analysis of alkaline phosphatase showed that sodium butyrate treatment affected both apparent K_m and V_{max}. The apparent K_m was lowered slightly from 3.1 ± 0.4 to 1.8 ± 0.1 mM ($p < 0.001$, $n = 4$) while the V_{max} was markedly enhanced from 4.9 ± 0.6 to 112.1 ± 3.6 units/mg protein ($p < 0.001$) after sodium butyrate treatment for 8 days. These data suggest that sodium butyrate exerts its effect on the catalytic efficiency of the enzyme and/or the content of the enzyme protein in HRT-18 cells rather than on enzyme's affinity for the substrate.

Next we examined the effect of protein synthesis inhibitors cycloheximide and

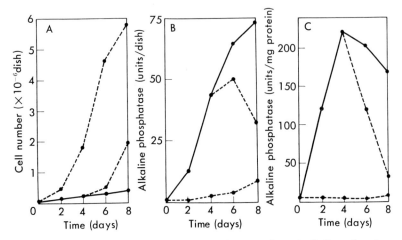

FIG. 1. Effect of sodium butyrate on cellular growth and alkaline phosphatase
activity of HRT-18 cells. Effect of sodium butyrate (2 mM) on cellular growth
(A) and total (B) and specific alkaline phosphatase activity (C). Solid line, in the
presence of sodium butyrate; dotted line, in the absence of sodium butyrate.
Culture medium was changed on fourth day. Each point represents the mean of
three experiments. (see Ref. 19)

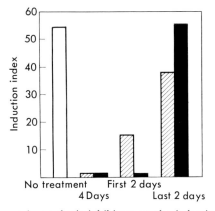

FIG. 2. Effect of protein synthesis inhibitors on the induction of alkaline phosphatase by sodium butyrate in HRT-18 cells. Cycloheximide (2 μg/ml) or actinomycin D (0.2 μg/ml) were added to the culture medium for 4 days, the first 2 days,
the last 2 days or not at all (no treatment). Induction index is the ratio of experimental to control specific activity of alkaline phosphatase. Each bar represents the
mean of 4 experiments. ▨ cycloheximide; ■ actinomycin D. (see Ref. 19)

actinomycin D on the induction of alkaline phosphatase by sodium butyrate. The enhancement of alkaline phosphatase activity by sodium butyrate treatment was inhibited by
the addition of cycloheximide (2 μg/ml) or actinomycin D (0.2 μg/ml) when these
agents were present in the culture medium throughout the 4 days of the experimental
protocol (Fig. 2). This indicates that both RNA and protein synthesis are necessary for
the enhancement of alkaline phosphatase activity by sodium butyrate in HRT-18 cells.
However as shown here, some differences in the mode of action were noted between
these two agents. When cycloheximide was removed from the culture after the first 2

days, there was a 15-fold enhancement of enzyme activity at the end of 4 days suggesting that the effect was partially reversible. This was not observed with actinomycin D. Furthermore, when cycloheximide was included in the culture medium after 2 days of sodium butyrate treatment, induction of alkaline phosphatase was partially inhibited, while under the same conditions actinomycin D showed no effect.

Thus the induction of alkaline phosphatase in HRT-18 cells by sodium butyrate requires new RNA and protein synthesis, since cycloheximide and actinomycin D inhibit the effect of sodium butyrate. It is likely that sodium butyrate acts at the transcriptional rather than translational level for the following reasons:
1) Actinomycin D did not block induction of alkaline phosphatase if included in the culture medium at the rapid phase of increase of enzyme activity suggesting that translation of preformed mRNA is unaffected. 2) Removal of cycloheximide from the culture medium after 2 days caused a 15-fold increase in enzyme activity, while only a 1.5-fold increase was observed with actinomycin D.
These data indicate that sodium butyrate-treated cells translate already-synthesized RNA into new alkaline phosphatase following removal of cycloheximide, while time is required for new RNA synthesis in the case of actinomycin D.

Although not shown here, further studies on biochemical and immunological characterization of the properties of alkaline phosphatase of HRT-18 cells before and after sodium butyrate treatment may be summarized as follows:
1) The enzyme became more sensitive to all amino acid and peptide inhibitors tested and more heat-stable compared to the enzyme in the control cells. 2) The butyrate-induced alkaline phosphatase could be completely precipitated by anti-placental alkaline phosphatase antibody while only 80% of the enzyme was immunoprecipitated in the control cells. 3) The electrophoretic pattern of the butyrate-induced enzyme was different from that of control cells. Butyrate treatment induced only the major heat-stable isozyme while it inhibited or had no effect on the heat-labile isozyme present in the control HRT-18 cells with an electrophoretic mobility similar to the major isozyme from human colonic cancer tissues.

The specificity of the sodium butyrate effect on HRT-18 cells was demonstrated by the inability of other short-chain fatty acids, such as acetate and caproic acid, at 2 mM to inhibit HRT-18 cell growth. Furthermore, unlike the marked induction of alkaline phosphatase by 2 mM sodium butyrate, neither acetate nor caproic acid at 2 mM had a significant effect on this enzyme.

Effect of Butyrate, DMSO, and Retinoic Acid on Glycoprotein Carcinoembryonic Antigen (CEA) of HRT-18 Cells

We next examined the effect of various differentiating agents on the content of CEA, a glycoprotein oncodevelopmental antigen in the HRT-18 cells which have a relatively low CEA level (30). With butyrate treatment, CEA content was increased 17-fold in the membrane fraction and 40-fold in the cytoplasmic fraction compared to control cells. By contrast, CEA content was reduced in DMSO-treated cells. Retinoic acid-treated cells showed no change (Table III).

The tissue CEA contents have been reported to vary depending on the degree of differentiation of human colorectal tumors with poorly-differentiated or anaplastic tumors generally having a lower CEA content than the well-differentiated colorectal tumors.

TABLE III. Effects on CEA Content of HRT-18 Cells

Conditions[a]	CEA (ng/mg protein)	
	Membrane fraction	Cytoplasmic fraction
Control	113 ± 22[b]	24 ± 6
Sodium butyrate	$1,918 \pm 1,585$	969 ± 356
DMSO	33 ± 26	9 ± 12
Retinoic acid	105 ± 81	21 ± 8

[a] Final concentrations in the media were: sodium butyrate, 2 mM; DMSO, 2%; retinoic acid, 3.3×10^{-5} M.

[b] Mean$\pm$S.D. of 4 experiments. (see Ref. 30)

Our data showed that butyrate and DMSO caused reversible changes in the CEA content of HRT-18 cells while retinoic acid had no effect. Butyrate caused a marked (20- to 40-fold) increase in the CEA content of HRT-18 cells. Since higher CEA content also seems to correlate with better-differentiated human colorectal tumor cell lines, these results may indicate the induction of a better-differentiated phenotype in the human rectal cancer cells by butyrate. Using immunofluorescent techniques, Hager et al. reported an increase in membrane-associated CEA of two human colon cancer cell lines following treatment with another polar solvent (N,N-dimethylformamide) (7).

Effect of Butyrate on Carbohydrate Content, Glycosyltransferase, Glycosidase, and Nucleotide Sugar Pyrophosphatase Activities

In our previous studies on human colon cancer tissues, we observed that the carbohydrate content of the membrane fraction of colon cancer tissues was markedly reduced compared to that of the adjacent normal colonic mucosa (8). This was also associated with a significant reduction in the activities of various glycosyltransferases while glycosidase activities remained unchanged (8). We therefore examined the effect of butyrate on carbohydrate content, glycosyltransferase, and glycosidase activities of HRT-18 cells.

Although the date are not shown here, our results to date indicate that all the monosaccharide consituents of membrane glycoproteins are increased in the butyrate-treated HRT-18 cells. The activities of all five glycosyltransferases, (2 galactosyltransferases, 2 sialyltransferases, and a polypeptidyl N-acetylgalactosaminyltransferase) were increased considerably in butyrate-treated cells while glycosidase activities (β-N-acetylglucosaminidase, β-N-acetylgalactosaminidase, and β-galactosidase), assayed using synthetic substrates, showed no changes with butyrate treatment. Nucleotide pyrophosphatase activity was increased in butyrate-treated cells. This is of interest since Dr. Don Carlson and his coworkers have recently reported that nucleotide pyrophosphatase activity was markedly increased in well-differentiated upper intestinal villus cells when compared to immature lower intestinal crypt cells (12).

Effect of Butyrate on Cell Surface Membrane Proteins of HRT-18 Cells

Since significant qualitative or quantitative alterations in cell surface glycoproteins have been reported to occur in association with normal processes of cellular differentiation or during in vitro differentiation of mouse embryonal carcinoma cells or mouse neuro-

100 Y. S. KIM ET AL.

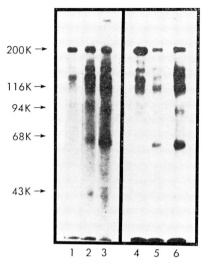

FIG. 3. Autoradiograms of ¹²⁵I-labeled surface membrane proteins of butyrate-treated and control HRT-18 cells. Cells were cultured for 8 days. Lanes 1, 2, and 3, the same amount of protein applied; Lanes 4, 5, and 6, the same amount of radio-activity applied. Lanes 1 and 4, control; Lanes 2 and 5, sodium butyrate (2 mM); Lanes 3 and 6, sodium butyrate (5 mM). (see Ref. *30*)

blastoma cells (*20*), we examined the effect of differentiating agents on cell surface protein using a lactoperoxidase-catalyzed iodination method (*9, 28*). The autoradiograms of ¹²⁵I-labeled surface membrane proteins of butyrate-treated and control HRT-18 cells are shown in Fig. 3. The most striking change with butyrate treatment was the appearance of a new protein band having an apparent molecular weight (M.W.) of 60,000. The glycoprotein nature of this band was determined by the lectin-affinity chromatography of iodinated surface membrane proteins of butyrate-treated HRT-18 cells using concanavalin A (ConA), *Recinus communis* agglutinin (RCA), wheat germ agglutinin (WGA), and peanut agglutinin (PNA) Sepharose columns. Since the protein with 60,000 M.W. bound specifically to ConA-, RCA-, and WGA-Sepharose columns, it would appear that it contains a glycoprotein. Although further studies are necessary before definitive conclusions can be drawn, it is possible that the cell surface glycoprotein with

TABLE IV.   Effect of Sodium Butyrate on HRT-18 Cells

1. Alkaline phosphatase	↑↑	1. Villus cells > Crypt cells
γ-Glutamyltranspeptidase	↑	Normal colon cells > Colon cancer cells
Sucrase	↑	
2. CEA	↑↑	2. Well differentiated colon cancer cells > Poorly differentiated colon cancer cells
3. Membrane carbohydrate content	↑	3. Normal colonic mucosal membrane > Cancerous colonic tissue membrane
4. Glycosyltransferases	↑	4. Normal colonic mucosa > Cancerous colonic mucosa
5. Glycosidases	=	5. Normal colonic mucosa = Cancerous colonic mucosa
6. Nucleotide pyrophosphatase	↑	6. Villus cells > Crypt cells
7. Appearance of 60,000 M. W. glycoprotein		

(see Refs. *8, 12, 16, and 18*)

a M.W. of 60,000 may be closely related to the mechanism by which butyrate causes the colon cancer cells to assume a more normal phenotype.

These data are summarized in Table IV. In the case of butyrate-treated human rectal cancer cells, it appears that the changes in the activities of membrane associated enzymes, membrane antigens, carbohydrate content, glycosyltransferases and glycosidases, and nucleotide pyrophosphatase are what would be expected of more-differentiated phenotypes as suggested by the data obtained by various investigators (8, 12, 16, 18).

DISCUSSION

The effects of several putative differentiating agents such as polar solvents (dimethylformamide or DMSO), retinoic acid, and sodium butyrate on the biological and biochemical properties of human colorectal cell lines have been studied by several investigators including our group (4, 10, 29, 30, 31). All of these agents caused a marked reduction in the *in vitro* tumorigenicity of colorectal carcinoma cells, and this was a reversible process. These cells regained malignant growth properties when the inducers were removed. Thus, under the experimental conditions employed to date, these putative inducers do not allow human colorectal cancer cells to reach a commitment stage (4, 10, 30). Unlike the erythroleukemia and neuroblastoma cell models which may proceed to a commitment stage, it is probable that the phenomena we have observed with the differentiating agents in colorectal cancer cells represent "early events" in the course of induced cellular differentiation.

Butyrate and other short-chain fatty acids are natural fermentation products of bacterial flora in the colon. Moreover, the concentration of butyrate in the colonic lumen is likely to be as high, if not higher, than the concentrations used in our study. Whether or not intraluminal concentrations of short-chain fatty acids play a role in the development of colorectal cancer, in the degree of malignancy, or the rate of tumor growth remains to be determined. However, when the same cell line is treated with DMSO or retinoic acid, the CEA content is reduced by DMSO, alkaline phosphatase activity is decreased in cells grown in DMSO or retinoic acid, and γ-glutamyltranspeptidase activity is decreased in cells grown in retinoic acid.

If the changes in growth parameters and colony formation in soft agar observed in the present study are taken as indicators of normal cell growth, then all three agents are able to induce a better-differentiated phenotype. However since the three agents had differential effects on CEA content and membrane-associated enzyme activities, these biochemical parameters may not represent specific markers of colonic cell differentiation. Alternatively, each inducer may cause expression of different phenotypic markers of differentiation in colonic cells, or the progression from a malignant to a normal cell line may not be closely related to the process of differentiation. In the absence of well-characterized differentiation markers for colonic cells, it is not yet possible to determine which of these conclusions are valid.

The mechanisms by which various substances induce cellular differentiation are not well understood. Butyrate has been noted to affect nuclear histone composition and DNA structure (24, 26, 31). Although DMSO and other polar compounds alter membrane permeability and microviscosity and also cause single-stranded breaks in DNA to occur, the relationship between these two events remains unclear (2, 26). It is known that retinol or retinoic acid is required for the normal differentiation of epithelial tissues

(14). Retinoids also cause differentiation of embryonal carcinoma cells *(25)*. It is thought that retinoids may act like steroid hormones by forming a complex with a binding protein which is translocated into the cell nucleus causing alterations in gene expression, but firm supportive evidence is lacking.

It is apparent that further studies using "differentiating agents" may not only provide useful information on the identification of differentiation-associated and stage specific glycoprotein and glycolipid markers of human colorectal cells, but may also contribute to elucidation of the molecular events involved in their tumorigenicity and differentiation, and to the development of methods for modifying the malignant properties of colorectal cells to more benign ones.

Acknowledgments

The authors wish to thank Ms. T. Harrington for the outstanding editing and typing of this manuscript.

This work was supported by USPHS Grant CA-14905 from the National Cancer Institute through the National Large Bowel Cancer Project and the Veterans Administration Medical Research Service.

REFERENCES

1. Abelev, G. I. *Transplant. Rev.*, **20**, 3–37 (1974).
2. Arndt-Jovin, D. J., Ostertag, W., Eisen, H., Limek, F., and Jovin, T. M. *J. Histochem. Cytochem.*, **24**, 332–347 (1976).
3. Cushing, H. and Wolbach, B. *Am. J. Pathol.*, **3**, 203–220 (1927).
4. Dexter, D. L. and Hager, J. C. *Cancer*, **45**, 1178–1184 (1980).
5. Friend, C., Scher, W., Holland, J. G., and Sato, T. *Proc. Natl. Acad. Sci. U.S.*, **68**, 378–382 (1971).
6. Gold, P. and Freedman, S. O. *J. Exp. Med.*, **122**, 467–481 (1965).
7. Hager, J. C., Gold, D. V., Barbosa, J. A., Fligiel, Z., Miller, F., and Dexter, D. L. *J. Natl. Cancer Inst.*, **64**, 439–445 (1979).
8. Kim, Y. S., Isaacs, P., and Perdomo, J. *Proc. Natl. Acad. Sci. U.S.*, **71**, 4869–4873 (1974).
9. Kim, Y. S., Tsao, D., Hicks, J., and McIntyre, L. J. *Cancer*, **47**, 1590–1596 (1981).
10. Kim, Y. S., Tsao, D., Siddiqui, B., Whitehead, J. S., Arnstein, P., Bennett, J., and Hicks, J. *Cancer*, **45**, 1185–1192 (1980).
11. Kimhi, Y., Palfrey, C., Spector, I., Barok, Y., and Littauer, U. Z. *Proc. Natl. Acad. Sci. U.S.*, **73**, 462–466 (1976).
12. Lau, J.T.Y. and Carlson, D. M. *J. Biol. Chem.*, **256**, 7142–7145 (1981).
13. Leder, A. and Leder, P. *Cell*, **5**, 319–322 (1975).
14. Lotan, R. *Biochim. Biophys. Acta*, **605**, 33–91 (1980).
15. Markert, C. L. *Cancer Res.*, **28**, 1908–1914 (1968).
16. Martin, E. W., Kibbey, W. E., DiVecchia, L., Anderson, G., Catalano, P., and Minton, J. P. *Cancer* **37**, (Suppl.), 62–81 (1976).
17. Mintz, B. *In* "Cell Differentiation and Neoplasia," The University of Texas System 30th Annual Symposium on Fundamental Cancer Research, ed. G. F. Saunders, pp. 27–53 (1977). Raven Press, New York.
18. Moog, F. *In* "Developments of Mammalian Absorptive Processes," Ciba Foundation Symposium 70, pp. 31–44 (1979). Excerpta Medica, New York.
19. Morita, A., Tsao, D., and Kim, Y. S. *Cancer Res.*, in press.

20. Muramatsu, T., Gachelin, G., Nicolas, J. F., Condamine, H., Jakob, H., and Jakob, F. *Proc. Natl. Acad. Sci. U.S.*, **75**, 2315–2319 (1978).

21. Pierce, G. B. *Curr. Top. Dev. Biol.*, **2**, 223–246 (1967).

22. Rifkind, R. A., Fibach, E., Reuben, R. C., Gazitt, Y., Yamasaki, H., Weinstein, I. B., Medel, U., Sumida, I., Terada, M., and Marks, P. A. *In* "Differentiation of Normal, and Neoplastic Hematopoietic Cells," Cold Spring Harbor Conference on Cell Proliferation, Vol. 5, ed. B. Clarkson, P. A. Marks, and J. E. Till, pp. 843–858 (1978).

23. Sasak, W., DeLuca, L. M., Dion, L. D., and Silverman-Jones, C. S. *Cancer Res.*, **40**, 1944–1949 (1980).

24. Sealy, L. and Chalkley, R. *Cell*, **14**, 115–121 (1978).

25. Strickland, S. and Mahdavi, V. *Cell*, **15**, 393–403 (1978).

26. Terada, M., Nudel, U., Fibach, E., Rifkind, R. A., and Marks, P. A. *Cancer Res.*, **38**, 835–840 (1978).

27. Tompkins, W.A.F., Watrach, A. M., Schmale, J. D., Schultz, R. M., and Harris, J. A. *J. Natl. Cancer Inst.*, **52**, 1101–1106 (1974).

28. Tsao, D., Colton, D. G., Chang, J. S., Buck, R. L., Hudson, B. G., and Carraway, K. L. *Biochim. Biophys. Acta*, **469**, 61–73 (1977).

29. Tsao, D. and Kim, Y. S. *J. Biol. Chem.*, **253**, 2271–2278 (1978).

30. Tsao, D., Morita, A., Bella, A., Jr., Luu, P., and Kim, Y. S. *Cancer Res.*, **42**, 1052–1058 (1982).

31. Vidali, G., Boffa, L. C., Bradbury, E. M., and Allfrey, V. G. *Proc. Natl. Acad. Sci. U.S.*, **75**, 2239–2243 (1978).

IV. GLYCOCONJUGATE ALTERATIONS IN MALIGNANCY

ALTERED GLYCOPROTEIN CARBOHYDRATES IN MALIGNANT CELLS

Leonard WARREN[*1] and Giulio COSSU[*2]

*The Wistar Institute[*1] and Istituto Di Istologie ed Embryiologie Generale, Universita di Roma[*2]*

A number of differences have been discerned in the carbohydrate groups of glycoproteins of normal and malignant cells. We and others have shown that there is a characteristic enlargement of the carbohydrate groups of most glycoproteins in every membrane system of the cell as cells become malignant. Despite the widespread, virtual ubiquitous occurrence of this category of change in malignant cells, its significance and its consequences are unknown. We attempt in this discussion to provide a rationale for the origin of the change and for the link between structural changes and the malignant behavior of cells.

The synthesis of bound carbohydrates of glycoproteins is not guided by a template. This probably accounts for the observation that these carbohydrates are readily alterable by a variety of agents and in various conditions. Changes in the external environment of a cell can induce a shift in the population of the carbohydrates bound to a polypeptide chain. It is reasoned that in malignancy there is a change in the internal environment of the cell, probably metabolic in origin, that could ultimately lead to the common observed shift. The shift could also be due to a direct genetic alteration of an enzyme responsible for the synthesis of bound carbohydrates. The altered structures of glycoproteins throughout the malignant cell could result in multiple, non-lethal functional changes, most of which are of little importance. We propose that altered glycoproteins in the cell surface might result in disturbed interaction of cells, giving rise to essential malignant characteristics—loss of growth control and the ability of cells to metastasize.

The surface membrane of normal and cancer cells has been a focus of ever-increasing interest and study over the past few decades. This organelle appears to be involved in the control of growth, movement, adhesiveness, binding of growth factors and hormones, transport of nutrients and other important functions. Regardless of the initiating changes, derangements in some of these processes may be essential for the full expression of malignancy. The carbohydrate polymers bound to polypeptide or to lipid are important components of the surface structure. These structures are, in fact, heavily concentreated in the surface membrane with the carbohydrate component facing the external environment, interacting with other carbohydrate-containing molecules, either free or bound to other cells. Numerous studies have shown that the lipid- and protein-bound carbohydrates of malignant cells differ in several respects from their normal counterparts (2, 19,

---

[*1] Philadelphia, Pennsylvania 19104, U.S.A.

[*2] 00161 Rome, Italy.

29–31, 36). Shifts in the glycolipid composition of malignant cells are discussed elsewhere in this volume (see pp. 113–127 in this volume).

What sense can be made of this information? What are the causes of the multiple,
complex changes in these structures in the cancer cell and what are the consequences of
the changes? At the present time these important questions remain unanswered. We
briefly describe here our own work on altered glycoprotein carbohydrates in malignant
cells, and present an hypothesis based on certain, known characteristics of bound carbohydrates to explain, at least in part, the significance of the shifts in malignancy.

Changes of Protein-bound Carbohydrates in Malignancy

When a cell becomes malignant, more, larger carbohydrate groups are found in 80%
of all its glycoproteins (28) in every membrane system of the cell (4). Because of the
extensiveness of the phenomenon, it is probable that this particular category of change
results from an alteration in the basic glycosylation mechanism of the cell. The shift has
been found in transformed and malignant cells of human, rat, hamster, mouse, and
chicken (see Ref. 36), in culture, in solid tumors (24, 35) and in leukemic cells (30), in
cells of fibroblastic, lymphocytic, and epithelial nature. There is good evidence that
the increase in size of the carbohydrate groups of the glycoproteins of malignant cells
is due to the fact that they bear an increased number of trisaccharide units of N-acetyl-
glucosamine-galactose-sialic acid (1, 11, 19, 20, 26) (see also pp. 177–195 in this volume).
This suggests that the malignant cell may acquire an enhanced ability to transfer one or
more molecules of N-acetylglucosamine to mannose residues already on glycoproteins
in the endoplasmic reticulum and the Golgi membranes. Once in place, a galactose and
then a sialic acid residue is added in succession to form a trisaccharide antenna. The
entire antenna-building process, though certainly not unique to the malignant cell,
may be exaggerated in this pathological cell.

The consequences of this general shift on the activity and interactions of a specific
glycoprotein or on whole populations of glycoproteins are unknown. However the shift
is closely associated with the tumorigenicity of cells. Cells transformed by chemicals or
viruses which grow in soft agar but are not tumorigenic do not undergo changes in their
protein-bound carbohydrates. On the other hand, those transformed cells that undergo
characteristic changes in bound carbohydrate, either immediately or after a period of
culture in flasks, are tumorigenic in appropriate hosts. It would appear that the carbohydrate change is more closely associated with tumorigenicity than with *in vitro*
criteria of transformation (12, 13, 23).

The basis for the phenotypic changes just described is unknown. They could arise
from an altered N-acetylglucosaminyl transferase activity as described above originating
from a genetic alteration. The consistency and the ubiquity of the change in bound
carbohydrate in malignant cells suggests that this change is not merely casually associated.
Yet the unknown link between the critical nuclear and the carbohydrate changes could
be quite remote. Direct links can be suggested, such as the synthesis of new sugar transferases or the activation or deactivation of existing transferases by phosphorylation and
dephosphorylation. The transferases are probably glycoproteins and alterations of their
sugar components might be a method of modulation. Transferases are embedded in
membranes, the lipid and glycolipid components of which could be modified, possibly
with numerous specific consequences.

Potential for Change of the Bound Carbohydrates

The bound carbohydrates of glycoprotein are complex; yet their synthesis is not guided or controlled by a template. As a result, the process of glycosylation is effected by a series of reactions dependent on the specificity of enzymes, whose activities can to some extent be modified by varying conditions existing at the time of synthesis. It has been found that the carbohydrates of some but not all glycoproteins vary depending on whether cells are growing on surfaces of glass, plastic or collagen-coated plastic (37) or whether they are growing at 23° or 33° (39). The glycoprotein carbohydrate groups of tumor cells grown in culture vary depending on the composition of the medium and the nature of the buffer (15). Chick embryo chondroblasts synthesize different populations of protein-bound carbohydrates depending on whether they are surrounded by a matrix of cartilage or are in culture (7).

Changes in bound carbohydrates can be induced by exposure of cells to a number of drugs and agents such as ethidium bromide (25), acriflavin (unpublished), adriamycin (14), sodium butyrate (22, 33), cyclic AMP (32), and tunicamycin (10). Deficiency of retinoic acid in culture (21) and in the whole animal (41) leads to alteration of bound carbohydrates.

Bound carbohydrates have been found to differ depending on the state of growth of the cell (3, 5). It is possible that the changes in glycoprotein carbohydrates seen in malignancy reflect, at least in part, an exaggeration in degree and persistence of the normal changes that occur during growth. Enlargement of glycopeptides may occur in the cell in any phase of the cell cycle while smaller carbohydrate structures with fewer antennae might characterize the resting cell (G_0 phase).

Radical changes in the bound carbohydrates of cells mutant in various glycosyl transferases have been described. These mutants are frequently detected by their loss of susceptibility to toxic lectins, since altered sugar structure and composition results in loss of affinity of the lectins for cells (26).

The carbohydrates of individual glycoproteins and glycolipids change during differentiation. It was shown by Muramatsu *et al.* (16; see pp. 157–167 in this volume) that undifferentiated mouse teratocarcinoma cells produce glycoproteins with large carbohydrate structures of molecular weight (M_r)>10,000 consisting mostly of alternating units of D-galactose and N-acetyl-D-glucosamine (lactosaminoglycan). When teratocarcinomas differentiate spontaneously or are induced to differentiate by exposure to retinoic acid or cyclic AMP, synthesis of these structures is sharply reduced (16–18). This change also occurs in human erythroleukemic cells that have been induced to form macrophages by treatment with a phorbol ester (6). Recently it has been found that the fibronectin of mouse (9) and human (8) teratocarcinoma cells bear covalently bound molecules of heparan sulfate and lactosaminoglycan and have an M_r 250,000. The differentiated counterparts of these cells produce fibronectin of M_r 220,000, devoid of these carbohydrate structures. However they retain the carbohydrate structures usually associated with "adult" fibronectin.

From the above discussion it would appear that the composition and structure of the carbohydrate groups of glycoproteins can, within limits, change depending on many factors and conditions. Further, it appears that most glycoproteins are heterogeneous in their carbohydrate component, *i.e.*, they are polymorphic (see Ref. 38 for discussion). With the changing of bound carbohydrates in so many situations, we may be dealing with a constantly shifting polymorphism that takes place normally in response to changes of environmental conditions, to drugs, and to normal and pathological states of the cell. The shifts may be modest, not necessarily affecting all glycoproteins and they may not be lethal or debilitating; changes in the structure of template-determined polymers are usually very harmful.

To continue this speculative discussion, the question arises whether the shift in protein-bound carbohydrates in the malignant cell is due to an "environmental" change within the cell. A condition would exist that promotes increased transfer of N-acetylglu-cosamine to carbohydrate structures. The altered state may be related to mitochondrial dysfunction with changes in pH, oxidation-reduction potential, concentrations of ATP, various metabolites, free and/or bound divalent cations, and other cell constituents (*34*, *40*). The composition of the lipid membranes in which the transferases are embedded could be altered. All or any of these changes, alone or in sequence, could shift the array of end products on the polypeptides without seriously harming the cell.

Shifts could also result from over- or underproduction of enzymes such as glycosyl transferases and glycosidases responsible for the synthesis of carbohydrate polymers. Ultimately the crucial change in the malignant cell involves the nucleus and the genetic apparatus. However changes in bound carbohydrates due to altered levels of biosynthetic enzymes would involve the nucleus more fully and directly than would changes of the "internal environment" of the cell. The latter might be a distant reponse to nuclear events.

It is proposed that the bound carbohydrates are allosteric modulators of the activity and interactions of the polypeptide moiety of the glycoprotein. They might act singly or in combination by modifying mobility and conformation of polypeptides. Their activi-ties would be mainly indirect rather than by direct participation in specific mechanisms. This might account for the fact that modification of sugars of most glycoproteins does not result in radical change in activity. Perhaps in those cases where radical change in function is observed, the carbohydrate structure participates in a specific mechanism, rather than modulating from a distance.

A persistent change in the structure of most glycoproteins, in every membrane system of the malignant cell, could result in a cascade of small changes in numerous activities. None of these changes would be lethal, nor would most of them be of any consequence. However it is suggested that certain changes in the glycoproteins of the cell surface would permit cells to cease interacting with one another in an appropriate manner and to divide persistently. These cells would also be capable of separating from their neighbors, spreading to remote sites in the body where they would commence dividing. Changes in other glycoproteins might result in alterations of transport of nutrients that would favor the survival of malignant cells. The proposed changes in bound carbohydrates would not be primary. Rather, they would occur during the devel-opment of the effectively malignant cell.

If the presence of a specific population of bound carbohydrates is one of several requirements for a cell to display malignant behavior, then it is possible that suppression of this population might prevent the development of malignant behavior. Agents capable of such action might not be lethal or toxic, because the cell appears to tolerate great variation in its bound carbohydrates. Therapeutic agents would have to be administered chronically, taming rather than killing malignant cells. The rationale differs from the conventional form which exploits the difference between normal and malignant cells to eradicate the malignant cell, usually with highly toxic damaging agents.

Acknowledgments

This work was supported by grants CA-19130, CA-10815 and CA-21069 from the U.S. Public Health Service and PRP-28 from the American Cancer Society. G. Cossu was the recipient of Fellowship TW-03012 from the U.S. Public Health Service. We wish to thank H. Schorr and M. Hoffman for editorial assistance.

REFERENCES

1. Blithe, D. L., Buck, C. A., and Warren, L. *Biochemistry*, **19**, 3386–3395 (1980).
2. Buck, C. A., Glick, M. C., and Warren, L. *Biochemistry*, **9**, 4567–4576 (1970).
3. Buck, C. A., Glick, M. C., and Warren, L. *Biochemistry*, **10**, 2176–2180 (1971).
4. Buck, C. A., Fuhrer, J. P., Soslau, G., and Warren, L. *J. Biol. Chem.*, **249**, 1541–1550 (1974).
5. Ceccarini, C., Muramatsu, T., Tsang, J., and Atkinson, P. H. *Proc. Natl. Acad. Sci. U.S.*, **72**, 3139–3143 (1975).
6. Cossu, G., Kuo, A. L., Pessano, S., Warren, L., and Cooper, R. A. *Cancer Res.*, **42**, 484–489 (1982).
7. Cossu, G., Warren, L., Boettiger, D., Holtzer, H., and Pacifici, M. *J. Biol. Chem.*, **257**, 4463–4468 (1982).
8. Cossu, G., Andrews, P. W., and Warren, L. *Biochem. Biophys. Res. Commun.*, **111**, 952–957 (1983).
9. Cossu, G. and Warren, L. *J. Biol. Chem.*, **258**, 5603–5607 (1983).
10. Damsky, C. H., Levy-Benshimol, A., Buck, C. A., and Warren, L. *Exp. Cell Res.*, **119** 1–13 (1979).
11. Glick, M. C. *Biochemistry*, **18**, 2525–2532 (1979)
12. Glick, M. C., Rabinowitz, Z., and Sachs, L. *Biochemistry*, **12**, 4864–4869 (1973).
13. Glick, M. C., Rabinowitz, Z., and Sachs, L. *J. Virol.*, **13**, 967–974 (1974).
14. Kessel, D. *Mol. Pharmacol.*, **16**, 306–312 (1979).
15. Megaw, J. M. and Johnson, L. D. *Proc. Soc. Exp. Biol. Med.*, **161**, 60–65 (1979).
16. Muramatsu, T., Gachelin, G., Nicolas, J. F., Condamine, H., Jakob, H., and Jacob, F. *Proc. Natl. Acad. Sci. U.S.*, **75**, 2315–2319 (1978).
17. Muramatsu, H. and Muramatsu, T. *Dev. Biol.*, **90**, 441–444 (1982).
18. Muramatsu, H. and Muramatsu, T. *Cancer Res.*, **42**, 1749–1752 (1982).
19. Ogata, S. I., Muramatsu, T., and Kobata, A. *Nature*, **259**, 580–582 (1976).
20. Santer, U. V. and Glick, M. C. *Biochemistry*, **18**, 2533–2540 (1979).
21. Sasak, W., Deluca, L. M., Dion, L. D., and Silverman-Jones, C. S. *Cancer Res.*, **40**, 1944–1949 (1980).
22. Simmons, J. F., Fishman, P. M., Freese, L., and Brady, R. O. *J. Cell Biol.*, **66**, 414–424 (1975).
23. Smets, L. A., Van Beek, W. P., and Rooij, van H. *Int. J. Cancer*, **18**, 462–468 (1976).
24. Smets, L. A., Van Beek, W. P., and Van Nie, R. *Cancer Lett.*, **3**, 133–138 (1977).
25. Soslau, G., Fuhrer, J. P., Nass, M.M.K., and Warren, L. *J. Biol. Chem.*, **249**, 3014–3020 (1974).
26. Stanley, P. *In* "The Biochemistry of Glycoproteins and Proteoglycans," ed. W. J. Lennarz, Chap. 4, p. 161 (1980). Plenum Press, New York.
27. Takasaki, S., Ikehira, H., and Kobata, A. *Biochem. Biophys. Res. Commun.*, **92**, 735–742 (1980).

28. Tuszynski, G. P., Baker, S. R., Fuhrer, J. P., Buck, C. A., and Warren, L. *J. Biol. Chem.*, **253**, 6092–6099 (1979).

29. Van Beek, W. P., Smets, L. A., and Emmelot, P. *Cancer Res.*, **33**, 2913–2922 (1973).

30. Van Beek, W. P., Smets, L. A., and Emmelot, P. *Nature*, **253**, 457–460 (1975).

31. Van Nest, G. A. and Grimes, W. J. *Biochemistry*, **16**, 2902–2908 (1977).

32. Van Veen, G. A., Noonan, K. D., and Roberts, R. M. *Exp. Cell Res.*, **103**, 405–413 (1976).

33. Via, D. P., Sramek, S., Sarriba, G., and Steiner, S. *J. Cell Biol.*, **84**, 225–234 (1980).

34. Warburg, O. *Science*, **123**, 309 (1956).

35. Warren, L., Zeidman, I., and Buck, C. A. *Cancer Res.*, **35**, 2186–2190 (1975).

36. Warren, L., Buck, C. A., and Tuszynski, G. P. *Biochim. Biophys. Acta*, **516**, 97–127 (1978).

37. Warren, L., Blithe, D. L., and Cossu, G. *J. Cell Physiol.*, **113**, 17–22 (1982).

38. Warren, L., Baker, S. R., Blithe, D. L., and Buck, C. A. *In* "Biomembranes," ed. A. Nowotny, Vol. 11, pp. 53–78 (1983). Plenum Publishing, New York.

39. Warren, L. and Clark, H. F. Unpublished.

40. Weinhouse, S. *Adv. Cancer*, **3**, 269 (1955).

41. Wolf, G., Kiorpes, T. C., Masushige, S., Schrieber, J. B., Smith, M. J., and Anderson, R. S. *Fed. Proc.*, **38**, 2540–2543 (1979).

GANN Monograph on Cancer Research 29, 1983

TUMOR-ASSOCIATED GLYCOLIPID MARKERS IN EXPERIMENTAL AND HUMAN CANCER

Sen-itiroh HAKOMORI

*Division of Biochemical Oncology, Fred Hutchinson Cancer Research Center and University of Washington**

Glycolipid changes associated with oncogenic transformation *in vitro* and tumor growth *in vivo* have been summarized in this paper. Four types of glycolipid changes are: i) incomplete synthesis, ii) neosynthesis, iii) a shift of glycolipid synthesis from one series to another, and iv) the change of glycolipid organization in membranes. Incomplete synthesis results in precursor accumulation. Therefore, both incomplete synthesis and neosynthesis induce the appearance of glycolipid markers which are distinct for tumor cells and can be defined by monoclonal antibodies. Glycolipids with the X determinant, particularly those with di- or tri-fucosylated structures, have been found in a large variety of human adenocarcinoma. GD_3 ganglioside in human melanoma and ceramide trihexoside in Burkitt lymphoma are well-defined markers by monoclonal antibodies. Alterations of blood group antigens, such as deletion of A and B determinants and neosynthesis of A-like antigen in tumors of blood group O or B individuals and PP_1-like antigen in p hosts, have also been characterized. These glycolipid markers can be useful targets for diagnosis and therapy of human cancer.

There is increasing evidence that cancer is associated with abnormalities in gene regulation expressed in multiple molecules at the cell surface membranes, and abnormal gene regulation may direct a blockage or deviation in synthesis and organization of cell surface molecules that mediate cellular interaction, development, and differentiation (26, 43). Glycosphingolipids are ubiquitous plasma membrane components, showing clear changes associated with oncogenesis and ontogenesis. Studies along this line have been greatly catalyzed by a few technological revolutions, such as i) separation of membrane glycolipids on high performance chromatography, and structural analysis based on methylation, mass spectrometry, and enzymatic degradation (*e.g.*, Ref. *46*); ii) hybridoma technique and production of monoclonal antibodies (*49*); and iii) immunostaining of glycolipids separated on thin-layer chromatography (*57*). The chemical quantity of glycolipids, their organization in membranes, and their reactivity to specific ligands are not only defined according to their genetic backgrounds but also are controlled by epigenetic conditions such as growth condition, environment, cell cycle, and cell contacts (*9, 21, 23, 71, 84*). Their overall expression, therefore, reflects the stage of differentiation and oncogenesis. Recently, a number of new glycolipids have been discovered, particularly those belonging to lacto series, by improved techniques in separation and structural characterization (*26, 56*). Accordingly, the changes of glycolipid patterns once described should be re-evaluated in various tumor systems.

---

* Seattle, Washington 98104, U.S.A. (箱守仙一郎).

Dramatic changes in glycolipid composition and metabolism have been observed not only in virally or chemically transformed cells but also in spontaneous tumors, including a large variety of human cancers. Since we first observed this phenomenon in virally transformed cells in 1968, it has been the focus of a number of studies; consequently, a specific role of glycolipids in defining membrane phenotype associated with oncogenesis has been sought. Early efforts on this topic have been reviewed repeatedly (2, 19, 24, 25) and will not be treated in this article. This review will focus on the tumor-associated glycosphingolipid markers and their implication in diagnosis and treatment of human cancer.

Types of Glycolipid Changes in Tumors

Since each type of cell has a specific profile of glycolipid composition, the change of glycolipids in each cell type differs greatly when it is transformed. Four types of glycolipid changes have been observed as shown in Table I, *i.e.*, i) incomplete synthesis of higher glycolipids due to a block of a single or multiple glycosyltransferase(s); ii) synthesis of glycolipids unique to the tumor, such as incompatible blood group antigens and unusual structures which are absent in normal cells; iii) a shifting of glycolipid synthesis from one series of glycolipid to another, *i.e.*, cells synthesizing ganglio-series glycolipid are converted to those synthesizing globo-series glycolipid or lacto-series glycolipid associated with oncogenic transformation; and iv) the change of glycolipid organization in membranes.

1. Blocked synthesis with accumulation of precursor

In early investigations, cultured fibroblastic cells and their viral transformants were compared for their glycolipid composition in which a relatively simple pattern was demonstrated, *i.e.*, incomplete synthesis of a higher glycolipid due to a block of a single or multiple transferase(s). Typical examples included GM_3 in hamster BHKpy cells, Gb_3, Gb_4, and Gb_5 in NIL cells, and higher gangliosides (GD, GT, GQ) in mouse fibroblast, rat mammary carcinoma, and hepatoma. For spontaneous tumors and human cancers, comparable normal cells and tissues are unavailable, nevertheless the glycolipid composition of human leukemic lymphocytes, brain tumors, kidney tumors, and gastrointestinal cancer were studied in comparison with normal tissues. The results indicated that blocked synthesis and precursor accumulation may indeed by occurring in these human cancers as well (see for reviews Refs. 2, 19, 24, 25).

2. Neosynthesis

Some tumors accumulate a large quantity of glycolipids which are absent or present

TABLE I.   Types of Glycolipid Alterations in Oncogenic Transformants

1. Incomplete synthesis with or without precursor accumulation (see review articles, Refs. 2, 19, 24, 25)
2. Neosynthesis: activation of new glycolipid synthesis characteristic of transformed cells (see Table II)
3. Shifting of glycolipid synthesis from one series to another (21, 38, 52, 76)
4. The change of glycolipid organization: loss of crypticity and cell cycle dependency (21, 30, 55)

in very small quantity in normal cells or tissues. Such examples are listed in Table I and are extensively discussed in the next section. The accumulation of glycolipids is essentially due to the enhanced synthesis of glycolipids, which in many cases can be called "neoglycolipids." Some tumors display a combination of blocked synthesis and neosynthesis, and therefore the pattern of glycolipids is highly complex.

3. Shifting of glycolipid synthesis from one series to another

Each type of cell or cell line is defined by a characteristic composition of three series of glycolipids, globo, lacto, and ganglio series. One type of cell is usually characterized by a predominance of one series of glycolipid, while other types of cells have two series. A shifting of glycolipid synthesis from one series to another can be seen upon oncogenic transformation. Non-transformed NIL cells had three components of globo series, Gb_3, Gb_4, and Gb_5. NILpy cells were characterized by a depletion of all three globo-series components and by neosynthesis of a lacto series, paragloboside (21). Normal myelocytes were characterized by the major component nLc_4, paragloboside. In contrast, myelomonoblastic leukemia cells contained about equal quantities of nLc_4 and Gb_4 (52). In both cases, glycolipid synthesis of one series shifted to another series on on-cogenic transformation. This type of shifting is also obviously associated with expression of the degree of malignancy (38, 76) and with differentiation of M_1 cells (46).

4. The change of glycolipid organization in membranes

Glycolipids not only alter their chemical composition and metabolism but also their state of organization associated with oncogenic transformation (21, 30). In many trans-formed cells, glycolipids in membranes become more exposed and accessible to exo-genous ligands. Cell cycle dependent changes of glycolipid exposure were also modified in various transformed cells (55). This is an important basis in considering glycolipid antigenicity in tumors.

Glycolipid Tumor-associated Markers or Antigens

A blocked synthesis of a glycolipid in tumors is often accompanied by the accumula-tion of its precursor, and a neosynthesis results in the appearance of a new glycolipid, i.e., "neoglycolipid." Either mechanism induces an accumulation of a glycolipid which is characteristic of tumor cells but absent or present in small quantity in non-transformed progenital cells. These glycolipid markers are hardly immunogenic to syngenic hosts; therefore, they are distinctive from a classically known tumor-associated antigen. In this sense, "tumor-associated markers" could be more appropriate to designate this new class of tumor markers. For detection of such molecules, two approaches have been undertaken. In the first, glycolipid components of transformed cells or tumors are chemically compared with their progenitors and normal cells. The comparison includes high performance chromatography, methylation, and mass spectrometry. If a unique component for the tumor is found, the antibody directed to this component is produced which is used to characterize the antigen distribution and quantity as well as the effect of antibodies on tumor growth. The second approach depends on the identification of glycolipid antigens recognized by established tumor-specific monoclonal antibodies, an approach made possible only by the development of such antibodies.

The tumor-associated glycolipids are immunologically distinct for tumor cells, but in many cases the same antigens are chemically detectable in small quantity in normal cells and are usually cryptic at the cell surface membranes. Another feature of glycolipid antigens is their presence at certain stages of differentiation and development. They are, therefore, essentially oncofetal or oncodifferentiation markers. We will discuss in this chapter three categories of tumor-associated glycolipid markers: i) glycolipid markers for experimental animal cancer; ii) human cancer antigens defined by monoclonal antibodies and chemical characterization; and iii) human cancer antigens arising from modification of blood group antigens (human allogenic antigens).

1. Glycolipid markers for experimental animal cancers

During the past few years, a few lines of evidence have indicated that some glycolipids of transformed cells are unique for certain types of experimental tumor cells and could be distinctive markers for specific types of animal cancer (see Table II). The presence of nLc$_4$ (lacto-N-neotetraosylceramide; paragloboside) in hamster NILpy tumors, and its absence in normal hamster NIL or BHK fibroblasts is one example (21). NILpy tumors grown in hamsters contained this glycolipid in significant quantity. Interestingly, antibody response to this glycolipid was observed in hamsters bearing NILpy tumors (75).

TABLE II.   Neoglycolipids in Experimental Tumors and Human Cancer

A. Experimental tumors		
Gg$_3$ (asialo GM$_2$)	GalNAcβ1 → 4Galβ1 → 4Glcβ1 → 1Cer	Mouse lymphoma (Young and Hakomori, 86) Mouse KiMSV-sarcoma (Rosenfelder et al., 70)
nLc$_4$ (paragloboside)	Galβ1 → 4GlcNAcβ1 → 3Galβ1 → 4Glcβ1 → 1Cer	Hamster NILpy tumor (Gahmberg and Hakomori, 21, Sundsmo and Hakomori, 75)
Galactosyl fucosyl GM$_1$	Fucα1 → 2Galβ1 → 3GalNAcβ1 → 4Galβ1 → 4Glcβ1 → 1Cer 3 3 ↑ ↑ Galα1 . NeuAcα2	Rat hepatoma and precancer liver (Holmes and Hakomori, 40)
B. Human cancer		
Fucosyl ceramide	Fucα1 → 1Cer	Colonic adenocarcinoma (Watanabe et al., 77)
A-like antigen	GalNAcα1 → 3Galβ1 → HexN → (Hex)$_n$ → Hex → Cer	Hepatocarcinoma (Yokota et al., 83)
P-like antigen in tumor of pp individual	GalNAcβ1 → 3Galβ1 → 4GlcNAcβ1 → 3Galβ1 → 4Glcβ1 → 1Cer	Gastric cancer of a patient (Mrs. J) with genotype pp (Levine, 53; Kannagi et al., 45)
Forssman antigen in	GalNAcα1 → 3GalNAcβ1 → 3Galα1 → 4Galβ1 → 4Glcβ1 → 1Cer	Colonic cancer of F− (fsfs) tissue (Hakomori et al., 32; Yokota et al., 83)
F− (fsfs) tumor	GalNAcα1 → 3GalNAcβ1 → Hex → Cer	
Sialyl Le^a	See Table III	
Fucosyl type	See Table III	

KiMSV, murine sarcoma virus Kirsten strain.

Tumors in Balb/c mice which arose from inoculation of 3T3 cells transformed by murine sarcoma virus Kirsten strain (70) as well as mouse lymphoma L5178 in DBA/2 mice (87) contained a large quantity of Gg_3 (ganglio-triaosylceramide). Various organs of Balb/c or DBA/2 mice did not contain appreciable quantities of this glycolipid. The glycolipid, therefore, can be regarded as a tumor-associated cell surface marker and has been found to be useful in immunotherapy with monoclonal antibodies directed to it (86).

Vesicular stomatitis virus (VSV) obtained from the simian virus 40 (SV40) transformed hamster cell line acquires a tumor specific transplantation antigen activity which causes SV40 tumor rejection. A glycolipid fraction prepared from VSV from SV40 transformed tumor incorporated into liposomes was shown to be immunogenic and is capable of suppressing tumor growth. Antiserum directed to liposomes containing the polar glycolipids of SV40 transformed hamster tumor cells, after being absorbed with normal hamster tissue, specifically reacts with the SV40 transformed cells (1, 42). These results imply that a specific glycolipid acts as an SV40 induced antigen in hamster cells. In these studies, however, a pure glycolipid was neither isolated nor characterized. Since the amphipathic polypeptides can be associated and co-purified with a polar glycolipid fraction, and such polypeptides can be highly immunogenic (78), great care is needed to distinguish glycolipid and amphipathic polypeptides present in the glycolipid fraction.

2. *Human cancer antigens defined by monoclonal antibodies*

Biochemical properties of "tumor-associated antigens" have been increasingly known by application of the hybridoma technology established by Köhler and Milstein (49). More than a few glycolipids have been identified as tumor-associated markers defined by monoclonal antibodies, although their biological significance is not well established.

1) *Glycolipid antigens of colorectoadenocarcinomas*

A number of monoclonal antibodies directed to colorectoadenocarcinomas have been prepared by Koprowski and associates (50). Four monoclonal antibodies produced

TABLE III. Structures of Unique Glycolipids with High Incidence
Shared by Various Cancers

A. Monosialoganglioside defined by monoclonal antibody N-19-9 (Koprowski *et al.*, 50) of human colonic, gastric, and pancreatic cancer

NeuAc2 → 3Galβ1 → 3GlcNAcβ1 → 3Galβ1 → 4Glcβ1 → 1Cer
$$4$$
$$\uparrow$$
Fucα1
Magnani *et al.* (58, 59)

B. Difucosyl or trifucosyl-polylactosaminolipids of human adenocarcinoma of colon, liver, and lung

Galβ1 → 4GlcNAcβ1 → 3Galβ1 → 4GlcNAcβ1 → 3Galβ1 → 4Glcβ1 → 1Cer
$$\quad\quad\quad 3 \quad\quad\quad\quad\quad\quad\quad\quad\quad 3$$
$$\quad\quad\quad \uparrow \quad\quad\quad\quad\quad\quad\quad\quad\quad \uparrow$$
$$\quad\quad\quad Fuc\alpha1 \quad\quad\quad\quad\quad\quad Fuc\alpha1$$
Galβ1 → 4GlcNAcβ1 → 3Galβ1 → 4GlcNAcβ1 → 3Galβ1 → 4GlcNAcβ1 → 3Galβ1 → 4Glcβ1 → 1 Cer
$$\quad 3 \quad\quad\quad\quad\quad\quad 3 \quad\quad\quad\quad\quad\quad\quad 3$$
$$\quad \uparrow \quad\quad\quad\quad\quad\quad \uparrow \quad\quad\quad\quad\quad\quad\quad \uparrow$$
$$\quad Fuc\alpha1 \quad\quad\quad\quad Fuc\alpha1 \quad\quad\quad\quad\quad Fuc\alpha1$$
Hakomori *et al.* (37)

by hybridomas obtained from a mouse immunized with a human adenocarcinoma cell line, SW1116 (50), have been characterized as being directed to Le^b structure (5). An apparent specificity of antibody for colorectoadenocarcinoma cell line described by Koprowski *et al.* (51) may reflect the high concentration of Le^a and Le^b glycolipids that co-exist in some adenocarcinomas regardless of the Lewis blood group status of the donor (28).

The hybridoma antibody, N-19-9, was found to be highly specific not only for colorectoadenocarcinoma but also gastric and pancreatic cancer. The binding of the antibody to carcinoma tissue extract was inhibited by serum from patients with adenocarcinoma of colon, but not by serum from patients with other bowel diseases or from healthy volunteers (51). The specific antigen defined by this monoclonal antibody was found in a ganglioside fraction of tumor and meconium but not in normal tissue, and was identified as monosialoganglioside (58). The structure of the antigen was recently determined as sialosyl-Le^a by Magnani *et al.* (59) (see Table III, item A). Antigen was found in meconium which essentially consists of fetal intestinal epithelial membranes.

TABLE IV. Structure of Glycolipids Bearing Le^x Determinant and Internally Located Fucα1 → 3GlcNAc Residues from Tumors and Normal Tissue

	Structure	Normal (RBC, liver, and colonic mucosa)	Adeno-carcinoma (liver and colon

1.	Galβ1 → **4GlcNAcβ1** → **3Galβ1** → **4Glcβ1** → **1Cer**
	    3
	    ↑
	    Fucα1
		−	⧻

2.	Galβ1 → 4GlcNAcβ1 → 3Galβ1 → 4GlcNAcβ1 → 3Galβ1 → 4Glcβ1 → 1Cer
	    3
	    ↑
	    Fucα1
		+	+

3.	Galβ1 → 4GlcNAcβ1 → 3Galβ1 → **4GlcNAcβ1** → **3Galβ1** → **4Glcβ1** → **1Cer**
	    3 3
	    ↑ ↑
	    Fucα1 **Fucα1**
		−	⧻

4.	Galβ1 → 4GlcNAcβ1 → 3Galβ1 → 4GlcNAcβ1 → 3Galβ1 → 4GlcNAcβ1 → 3Galβ1 → 4Glcβ1 → 1Cer
	    3
	    ↑
	    Fucα1
		+	+

5.	Galβ1 → 4GlcNAcβ1 → 3Galβ1 → 4GlcNAcβ1 → 3Galβ1 → 4GlcNAcβ1 → 3Galβ1 → 4Glcβ1 → 1Cer
	    3 3
	    ↑ ↑
	    Fucα1 Fucα1
		+	+

6.	Galβ1 → 4GlcNAcβ1 → 3Galβ1 → 4GlcNAcβ1 → 3Galβ1 → **4GlcNAcβ1** → **3Galβ1** → **4Glcβ1** → **1Cer**
	    3 3 3
	    ↑ ↑ ↑
	    Fucα1 Fucα1 **Fucα1**
		−	+

1. Lacto-N-fucopentaosyl (III) ceramide (Yang and Hakomori, 1971).   2. Y$_2$ (Kannagi *et al.*, 1982).
3. Difucosyllacto-N-norhexaosylceramide.   4. Z$_1$ (Kannagi *et al.*, 1982).   5. Z$_{2a}$ (Kannagi *et al.*, 1982).
6. Trifucosyllacto-N-noroctaosylceramide. 1, 3, 6. (Hakomori, Nudelman, Kannagi, Levery, unpublished; structure 6 is tentative).
⧻ 30–100 μg/10 mg tissue protein ;   ╫ 10–30 μg/10 mg tissue protein ;   + 1–10 μg/10 mg tissue protein ;
− <1 μg/10 mg tissue protein.

2) Monoclonal antibodies directed to the carbohydrate sequence Le^x (Galβ1 → 4[Fucα1 → 3] GlcNAc), showing an apparent tumor specificity

One hybridoma antibody (WGHS 29–1) which resulted from immunization with gastric cancer cells and three (ZWG13, ZWG14, ZWG111) which resulted from immunization with cells from a liver metastasis of a colon adenocarcinoma were all recently found to be directed to Le^x structure (Galβ1→4[Fucα1→3]GlcNAc) (*6*). The embryonic antigen, SSEA-1, defined by its monoclonal antibody has been identified as Le^x structure (*22*), although SSEA-1 antibody does not react well in a solid-phase radioimmunoassay with lacto-N-fucopentaosyl(III)ceramide (*34*) under the same conditions which allow it to react with the Le^x structure carried by a long type 2 chain such as Y2, Z1, Z2a (*46*). One of the antibodies (WGHS-29) reacts with lacto-N-fucopentaosyl(III)ceramide better than with other Le^x glycolipids having longer carbohydrate chains (*6*).

Another set of monoclonal antibodies was produced by hybridomas obtained from mice immunized with a human small cell lung cancer cell line that has an apparent specificity for human small cell carcinoma, adenocarcinoma, and squamatous carcinoma of lung (*10*). The antibodies had been identified as having an apparent specificity with Le^x structure (*41*). The monoclonal antibodies all react with a series of glycolipids accumulated in various lung cancer tissues. The major glycolipid reacting to these antibodies had the same thin layer chromatogram (TLC) mobility as lacto-N-fucopentaosyl (III)ceramide (*41*) which was first found to be accumulated in some, if not all, human adenocarcinoma (*80*). Other slower migrating glycolipids from lung tumors, detected by these antibodies on TLC, may include di- or tri-fucosylated derivatives.

Recently, a systematic study on the Le^x glycolipids of normal and tumor tissues has been undertaken (*34, 37*). The presence of an unusual di- or tri-fucosylated polylactosamine glycolipid accumulating in a large variety of human adenocarcinomas has been particularly noticeable (see Table III, item B). Six structures with Le^x determinant have been identified. Glycolipids having a common structure as shown below and as printed in bold print in Table IV accumulate in large quantities in many cases of human adenocarcinoma, including colonic, gastric, lung, and liver cancer.

$$R \rightarrow 4GlcNAc\beta1 \rightarrow 3Gal\beta1 \rightarrow 4Glc\beta1 \rightarrow 1Cer \quad (A)$$
$$\underset{\underset{Fuc\alpha1}{\uparrow}}{3}$$
$$(I)$$

$$R \rightarrow GlcNAc\beta1 \rightarrow 3Gal\beta1 \rightarrow 4GlcNAc\beta1 \rightarrow 3Gal\beta1 \rightarrow 4Glc\beta1 \rightarrow 1Cer \quad (B)$$
$$\underset{\underset{Fuc\alpha1}{\uparrow}}{3} \qquad\qquad \underset{\underset{Fuc\alpha1}{\uparrow}}{3}$$
$$(III) \qquad\qquad (II)$$

However, glycolipids with Le^x determinant at the terminus of a long type 2 chain, as shown below (C and D), are present in normal tissues and do not accumulate in tumor tissue (*37*).

$$Gal\beta1 \rightarrow 4GlcNAc\beta1 \rightarrow 3Gal\beta1 \rightarrow 4GlcNAc\beta1 \rightarrow 3Gal\beta1 \rightarrow 4Glc\beta1 \rightarrow 1Cer \quad (C)$$
$$\underset{\underset{Fuc\alpha1}{\uparrow}}{3}$$

$$Gal\beta1 \rightarrow 4GlcNAc\beta1 \rightarrow 3Gal\beta1 \rightarrow 4GlcNAc\beta1 \rightarrow 3Gal\beta1 \rightarrow 4GlcNAc\beta1 \rightarrow 3Gal\beta1 \rightarrow 4Glc\beta1 \rightarrow 1Cer \quad (D)$$
$$\underset{\underset{Fuc\alpha1}{\uparrow}}{3}$$

It is possible that a specific fucosyltransferase for synthesis of the fucosylresidues (I), (II), and (III) above could be greatly enhanced in various human adenocarcinoma. In contrast, a fucosyltransferase for synthesis of a fucosyl residue at the penultimate GlcNAc residue of a long type 2 chain may not be altered by cancer. So far, all monoclonal antibodies directed to Le^x are directed to the terminal structures. If we could select an antibody directed to the difucosyl structure in B or its analog, such an antibody may have higher specificity to human adenocarcinoma.

3) Melanoma antigen

Two monoclonal antibodies specifically directed to human melanoma cells have been identified as being directed to a glycolipid. The antigen defined by IgG3 antibody (R24) (16) was identified as a ganglioside with the same TLC mobility and carbohydrate composition as GD$_3$ gangliosides (67). The antigen specifically reacting to IgM antibody (4.2 antibody) (81) was characterized by methylation and enzymatic degradation as GD$_3$ (Table V). In contrast to brain GD$_3$ ganglioside, melanoma GD$_3$ contained a much higher proportion of long chain fatty acids, C22 and C24. The 4.2 antibody did not react with various other gangliosides, including GT$_{1a}$ and GQ$_{1b}$, which have the same terminal sequence as GD$_3$, i.e., NeuAc$\alpha2 \rightarrow 8$NeuAc$\alpha2 \rightarrow 3$Gal (63). GD$_3$ ganglioside is known to be present in small quantity in the brain and in various tissues and organs. A relative abundance of this glycolipid in retina (39) and kidney (68) was described, nevertheless, the reactivity of the antibody was found to be highly restricted to human melanoma cells and tissues. Normal melanocytes and nevus did not show the reactivity. An association of GD$_3$ with human melanoma was previously claimed by Portoukalian et al. (66). The apparent melanoma specificity of GD$_3$ gangliosides could be due to their very high concentration and also due to a specific organization of GD$_3$ at the melanoma cell surface.

4) The Burkitt lymphoma antigen

The hybridoma secreting the rat monoclonal IgM antibody directed to Burkitt lymphoma (Daudi) was established (79). The antibody defined the antigen specifically expressed on Burkitt tumor cells irrespective of their possessing Epstein-Barr virus (EBV) genome. The antigen was not detectable on the EBV-positive lymphoblastoid cell line, mitogen-activated lymphocytes, or fresh malignant cells from patients affected by a variety of lymphoproliferative disorders (79). It was identified as a simple glycolipid ceramide trihexoside (Gb$_3$), Gal$\alpha1 \rightarrow 4$Gal$\beta1 \rightarrow 4$Glc$\beta1 \rightarrow 1$Cer (64), whose structure was established in 1971 (31). On chemical analysis, only Burkitt lymphoma cell lines had

TABLE V. Glycolipid Antigens of Two Special Types of Human Malignancy, Melanoma and Burkitt Lymphoma, Defined by "Specific" Monoclonal Antibody

---

A. Melanoma antigen, defined by monoclonal antibody

NeuAc$\alpha2 \rightarrow 8$NeuAc$\alpha2 \rightarrow 3$Gal$\beta1 \rightarrow 4$Glc$\beta1 \rightarrow 1$Cer (ceramide contained C20–24 fatty acids)

Pukel et al. 1982 (67)

Nudelman et al. 1982 (63)

(No reaction with NeuAc$\alpha2 \rightarrow 8$NeuAc$\alpha2 \rightarrow 3$Gal$\beta1 \rightarrow 3$GalNAc$\beta1 \rightarrow 4$[NeuAc$\alpha2 \rightarrow 3$]Gal$\beta1$ $\rightarrow 4$Glc$\beta1 \rightarrow 1$Cer; 63)

B. Burkitt lymphoma antigen, defined by monoclonal antibody "38–13" (79)

Gal$\alpha1 \rightarrow 4$Gal$\beta1 \rightarrow 4$Glc$\beta1 \rightarrow 1$Cer

Nudelman et al. 1983 (64)

(No reaction with Gal$\alpha1 \rightarrow 3$Gal$\beta1 \rightarrow 4$Glc$\beta1 \rightarrow 1$Cer; 64)

a large quantity of this glycolipid (200–800 $\mu g/10$ mg cell residue); however, a small quantity is widely distributed in various tissues and cells. Human erythrocytes have this glycolipid in moderate amount (5–10 $\mu g/10$ mg), but erythrocytes were not reactive to anti-P[k] antibodies (60). In a very rare genetic trait, blood group P[k] individuals, the chemical quantity of this glycolipid in erythrocytes was many times higher than normal; therefore P[k] erythrocytes reacted very well with anti-P[k] antibodies, although normal human erythrocytes of P_1 or P_2 populations did not react with anti-P[k] antibodies (60). It is possible that a small quantity of ceramide trihexoside in various normal cells in normal tissues may be cryptic.

3. Modification of blood group ABH, Ii, P, and Lewis antigens in human cancer

Glycolipids constitute an essential part of the blood group antigens present at the cell surface membranes (27). In human tumors, blood group antigens change in the same general direction as other glycosphingolipids do in tumors, i.e., i) incomplete, or blocked synthesis and accumulation of their precursor structures, and ii) neosynthesis of blood group determinants which results in the appearance of illegitimate or incompatible blood group antigens. These changes will be discussed in this section. The major blood group changes in human cancer are listed in Table VI.

1) The deletion of A and B determinants

The most frequent and remarkable change in blood group determinants associated with human cancer is the deletion of blood group A/or B antigen, since it was first observed by Masamune and his co-workers (61, 62, 65). Extensive studies were also performed by Davidsohn and associates on this phenomenon (14, 15). The early studies on this topic have been reviewed extensively (29).

The deletion of A and B antigens can also be found in premalignant dysplasia of oral epithelial tissue which is associated with disorganization structure (11, 12). Similarly, Feizi and associates (47) observed that A/H antigens in secretors and I-antigen (Ma) in non-secretors were lost in the mucosa of patients with intestinal metaplasia, some of which represent a precancerous state. These studies suggest strongly that the change of blood group A/or B determinants can be useful in detection of premalignancy.

To define the cause of these sensitive changes of A and B determinants, enzymatic studies on their synthesis were carried out. The results indicated that the A transferase which converts H-glycolipid to A-glycolipid decreased significantly in tumors as compared with normal mucosa from the same individual (74). The hydrolase activity for A-glycolipid of normal mucosa tissue was nearly identical to that of carcinoma. Thus, the deletion of A and B determinants in epithelial tumor is due to a deficiency of glycosyltransferase for synthesis of these determinants, but not to enhanced hydrolase activity.

TABLE VI. Important Changes of Blood Group Determinants in Human Cancer

a. Deletion of A, B determinant (14, 15, 62, 65).
b. Enhanced reactivity of its precursors.
    H, Ii (type 2 chain) (8, 13, 18, 73)
    Type 1 chain (44)
c. Increased Le[a], Le[b] and their co-existence (5, 28).
d. P_1P-like structure in tumors of an individual with genotype pp (45, 53, 54).
e. Forssman antigen in tumors from F[-] (fsfs) tissues (32, 48, 82).
f. A-like antigen in tumors from blood group O or B tissue (3, 83).

2) *Precursor accumulation*

The precursor structure for the type 2 chain blood group ABH antigen is represented by Ii structure (*17*), although Ii structure can also be regarded as the precursor of the sialosyl derivative (*27*). An incomplete synthesis of the blood group ABH antigens or sialosyl derivative may result in accumulation of Ii structure. Simmons and Pearlman first described the presence of I-specific determinant in "carcinoembryonic antigens" (CEA) and assumed that CEA may represent incomplete blood group antigens (*73*). Later studies indicated that Ii activity of tumor glycoproteins was separated from the major CEA activity, but its presence still represents a feature of immunological specificity of normal human glycoprotein (*8*). Subsequently, Feizi *et al.* (*18*) reported Ii activity of glycoprotein in two cancer cases. Glycoprotein from both cases showed I (Step) and i (McDon) activity, whereas only one patient displayed I (Ma) activity. Subsequent immunohistochemical studies (*47*) indicated that Ii reactivity of mucosa is closely related to secretor or non-secretor status in addition to malignancy, *i.e.*, a majority of the carcinomas from "secretors" showed foci of substantial staining with anti-I(Ma) in contrast to normal "secretor" mucosa which had no staining with anti-I(Ma). This is probably due to incomplete synthesis of A/H determinants. No substantial staining with anti-I(Ma) was observed in non-secretor mucosa or in non-secretor tumors.

A well organized pattern of carbohydrate architecture in oral mucosa is disarranged, *i.e.*, dislocation of H and loss of A-antigen is obvious in the spinous layer of dysplastic mucosa (*13*).

Incomplete synthesis of blood group ABH antigen with type 1 chain may result in the accumulation of structures with other specificities unrelated to Ii. Recently a case of bronchogenic cancer with an incidental gammopathy was reported (*44*). The serum of the patient was found to contain a monoclonal IgM (designated IgM^{woo}) which was shown to react with lacto-N-tetraosyl structure (Galβ1 → 3GlcNAcβ1 → 3Galβ1 → R). The specificity was not directed to Ii determinant, whereas this antibody was directed to the type 1 chain precursor. The lung cancer was reduced presumably because the patient had a concurrent gammopathy, although he also had received X-ray therapy. One interpretation was that concurrent IgM directed to the type 1 chain precursor suppressed the tumor growth, since the corresponding antigen structure could be accumulated in this tumor.

3) *Incompatible blood group antigens in human tumors*

A-like antigen: Early studies on the presence of A-like antigen in human cancer of blood group O or B individuals have been extensively reviewed (*29*). There is a question, however, about the identity of A-like antigen with Forssman antigen. An A-like glycolipid weakly reactive with only one of the commercial anti-A sera but not reactive with other anti-A sera was found in one human cancer of a host whose blood group was Type B. The glycolipid was identified to be a ceramideheptasaccharide with difucosylated A structure (*3*). We isolated a blood group glycolipid showing a clear inhibition of A-hemagglutination from a case of hepatocarcinoma of a patient with blood group O (*83*). The glycolipid had no Forssman activity, showed a single spot on thin-layer chromatography, and was degraded by hog liver α-N-acetylgalactosaminidase. The enzyme-treated product had no A-like activity. Direct probe mass spectrometry of the fraction after permethylation indicated the presence of the sequence GalNAcα → Hex → N → R, but the absence of the usual A determinant with a fucosyl residue. It is of interest to know that in this case the tissue of the tumor also contained Forssman determinant in a short carbohydrate chain. It is assumed that human adenocarcinomas may produce an unusual αGalNAc transferase with less restricted substrate specificity so that αGalNAc residue could be added to the unusual structure.

Forssman antigen: Immunological distinction between A-like and Forssman antigens was difficult in the early studies until the Forssman antigen was identified as glycolipid and its structure was established (72). Although considerable interest has been aroused in a possible human tumor antigen suggested by early studies (32, 48), it is premature to draw any final conclusion. Normal human erythrocytes do not contain Forssman antigen, but the tissue of some populations (20 to 30% of gastrointestinal mucosa) contains a relatively high level of Forssman glycolipid, while normal tissue of the majority of the human population has a very low, or undetectable, level (1 μg/10 g). Many tumors contain a much higher level of Forssman glycolipid derived from Forssman-negative tissue (32, 82). On the other hand, the isoantigenic property of Forssman in human sera showed a significant level of anti-Forssman antibody as determined by Forssman liposome lysis, whereas the minority (20 to 30% sera) showed a very low, or undetectable, level of anti-Forssman antibody (85), and anti-Forssman levels altered significantly in sera of tumor patients.

PP_1-antigen: Another striking example of the presence of an incompatible blood group antigen in gastric cancer came from the work of Levine and associates (53, 54). In 1951, Levine *et al.* (54) reported the case of a sixty-six year old woman who had gastric adenocarcinoma. Her serum contained an agglutinin termed "anti-Tj[a]," which reacted on random populations of human erythrocytes. In desperation, she was given a 25 ml trial intravenous injection of O blood before surgery. She had an immediate, severe reaction; but as a result, her anti-Tj[a] titer increased from 8 to 512. A few days later, surgery was performed without further blood transfusion. The patient survived for twenty-two years and died of a brain hemorrhage without any obvious sign of metastasis. The anti-Tj[a] serum has now been identified as anti-P_1PP^k specific. The patient obviously belonged to the rare genotype "pp." Recent analysis of her tumor glycolipid and glycoprotein has shown that the major glycolipid was identified as β-GalNAc attached to paragloboside, whose terminal structure was identical to P-antigen (globoside). A neutral glycolipid with P_1 activity was also demonstrated (45). Thus, the glycolipid alteration in this tumor of a rare pp genotype may involve synthesis of incompatible blood group P_1 and P-like antigens.

CONCLUSIONS AND PERSPFCTIVES

Glycolipids of cell surface membranes alter their chemical composition and organization upon oncogenic transformation *in vitro* and in tumors *in vivo*. The changes can be observed in tumors caused by DNA and RNA tumor viruses and chemical carcinogens, and spontaneous tumors, including human cancer. Three types of changes have been described: i) blocked synthesis with accumulation of precursor; ii) neosynthesis, including shifting of glycolipid synthesis from one series of glycolipid to the other; and iii) the change of glycolipid organization in membranes. Blocked synthesis is due to a suppressed (or repressed) glycosyltransferase, and neosynthesis is caused by activation (or de-repression) of an unusual enzyme with less restricted substrate specificity. Some of these changes occur as a consequence of transforming gene activation as typically observed in virally transformed cells with temperature-sensitive mutant (20, 33). The mechanism of activation (de-repression) and repression of glycosyltransferase associated with the transforming gene activation will be an important topic in the immediate future. Some, if not all, glycolipid changes in tumors probably represent a frozen program of differentiation and development; a number of anachronistic expressions of glycolipid synthesis have been observed in various tumors (*55*). A correlation between a frozen program of development and transforming gene activation is an important link for understanding the biological significance of transforming genes.

The question of why cells alter their glycolipid profile on oncogenic transformation is a basic one involving functions of cell surface carbohydrates in general. Two important notions, one for cell recognition (*7, 69*) and the other for regulation of membrane receptor function (*4*), have been considered. Further extensive studies in these two areas will obviously deepen our knowledge of how glycolipid changes are coupled with the mechanism of oncogenesis and differentiation.

Whatever the mechanism and biological significance of glycolipid changes, neoglycolipids accumulated in a specific type of tumor can be an excellent target useful for diagnosis and therapy of human cancer in the immediate future as we have discussed (*35, 86*). An optimistic way to this goal has been opened by the monoclonal antibody approach (*86*) and modern technology for glycolipid characterization. There are, however, expected drawbacks in this approach which have been described previously (*35, 86*). If a regulating mechanism of glycolipid synthesis could be aberrant in malignancy, we are in a position to isolate genes and correct defective enzymes. Genetic technology for glycolipid synthesis and degradation will give us important clues to the control of malignancy.

Acknowledgment

The author's own studies cited in this paper have been supported by grants from the National Institutes of Health, CA20026, CA19224, GM 23100 and from the American Cancer Society grant BC9M.

REFERENCES

1. Ansel, S. and Huet, C. *Int. J. Cancer*, **25**, 797–803 (1980).
2. Brady, R. O. and Fishman, P. *Biochim. Biophys. Acta*, **335**, 121–148 (1974).
3. Breimer, M. E. *Cancer Res.*, **40**, 897–908 (1980).
4. Bremer, E. G. and Hakomori, S. *Biochem. Biophys. Res. Commun.*, **106**, 711–718 (1982).
5. Brockhaus, M., Magnani, J. L., Blaszczyk, M., Steplewski, Z., Koprowski, H., Karlsson, K.-A., Larson, G., and Ginsburg, V. *J. Biol. Chem.*, **256**, 13223–13225 (1981).
6. Brockhaus, M., Magnani, J. L., Herlyn, M., Blaszczyk, M., Steplewski, Z., Koproswki, H., and Ginsburg, V. *Arch. Biochem. Biophys.*, **217**, 647–651 (1982).
7. Carter, W. G., Rauvala, H., and Hakomori, S. *J. Cell Biol.*, **88**, 138–148 (1981).
8. Cooper, A. G., Brown, M. C., Kirsh, M. E., and Rule, A. H. *J. Immunol.*, **113**, 1246–1251 (1974).
9. Critchley, D. R. and MacPherson, I. *Biochim. Biophys. Acta*, **296**, 145–159 (1973).
10. Cuttitta, F., Rosen, S., Gazdar, A. F., and Minna, J. D. *Proc. Natl. Acad. Sci. U.S.*, **78**, 4591–4595 (1981).
11. Dabelsteen, E. *Acta Pathol. Microbiol. Scand. Sect. A*, **80**, 847–853 (1972).
12. Dabelsteen, E. and Fejerskov, O. *Scand. J. Dent. Res.*, **82**, 206–211 (1974).
13. Dabelsteen, E., Vedtofte, P., Hakomori, S., and Young, W. W., Jr. *Cancer Res.*, **43**, 1451–1454 (1983).

14. Davidsohn, I., Kovarik, S., and Lee, C. L. *Arch. Pathol.*, **81**, 381–390 (1966).
15. Davidsohn, I., Kovarik, S., and Ni, Y. *Arch. Pathol.*, **87**, 306–314 (1969).
16. Dippold, W. G., Lloyd, K. O., Li, L.T.C., Ikeda, H., Oettgen, H. F., and Old, L. J. *Proc. Natl. Acad. Sci. U.S.*, **77**, 6114–6118 (1980).
17. Feizi, T., Kabat, E. A., Vicari, G., Anderson, B., and Marsh, W. L. *J. Exp. Med.*, **133**, 39–52 (1971).
18. Feizi, T., Turberville, C., and Westwood, J. H. *Lancet*, August 30, 391–393 (1975).
19. Fishman, P. H. and Brady, R. O. *Science*, **194**, 906–915 (1976).
20. Gahmberg, C. G., Kiehn, D., and Hakomori, S. *Nature*, **248**, 413–415 (1974).
21. Gahmberg, C. G. and Hakomori, S. *J. Biol. Chem.*, **250**, 2438–2446 (1975).
22. Gooi, H. C., Feizi, T., Kapadia, A., Knowles, B. B., Solter, D., and Evans, J. M. *Nature*, **292**, 156–158 (1981).
23. Hakomori, S. *Proc. Natl. Acad. Sci. U.S.*, **67**, 1741–1747 (1970).
24. Hakomori, S. *Adv. Cancer Res.*, **18**, 265–315 (1973).
25. Hakomori, S. *Biochim. Biophys. Acta*, **417**, 55–89 (1975).
26. Hakomori, S. *Annu. Rev. Biochem.*, **50**, 733–764 (1981).
27. Hakomori, S. *Semin. Hematol.*, **18**, 39–62 (1981).
28. Hakomori, S. and Andrews, H. *Biochim. Biophys. Acta*, **205**, 225–228 (1970).
29. Hakomori, S. and Young, W. W., Jr. *Scand. J. Immunol.* **6** (Suppl.), 97–117 (1978).
30. Hakomori, S., Teather, C., and Andrews, H. *Biochem. Biophys. Res. Commun.*, **33**, 563–568 (1968).
31. Hakomori, S., Siddiqui, B., Li, Y.-T., Hellerqvist, C. G., and Li, S.-C. *J. Biol. Chem.* **246**, 2271–2277 (1971).
32. Hakomori, S., Wang, S. H., and Young, W. W., Jr. *Proc. Natl. Acad. Sci. U.S.*, **74**, 3023–3027 (1977).
33. Hakomori, S., Wyke, J. A., and Vogt, P. K. *Virology*, **76**, 485–493 (1977).
34. Hakomori, S., Nudelman, E., Levery, S., Solter, D., and Knowles, B. B. *Biochem. Biophys. Res. Commun.*, **100**, 1578–1586 (1981).
35. Hakomori, S., Young, W. W., Jr., and Urdal, D. *In* "First Aubel Symposium on Drug Development," ed. T. August, pp. 177–199 (1982). American Society for Pharmaceutical and Experimental Therapeutics, Bethesda.
36. Hakomori, S., Fukuda, M., and Nudelman, E. *In* "Teratocarcinoma and Cell Surface," ed. T. Muramatsu and Y. Ikawa, Proceedings of First Hiei Symposium on Teratocarcinoma, pp. 179–200 (1982). Japan Sci. Soc. Press, Tokyo / Springer-Verglag, Heidelberg and New York.
37. Hakomori, S., Nudelman, E., Kannagi, R., and Levery, S. B. *Biochem. Biophys. Res. Commun.*, **109**, 36–44 (1982).
38. Hirabayashi, Y., Taki, T., Matsumoto, M., and Kojima, K. *Biochem. Biophys. Acta*, **529**, 96–105 (1978).
39. Holm, M., Mansson, J.-E., Vanier, M.-T., and Svennerholm, L. *Biochim. Biophys. Acta*, **280**, 356–364 (1972).
40. Holmes, E. H. and Hakomori, S. *J. Biol. Chem.*, **257**, 7698–7703 (1982).
41. Huang, L. C., Brockhaus, M., Magnani, J. L., Cuttitta, S. R., Minna, J. D., and Ginsburg, V. *Arch. Biochem. Biophys.*, in press.
42. Huet, C. and Ansel, S. *Int. J. Cancer*, **20**, 61–66 (1977).
43. Hynes, R. O. and Fox, C. F. "Tumor Cell Surface and Malignancy," Progress in Clinical and Biological Research Vol. 41 (1980). Allen R. Liss, New York.
44. Kabat, E. A., Liao, J., Shyong, J., and Osserman, E. F. *J. Immunol.*, **128**, 540–544 (1982).
45. Kannagi, R., Levine, P., Watanabe, K., and Hakomori, S. *Cancer Res.*, **42**, 5249–5254 (1982).

46. Kannagi, R., Nudelman, E., Levery, S. B., and Hakomori, S. *J. Biol. Chem.*, **257**, 14865–14874 (1982).

47. Kapadia, A., Feizi, T., Jewell, D., Keeling, J., and Slavin, G. *J. Clin. Pathol.*, **34**, 320–337 (1981).

48. Kawanami, J. *J. Biochem.*, **72**, 783–785 (1972).

49. Köhler, G. and Milstein, C. *Nature*, **256**, 495–497 (1975).

50. Koprowski, H., Steplewski, Z., Mitchell, K., Herlyn, M., Herlyn, D., and Fuhrer, P. *Somat. Cell Genet.*, **5**, 957–972 (1979).

51. Koprowski, H., Herlyn, M., Steplewski, Z., and Sears, H. F. *Science*, **212**, 53–54 (1981).

52. Lee, W.M.F., Westnick, M. A., and Macher, B. A. *J. Biol. Chem.*, **257**, 10090–10095 (1982).

53. Levine, P. *Semin. Oncol.*, **5**, 28–34 (1978).

54. Levine, P., Bobbit, O. B., Waller, R. K., and Kuhmichel, A. *Proc. Soc. Exp. Biol. Med.* **77**, 403–405 (1951).

55. Lingwood, C. and Hakomori, S. *Exp. Cell Res.*, **108**, 385–391 (1977).

56. Macher, B. A. and Sweeley, C. C. *Methods Enzymol.*, **50**, 236–251 (1978).

57. Magnani, J. L., Smith, D. F., and Ginsburg, V. *Anal. Biochem.*, **109**, 399–402 (1980).

58. Magnani, J. L., Brockhaus, M., Smith, D. F., Ginsburg, V., Blaszczyk, M., Mitchell, K. F., Steplewski, Z., Koprowski, H. *Science*, **212**, 55–56 (1981).

59. Magnani, J., Nilsson, B., Brockhaus, M., Zopf, D., Steplewski, Z., Koprowski, H., and Ginsburg, V. *Fed. Proc.*, **41**(4), 898 (1982).

60. Marcus, D. M., Naiki, M., and Kundu, S. K. *Proc. Natl. Acad. Sci. U.S.*, **73**, 3263–3267 (1976).

61. Masamune, H., Yosizawa, Z., and Masukawa, A. *Tohoku. J. Exp. Med.*, **58**, 381–398. (1953).

62. Masamune, H., Kawasaki, H., Sinohara, H., and Abe, S. *Tohoku J. Exp. Med.*, **72**, 328–337 (1960).

63. Nudelman, E., Hakomori, S., Kannagi, R., Levery, S., Yeh M.-Y., Hellström, K. E., and Hellström, I. *J. Biol. Chem.*, **257**, 12752–12756 (1982).

64. Nudelman, E., Kannagi, R., Hakomori, S., Lipinski, M., Wiels, J., Parsons, M., Fellous, M., and Tursz, T. *Science*, **220**, 509–511 (1983).

65. Oh-Uti, K. *Tohoku J. Exp. Med.*, **51**, 297–304 (1939).

66. Portoukalian, J., Zwingelstein, G., and Dore, J.-F. *Eur. J. Biochem.*, **94**, 19–23 (1979).

67. Pukel, C. S., Lloyd, K. O., Travassos, L. R., Dippold, W. G., Oettgen, H. F., and Old, L. J. *J. Exp. Med.*, **155**, 1133–1147 (1982).

68. Puro, K. *Biochim. Biophys. Acta*, **187**, 401–413 (1969).

69. Rauvala, H., Carter, W. G., and Hakomori, S. *J. Cell Biol.*, **88**, 127–137 (1981).

70. Rosenfelder, G., Young, W. W., Jr., and Hakomori, S. *Cancer Res.*, **37**, 1333–1339 (1977).

71. Sakiyama, H., Gross, S. K., and Robbins, P. W. *Proc. Natl. Acad. Sci. U.S.*, **69**, 872–876 (1972).

72. Siddiqui, B. and Hakomori, S. *J. Biol. Chem.*, **246**, 5766–5769 (1971).

73. Simmons, D.A.R. and Pearlman, P. *Cancer Res.*, **33**, 313–322 (1973).

74. Stellner, K., Hakomori, S., and Warner, G. A. *Biochem. Biophys. Res. Commun.*, **55**, 439–445 (1973).

75. Sundsmo, J. and Hakomori, S. *Biochem. Biophys. Res. Commun.*, **68**, 799–806 (1976).

76. Taki, T., Hirabayashi, Y., Matsumoto, M., and Kojima, K. *Biochim. Biophys. Acta*, **572**, 105–112 (1979).

77. Watanabe, K., Matsubara, T., and Hakomori, S. *J. Biol. Chem.*, **251**, 2385–2387 (1976).

78. Watanabe, K., Hakomori, S., Powell, M. E., and Yokota, M. *Biochem. Biophys. Res. Commun.*, **92**, 638–648 (1980).

79. Wiels, J., Fellous, M., and Tursz, T. *Proc. Natl. Acad. Sci. U.S.*, **78**, 6485–6488 (1981).
80. Yang, H.-Y. and Hakomori, S. *J. Biol. Chem.*, **246**, 1192–1200 (1971).
81. Yeh, M.-Y., Hellström, I., Abe, K., Hakomori, S., and Hellström, K. E. *Int. J. Cancer*, **29**, 269–275 (1982).
82. Yoda, Y., Ishibashi, T., and Makita, A. *J. Biochem.*, **88**, 1887–1890 (1980).
83. Yokota, M., Warner, G., and Hakomori, S. *Cancer Res.*, **41**, 4185–4190 (1981).
84. Yogeeswaran, G. and Hakomori, S. *Biochemistry*, **14**, 2151–2156 (1975).
85. Young, W. W., Jr., Hakomori, S., and Levine, P. *J. Immunol.*, **123**, 92–96 (1979).
86. Young, W. W., Jr. and Hakomori, S. *Science*, **211**, 487–489 (1981).
87. Young, W. W., Jr., Durdik, J. M., Urdal, D., Hakomori, S., and Henney, C. S. *J. Immunol.*, **126**, 1–6 (1981).

GANN Monograph on Cancer Research 29, 1983

STRUCTURAL CHANGES OF THE ASPARAGINE-LINKED SUGAR CHAINS OF PLASMA MEMBRANE AND SECRETORY GLYCOPROTEINS BY CELL TRANSFORMATION

Seiichi Takasaki, Katsuko Yamashita, and Akira Kobata

Department of Biochemistry, Kobe University School of Medicine*

The appearance or increase of fucose containing glycopeptides with apparently higher molecular weight is well known to be closely related to cell transformation. Using concanavalin A-Sepharose, we have obtained results which suggest that the key step leading to the large glycopeptide formation is not sialylation as suggested by several researchers, but N-acetylglucosaminylation which causes the formation of additional outer chain moieties in complex type asparagine-linked sugar chains. The validity of this interpretation was confirmed by the structural analysis of radioactive oligosaccharides released by hydrazinolysis from the cell surface glyco-peptides prepared from ^{3}H-fucose labeled normal and polyoma virus trans-formed baby hamster kidney cells. The oligosaccharides from normal cells have the following structure: ($\pm$sialic acid$\alpha \rightarrow$ Gal$\beta \rightarrow$ GlcNAc$\beta \rightarrow$)$_n$ (Man$\alpha \rightarrow$)$_2$Man$\beta \rightarrow$ GlcNAc$\beta \rightarrow$ (Fuc$\alpha \rightarrow$) GlcNAc in which n-values range from 2 to 4. Those from transformed cells also have the same general structure but the n-values range from 2 to 6 and are relatively rich in larger oligosaccharides with highly branched outer chains.

Interestingly, the sugar chains of secretory glycoproteins are deleted by malignant transformation. This reverse phenomenon was found by the comparative study of sugar chains of α-amylases purified from parotid gland and various cancer tissues.

One of the characteristic features of multicellular organisms is that they are com-posed of different types of cells, each of which is endowed with a recognition mechanism which controls its growth and behavior in a manner suitable for the cell society. Through this mechanism, the cells can construct a well organized society by communicating with each other. To solve the molecular mechanism of cell surface communication is therefore one of the most important subjects in biology and medicine.

It is well known that tumor cells grow rapidly without control and migrate out of tissue boundaries leading to invasion and metastasis. This abnormal behavior of tumor cells can be regarded as a deviation from the control of the social interactions of cells. Malignancy may be a disorder of cell-cell interaction, which requlates various functions such as growth, movement, adhesion, metabolism, and so on.

These disorders may undoubtedly be induced by changes of cell surface components. Therefore, it is of interest to investigate the structural changes of cell surface com-ponents after transformation. In view of the recent evidence that the sugar chains of cell

---

* Kusunoki cho 7-5-1, Chuo-ku, Kobe 650, Japan (高崎誠一, 山下克子, 木幡 陽).

surface glycoconjugates play a role as signals of cellular recognition, we have made a comparative study of the structures of sugar chains of control baby hamster kidney cells and their polyoma virus transformants.

Appearance of Large Glycopeptides by Transformation

Meezan *et al.* (*16*) were the first to make a detailed comparison of the glycoproteins and glycopeptides from normal and virus-transformed cells. Mouse 3T3 fibroblasts and their Simian virus-transformants (SV-3T3) were metabolically labeled with radioactive glucosamine. By comparing the gel filtration patterns of radioactive glycopeptides obtained from the subcellular fractions of the two cells by exhaustive pronase digestion, they found that SV-3T3 cells are more enriched in large glycopeptides than 3T3 cells. This observation propelled many investigators to analyze glycopeptides comparatively in other cell systems. Warren's group (*3, 4*) examined BHK_{21}/C_{13} cells, a hamster cell line, and the cells transformed with an RNA tumor virus, Rous sarcoma virus and two DNA tumor viruses, polyoma virus and SV40. They also analyzed mouse 3T3 cells and chick embryo fibroblasts (*4*) both of which had been transformed by Rous sarcoma virus. In every case, large glycopeptides from the cell surface of transformed cells were increased. As shown in Fig. 1 as a typical example, the difference was also observed when radioactive fucose was used for metabolic labeling. Since then, this phenomenon was found not only in virus-transformed cells but in chemically and spontaneously transformed cells (*22, 30*). The cells transformed with temperature-sensitive mutant of Rous sarcoma virus showed the presence of large glycopeptides at permissive temperature where the transformed phenotype is expressed; shift of the cells to nonpermissive temperature resulted in the disappearance of the transformed phenotype and the large glycopeptides (*31*). The same observation was extended to non-fibroblastic cells, including rat hepatoma cells (*28*), human leukemic cells (*29*), lymphoma cells (*29*), and neuroblastoma cells (*10*).

Based on the evidence so far described, it is strongly suggested that the increment

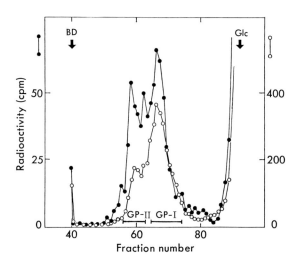

FIG. 1.   Gel filtration of fucose-labeled cell surface glycopeptides on Sephadex G-50 (*19*).

of large glycopeptides is a general phenomenon detected in transformed and tumorigenic cells regardless of cell species and the manner of transformation.

Correlation of the Appearance of Large Glycopeptides with Tumorigenicity

It is well known that transformed and tumorigenic cells lack contact inhibition of movement and growth, the ability to grow in soft agar, high saturation density in tissue culture, relatively low serum requirement and so on. A high correlation of glycopeptide changes with tumorigenicity has also been found (8, 9, 21). There have been a few reports that some transformed cells do not possess large glycopeptides in spite of their showing the phenotype of tumor cells as judged by *in vitro* criteria (5, 8, 21). However, these cells were unable to make tumors in nude mice (23). It was also found that the cells isolated from tumors, which were obtained by passage of less tumorigenic cells through animals such as nude mice (8, 21), contained large glycopeptides. Considerable evidence has indicated that the appearance of large glycopeptides is highly correlated with tumorigenicity.

Analysis of Large Glycopeptides by Concanavalin A (Con A)-Sepharose Column Chromatography

Extensive analyses have been performed on the change in elution profiles fo glycopeptides in gel filtration, but the structural basis for the change is not clear. Many people examined the possible involvement of sialylation in the appearance of large glycopeptides. In fact, the size difference of glycopeptides of normal and transformed cells almost vanished when the glycopeptides were exhaustively digested with sialidase before gel filtration. Based on this evidence, Warren suggested that the difference between large glycopeptides from transformed cells and small glycopeptides from normal cells should be ascribed only to the amount of sialic acid residue included in their sugar chains, and proposed that sialylation is a key step in the inducement of structural change of surface sugar chains by cellular transformation. The level of sialyltransferase activities in normal and transformed cells was compared in many laboratories in order to confirm the Warren hypothesis. However, the results were not favorable for the hypothesis: in some experiments, the enzyme level was higher while in others it was lower in transformed cells compared to normal (12, 32).

At that time, we were studying the behavior of various oligosaccharides and glycopeptides of known structure by Con A-Sepharose column chromatography. The results obtained in the study indicated that Con A-Separose column chromatography can be used as an invaluable tool to estimate the structures of complex type asparagine-linked sugar chains (18). It had already been confirmed by Goldstein that α-mannosyl residues, either free or only substituted at its C-2 position by other sugars can bind to Con A. However, we found that the presence of only one such residue in a molecule of sugar chain is not enough for the oligosaccharide and glycopeptide to bind to the Con A-Sepharose column. Such sugar chains are retarded but can be eluted with buffer. If a sugar chain contains two such α-mannosyl residues, it can bind to the column and is eluted only by a solution of 0.1 M α-methylmannoside.

In Fig. 2, typical fucose-containing asparagine-linked sugar chains are listed. In biantennary sugar chains so far reported, the two outer chains are linked only at the

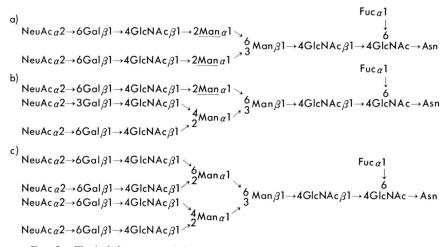

FIG. 2. Typical fucose-containing asparagine-linked sugar chains. Mannosyl residues which can interact with Con A-Sepharose are underlined.

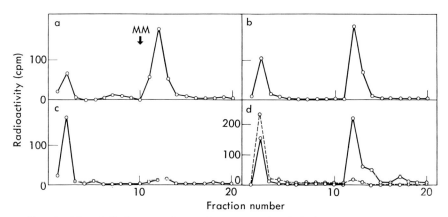

FIG. 3. Con A-Sepharose column chromatography (19). The column was first eluted with 0.01 M Tris-HCl buffer containing 0.1 M NaCl, pH 7.5, and then eluted with the same buffer containing 0.1 M α-methyl mannoside (MM). a, GP-I from BHK cells; b, GP-I from Py-BHK cells; c, GP-II from Py-BHK cells; d, GP-II from Py-BHK cells treated with neuraminidase alone (- - - -) or with neuraminidase, β-galactosidase and β-N-acetylhexosaminidase (——).

C-2 position of two α-mannosyl residues (a). Therefore this type of sugar chain can bind to a Con A-Sepharose column. However, triantennary sugar chains (b) contain only one α-mannosyl residue that binds to Con A. Therefore, these sugar chains are retarded but do not bind to Con A-Sepharose column. Tetraantennary sugar chains (c) pass through the column without any interaction with Con A because they do not contain any α-mannosyl residues which bind to the lectin.

This specificity of Con A-Sepharose column was used to analyze the structures of glycopeptides, GP-I and GP-II in Fig. 1 (19). When GP-Is obtained from normal and transformed cells were applied to a Con A-Sepharose column, most of them bound to the column and were eluted by 0.1 M α-methylmannoside solution (Fig. 3a, b). On the other hand, almost all GP-II passed through the column without retardation (Fig. 3c).

The elution profile of GP-II did not change even after sialidase digestion (Fig. 3d, dotted line) indicating that the difference between GP-I and GP-II cannot be ascribed only to the different amount of their sialic acid residues as proposed by Warren *et al.*

When asialo GP-II was further digested with jack bean β-galactosidase and β-N-acetylhexosaminidase and then applied to a Con A-Sepharose column, most of the glycopeptides bound to the column (Fig. 3d, solid line). That the glycopeptide at this stage had the structure: Manα1 → 6(Manα1 → 3)Manβ1 → 4GlcNAcβ1 → 4(Fucα1 → 6)GlcNAc → Asn was confirmed by its conversion to Fucα1 → 6GlcNAc → Asn after digestion with endo-β-N-acetylglucosaminidase D.

The series of results indicated that the structure of most of the GP-I must be the "a" as shown in Fig. 2 and GP-II mostly free from the biantennary structure.

Structural Analysis of Asparagine-linked Sugar Chains Obtained from Normal and Transformed Cells (24)

Hydrazinolysis is known to cleave the amide bond. This method had been used by several people to cleave the GlcNAc → Asn linkage (2, 7). However, the reaction also induces various modifications of the sugar chains and the recovery of the released oligosaccharides is far from quantitative. We have investigated the reaction in detail by using glycopeptides of known structure, and have finally established conditions for hydrazinolysis to quantitatively release the asparagine-linked sugar chains as oligosaccharides (25). This method can be applied not only to glycopeptides but also to intact glycoproteins.

We applied this newly established method to the structural analysis of the asparagine-linked sugar chains of surface glycoproteins of normal and transformed cells. Mixtures of glycopeptides (tube No. 53–77 in Fig. 1) obtained from BHK and Py-BHK cells, which were metabolically labeled with [³H]-fucose, were subjected to hydrazinolysis and the released oligosaccharides were reduced with NaBH₄. When the radioactive oligosaccharide mixtures were analyzed by paper electrophoresis at pH 5.4, both samples gave similar but not the same electrophoretograms (Fig. 4). More than 80% of both samples were sialylated. However, the acidic oligosaccharides of Py-BHK were more enriched in the A-3 fraction (26%) as compared to that of BHK cells (10%). Furthermore, an additional peak was detected in the A-2 fraction of Py-BHK cells as indicated by hatching in Fig. 4b.

The difference became more evident when the total oligosaccharide fractions were

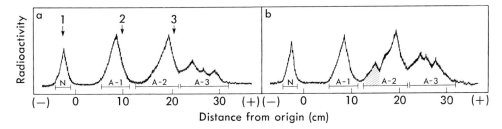

FIG. 4. Paper electrophoresis of hydrazinolysis products (24). Paper electrophoresis was carried out at 73 V/cm for 70 min using pyridine-acetate buffer, pH 5.4. Arrow 1 indicates the position of neutral oligosaccharide, and arrows 2 and 3 are those of monosialylated and disialylated oligosaccharides from human transferrin, respectively. a, BHK cells; b, Py-BHK cells.

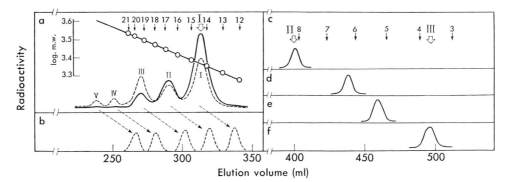

Fig. 5. Gel chromatography of desialylated oligosaccharides and their exoglycosidase digests on Bio-Gel P-4 (24). Black arrows and numbers indicate elution positions and number of glucose units in glucose oligomers used as internal standards.
White arrows I, II, and III indicate elution positions of $Gal_2 \cdot GlcNAc_2 \cdot Man_3 \cdot$
$GlcNAc$ (Fuc) N-acetylglucosaminitol, $Man_3 \cdot GlcNAc$ (Fuc) N-acetylglucosaminitol,
and Fuc-N-acetylglucosaminitol, respectively. a, Sialidase digests of the mixture of
acidic oligosaccharides (A-1, A-2, and A-3) from BHK cells (——) and Py-BHK
cells (- - - -); b, β-galactosidase digests of peaks I to V in a; c, β-galactosidase and
β-N-acetylhexosaminidase digests (in sequence) on peaks I to V in a; d, α-man-
nosidase digest of peak in c; e, β-mannosidase digest of peak in d; f, β-N-acetyl-
hexosaminidase digest of peak in e.

exhaustively digested with sialidase and then subjected to Bio-Gel P-4 column chromatography. As shown in Fig. 5, the desialylated oligosaccharides of BHK cells were
fractionated into three components (peaks I, II, and III), while two additional peaks
(IV and V) were found in those of Py-BHK cells. Moreover, the ratio of larger oligosaccharides in Py-BHK compared to BHK cells was increased. Therefore, the Py-BHK
cells were more enriched in higher molecular weight oligosaccharides than were BHK
cells. Sequential digestions with jack bean β-galactosidase and jack bean β-N-acetyl-
hexosaminidase converted all these components into a hexasaccharide: $(Man\alpha1 \rightarrow)_2$
$Man\beta1 \rightarrow GlcNAc\beta1 \rightarrow (Fuc\alpha1 \rightarrow)N$-acetylglucosaminitol. Since 2, 3, 4, 5, and 6 mol
each of galactose and N-acetylglucosamine were released respectively from components
I, II, III, IV, and V by sequential enzymatic digestion, these five components should
have the structures shown in Table I. The molar ratio of each component in BHK and
Py-BHK cells is also shown in Table I. These results explain well the behavior of the
glycopeptides from both types of cells on (Con A-Sepharose columns as described in

TABLE I. Summary of Asparagine-linked Sugar Chains in BHK and Py-BHK Cells

$$(\pm Sia \xrightarrow{\alpha} Gal \xrightarrow{\beta} GlcNAc \xrightarrow{\beta})_n \begin{matrix} Man \searrow^{\alpha} \\ \\ Man \nearrow_{\alpha} \end{matrix} Man \xrightarrow{\beta} GlcNAc \xrightarrow{\beta} \overset{\overset{\text{Fuc}}{\downarrow^{\alpha}}}{GlcNAc}$$

Components	n	BHK (%)	Py-BHK (%)
I	2	69	39
II	3	20	25
III	4	11	27
IV	5	0	5
V	6	0	4

the previous section and indicate that the N-acetylglucosaminylation step is the key to the structural change of surface carbohydrates in transformed cells.

Structural Changes of Sugar Chains in Secreted Glycoproteins by Cellular transformation

Several enzymes and hormones of glycoprotein nature have been reported to be produced in tumor tissues ectopically or in elevated amounts than normal tissues. Although these secretory glycoproteins produced in tumor tissues have been shown to be different from those in normal tissues in their physicochemical characteristics, the structural basis of their differences have never been presented. Our recent studies on the sugar chains of α-amylases presented for the first time the structural difference of the secretory glycoproteins of normal and tumor tissues.

Amylase, together with alkaline phosphatase, is known as one of the few enzymes produced ectopically in cancer tissues (*1, 6*). Weiss *et al.* (*33*) reported a case of bronchogenic carcinoma with increased serum amylase activity. Since then, many cases of hyperamylasemia in association with tumors such as that of the ovary and lung have been reported (*11, 15, 20, 27*). These amylases behave like parotid amylase but not like pancreatic amylase on agar gel electrophoresis (*17*) and diethylaminoethyl (DEAE)-column chromatography (*1*).

Studies of human α-amylases purified from parotid gland (*34*) and from two amylase-producing tumors—a serous papillary cystadenocarcinoma of the ovary and a bronchioloalveolar adenocarcinoma of the lung (*35*)—revealed that the sugar chains of normal and tumor enzymes are different. As summarized in Fig. 6, four structurally different

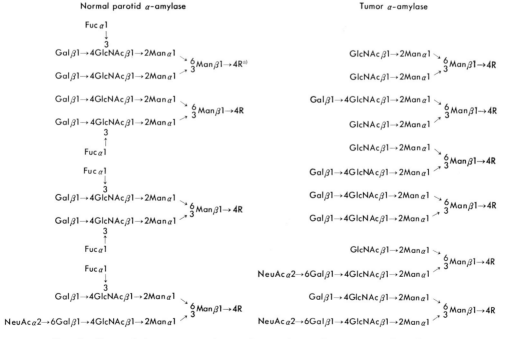

FIG. 6. Sugar chain structures of normal α-amylase and tumor α-amylases from a serous papillary cystadenocarcinoma of the ovary and a bronchioloalveolar adenocarcinoma of the lung (*34, 35*). a) R=GlcNAcβ1 → 4 (Fucα1 → 6) GlcNAc.

sugar chains were found in parotid α-amylase. In contrast, six different sugar chains were found to occur in the amylases purified from ovarian and lung cancers. Interestingly, these sugar chains include the structural characteristics of parotid α-amylase. First of all, they were all biantennary complex type sugar chains with an α-fucosyl residue linked at the C-6 position of the proximal N-acetylglucosamine residues. Secondly, the acidic sugar chains occur only in the monosialylated form. This structural characteristic should be considered very unusual because at least a part of the biantennary sugar chains of other glycoproteins except parotid α-amylase contain two sialic acid residues. Thirdly, the single sialic acid residue of the sugar chains of tumor amylase is linked only to the outer chain of the Manα1 $\rightarrow$ 3 side, as in the case of parotid α-amylase. Despite these similarities, the sugar chains of tumor amylase were different from those of parotid enzyme. The fucosyl residue found in the outer chain moieties of parotid α-amylase was completely missing in the sugar chains of tumor amylases. Furthermore, many of the sugar chains of tumor amylase contain incomplete outer chains. These results indicate that formation of the sugar chains of tumor enzymes are incomplete as compared to that of parotid enzyme.

CONCLUSION

Based on the evidence so far described we would like to propose that cellular transformation induces different changes in plasma membrane glycoproteins and secretory glycoproteins: in contrast to the asparagine-linked sugar chains of the plasma membrane glycoproteins which increase the number of their outer chains, those of the secretory glycoproteins become attenuated as widely reported in glycolipids (13). Further studies on many other glycoproteins are needed to confirm the validity of the hypothesis proposed here. We have recently found that the sugar chains of γ-glutamyl transpeptidase of rat hepatoma are also incomplete as compared to those of rat liver enzyme (Yamashita et al., submitted for publication). Although this enzyme is one of the plasma membrane glycoproteins, it has the following unusual feature. Most plasma membrane glycoproteins are anchored in the membrane close to their C-terminal region. This arrangement has been well explained by the recently proposed biosynthetic mechanism for membrane glycoproteins (14). In contrast, the heavy subunit of γ-glutamyl transpeptidase, which is the binding site to plasma membrane, anchors in membrane through its N-terminal portion (26). Therefore, the enzyme may not be a real membrane glycoprotein, but a secretory glycoprotein which has anchored to membrane by the hydrophobic portion located at its N-terminal.

REFERENCES

1. Amman, R. W., Berk, J. E., Fridhandler, L., Ueda, H., and Wegmann, W. *Ann. Intern. Med.*, **78**, 521–525 (1973).
2. Bayard, B. and Montreuil, J. In " *Méthodologie de la structure et du Métabolisme des Glycoconjugués,*" pp. 208–218 (1974). CNRS, Paris.
3. Buck, C. A., Glick, M. C., and Warren, L. A. *Biochemistry*, **9**, 4567–4576 (1970).
4. Buck, C. A., Glick, M. C., and Warren, L. A. *Science*, **172**, 169–171 (1971).
5. Ceccarini, C. *Proc. Natl. Acad. Sci. U.S.*, **72**, 2687–2690 (1975).
6. Fishman, L., Miyayama, H., Driscoll, S. G., and Fishman, W. H. *Cancer Res.*, **36**, 2268–2273 (1976).

7. Fukuda, M., Kondo, T., and Osawa, T. *J. Biochem.*, **80**, 1223–1232 (1976).
8. Glick, M. C., Rabinowitz, Z., and Sachs, L. *Biochemistry*, **12**, 4864–4869 (1973).
9. Glick, M. C., Rabinowitz, Z., and Sachs, L. *Virology*, **13**, 967–974 (1974).
10. Glick, M. C., Schlesinger, H., and Hummeler, K. *Cancer Res.*, **36**, 4520–4524 (1976).
11. Gomi, K., Kameya, T., Tsumuraya, M., Shimosato, Y., Zeze, F., Abe, K., and Yoneyama, T. *Cancer*, **38**, 1645–1654 (1976).
12. Grimes, W. J. *Biochemistry*, **12**, 990–996 (1970).
13. Hakomori, S. *Adv. Cancer Res.*, **18**, 265–315 (1973).
14. Lingappa, V. R., Katz, F. N., Lodish, H. F., and Blobel, G. *J. Biol. Chem.*, **24**, 8667–8670 (1978).
15. McGeachin, R. L. and Adams, M. R. *Cancer*, **10**, 497–499 (1957).
16. Meezan, E., Wu, H., Black, P., and Robbins, P. W. *Biochemistry*, **8**, 2518–2524 (1969).
17. Nakayama, T., Hayashi, Y., and Kitamura, M. *In* "Onco-Developmental Gene Expression," ed. W. H. Fishman, pp. 455–462 (1976). Academic Press, New York.
18. Ogata, S., Muramatsu, T., and Kobata, A. *J. Biochem.*, **78**, 687–696 (1975).
19. Ogata, S., Muramatsu, T., and Kobata, A. *Nature*, **259**, 580–582 (1976).
20. Shimamura, J., Fridhandler, L., and Berk, J. E. *Cancer*, **38**, 2121–2126 (1976).
21. Smets, L. A., Van Beek, W. P., and van, Rooij, H. *Int. J. Cancer.*, **18**, 462–468 (1976).
22. Smets, L. A., Van Beek, W. P., and Van Nie, R. *Cancer Lett.*, **3**, 133–138 (1977).
23. Stiles, C. D., Desmond, W. J., Sato, G., and Saier, M. H. *Proc. Natl. Acad. Sci. U.S.*, **72**, 4971–4975 (1975).
24. Takasaki, S., Ikehira, H., and Kobata, A. *Biochem. Biophys. Res. Commun.*, **92**, 735–742 (1980).
25. Takasaki, S. and Kobata, A. *Methods Enzymol.*, **83**, 263–269 (1982).
26. Tsuji, A., Matsuda, Y., and Katsunuma, N. *J. Biochem.*, **87**, 1567–1571 (1982).
27. Ueda, M., Kobayashi, M., Takeda, K., and Soto, J. *Clin. Chim. Acta*, **80**, 105–111 (1977).
28. Van Beek, W. P., Smets, L. A., and Emmelot, P. *Cancer Res.*, **33**, 2913–2922 (1973).
29. Van Beek, W. P., Smets, L. A., and Emmelot, P. *Nature*, **253**, 457–460 (1975).
30. Von Nest, G. and Grimes, W. J. *Biochemistry*, **16**, 2902–2908 (1977).
31. Warren, L., Critchley, D., and Macpherson, I. *Nature*, **235**, 275–278 (1972).
32. Warren, L., Fuhrer, P., and Buck, C. A. *Proc. Natl. Acad. Sci. U.S.*, **69**, 1838–1842 (1972).
33. Weiss, M. J., Edmondson, H. A., and Wertman, M. *Am. J. Clin. Pathol.*, **21**, 1057–1061 (1951).
34. Yamashita, K., Tachibana, Y., Nakayama, T., Kitamura, M., Endo, Y., and Kobata, A. *J. Biol. Chem.*, **255**, 5635–5642 (1980).
35. Yamashita, K., Tachibana, Y., Takeuchi, T., and Kobata, A. *J. Biochem.*, **90**, 1281–1289 (1981).

GLYCOCONJUGATE ALTERATIONS ASSOCIATED WITH MALIGNANT CELLS

Eugene A. Davidson, Veerasingham, P. Bhavanandan, Adel L. Barsoum, Yoshio Hatae, and Taiko Hatae

Department of Biological Chemistry, The Milton S. Hershey Medical Center, The Pennsylvania State University*

Studies carried out with cultured mouse melanoma cells identified a unique glycoprotein class as significantly elevated when compared to control cells. These glycoproteins were characterized by a high content of sialic acid, clustered O-linked oligosaccharides analogous to those present in human glycophorin and an affinity for wheat germ agglutinin (WGA) which was dependent on three dimensional array of the sialyl residues. The mouse tumor glycoproteins are shed from the cell surface, can be identified thereon with a suitable fluorescent antibody, appear in the circulation of a tumor-bearing host and are structurally altered in certain WGA-resistant variants which exhibit diminished tumorigenicity.

An extension of these investigations to cultured human melanoma and human mammary carcinoma cells showed that similar glycoproteins were produced by the transformed lines and in greatly diminished or undetectable amounts by control counterparts. Common characteristics included clustered O-linked sialylated oligosaccharides, lectin affinity properties and surface localization. Thus, monoclonal antibodies directed against the exterior portion of human erythrocyte glycophorin were reactive with several cultured tumor cell surfaces suggesting similar epitopes in the saccharide attachment region.

Based on the physical and chemical properties of these glycoproteins, a search was instituted for comparable molecules in the plasma of patients with extensive metastatic disease. A glycoprotein was isolated with a high correlation with the presence of malignancy. The apparent molecular weight (52,000), isoelectric point (4.4), solubility characteristics and interaction with WGA differentiate it from previously defined circulating components or the tumor markers, carcinoembryonic antigen and α-fetoprotein. Antibodies were developed in rabbit which permitted establishment of a quantitative radioimmunoassay. This technique was employed to analyze blood samples from a variety of patients for glycoprotein as well as total and perchloric acid-soluble sialic acid. The glycoprotein levels (p *vs.* normal <0.0001) correlate well with disease status based on clinical criteria. Adjunct and cured patients have values not significantly different from a well clustered normal set which exhibited a very low incidence of false positives. Increases were observed in necrotizing infections which reflect cross-reactivity with α1-acid glycoprotein, the only acute phase reactant that is immunologically recognized. The association with a variety of cancer types suggests that the glycoprotein may be produced by

* Hershey, Pennsylvania 17033, U.S.A.

circulating or formed normal cellular elements (*e.g.*, lymphocytes or liver) as well as tumor cells.

Monoclonal antibodies raised against the isolated glycoprotein should assist in better defining structural features relevant to malignancy.

It is generally agreed that the first event in malignant transformation affects the genetic apparatus of the cell. The resultant change allows that particular cell to escape the normal constraints on growth control. This may occur spontaneously, as a result of an external stimulus such as short wave-length radiation or a particular chemical, or as a result of integration of elements from a virus. Regardless of the nature of the stimulus, it is quite likely that these occur with a considerable frequency given that all possible sources of such events cannot be removed from the environment. The initial response of the host determines the frequency with which malignancy results. It is likely that the bulk of changes which occur in DNA are repaired without incident or are lethal. Few alterations are likely to affect regions of the DNA which will allow the cell to undergo new cycles of division and transmit this same capability to daughter cells. In the event that cells escape from the non-proliferating pool, recognition by the host immune system of an abnormal structure may occur. This is likely since continually cycling cells will exhibit alterations in surface macromolecules. It is impossible to estimate the quantitative role of the immune system in controlling runaway cells. This is a substantial regulatory mechanism since the associated alteration of the cell surface increases the probability that the cell will be recognized as abnormal. Escape from both the non-proliferative pool and host immune surveillance are required before abnormal cells accrue in significant numbers. These early events are invariably not detected; in fact, the multiplication of cells will not be noticed until the cellular mass becomes of sufficient magnitude to be physically detectable or to interfere with normal physiologic function. Metastasis is the life threatening event since local disease rarely causes a lethal physiologic alteration. Recent work has shown that metastatic cells arise spontaneously or at random from within the local population of tumor cells and that control of this secondary event is unlikely to be successful (*17*, *19*). It remains most advantageous for the patient to provide a reliable means for early diagnosis.

A number of laboratories are working on tumor unique products. There are two broad strategies which can be adopted: The first involves isolation of unique molecules from tumor cells themselves (that is, from tumor explants or cultured tumor cells) or from the blood of individuals with malignant disease. Generally, it must be shown that this product is unique to the tumor cells. The second approach involves the use of monoclonal antibodies. The antibodies produced by the hybridoma technique generally, although not exclusively, recognize single product molecules and can be used as the basis of a screening procedure to search for such molecules. Generally, the focus is on products associated with the surface of tumor cells not represented on normal cells. This technique depends to a large extent on the immunogenic properties of the individual cell surface components and on the very high structural discrimination of monoclonal antibodies.

There are difficulties with both approaches. Model systems (cultured cells or human tumors growing in athymic mice) may not accurately reflect the *in vivo* process in man; this is particularly true where only cultured cells have been studied. The specificity of monoclonal antibodies is high but it is not absolute and many cell surface macromolecules have similar determinant regions (epitopes) allowing cross reaction with monoclonal antibodies. The use of cells or membranes for development of monoclonal antibodies does not insure that circulating molecules of interest will be detected. It is assumed that molecules present on the surface of cells will appear in the circulation either unmodified or insufficiently modified so as to still permit antibody detection.

Mucin Type Glycoproteins of Malignant Cells

Work in our laboratory has followed mainly the first approach, that is, isolation and characterization of cell surface components by biochemical and immunologic means. These products are isolated from animal models and cultured cells as well as from patient material. Most of our studies have focused on glycoproteins. An important point to recognize about cell surface glycoproteins is that association with the plasma membrane generally results in the carbohydrate-containing domain being externally directed because of the hydrophilicity of the saccharide units. Defined glycoprotein functions include protection from antibody surveillance as is the case for a well studied mouse mammary carcinoma (8).

In preliminary studies with cultured cells or whole animals, we provide appropriate radiolabeled precursors to allow incorporation into glycoconjugates for ease in subsequent biochemical workup. The general strategy is to incubate cultured cells in low glucose medium, serum free if possible, with appropriate radiolabeled precursors (^{3}H-glucosamine, ^{14}C-leucine) for a sufficient time period to equilibrate the label. The spent medium and cells are separated and the glycoconjugates isolated and characterized. Early work from our laboratory with the B16 mouse melanoma led to the identification of an unusual glycopeptide isolated after exhaustive proteolysis of spent medium macromolecules. This fragment was characterized by several rather specific properties: a high sialic acid content, the saccharide units were linked O-glycosidically to the polypeptide backbone, precipitability with cetyl pyridinium chloride and affinity for wheat germ agglutinin (WGA)-Sepharose which was dependent on the number and spatial arrangement of the sialyl residues (2, 3, 15, 16). Detailed studies on the nature of the saccharide residues present in the glycopeptide showed composition to be (sialic acid)$_2$-galactose-N-acetylgalactosamine. Based on exclusion chromatography results, a molecular weight of approximately 10,000 was assigned to the glycopeptide, which was resistant to further proteolytic degradation. Degradation by alkali catalyzed elimination in the presence of sodium borohydride allowed us to establish GalNAc as the linkage sugar and confirmed the O-glycosidic attachment of the saccharide moieties to the polypeptide. As many as eight sugar units are present.

The glycoprotein from which this fragment was derived was isolated from the solid tumor by a combination of ion exchange and affinity methods. A nominal molecular weight of 100,000 was assigned based on exclusion behavior. This macromolecule, which does not contain glucosamine was shown to be shed from both cultured B16 cells and the solid tumor growing in an appropriate host mouse.

Comparable experiments with a human melanoma line and a control population of human fetal melanocytes were carried out (5, 18). In contrast to the B16 system, the glycopeptides isolated from the human melanoma cells were entirely soluble in the presence of cetyl pyridinium chloride. However, it was demonstrated that those glycopeptides which bound to WGA-Sepharose had structural features similar to those

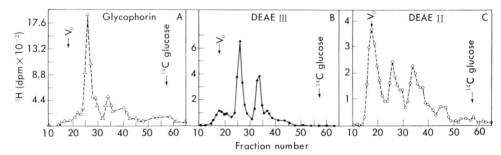

Fig. 1. Chromatography on BioGel P4 of products obtained after alkali catalyzed elimination performed in the presence of NaB³H₄. A, human glycophorin; B, wheat germ-binding glycoprotein III from human melanoma; C, wheat germ-binding glycoprotein II from human melanoma.

observed from the murine material. These included high sialic acid content and O-linked, clustered saccharide units. It is important to note that the structure of the sugar segments is identical to that present in the mouse glycoprotein but that their arrangement (clustering) on the polypeptide chain is different.

An extension of these studies to intact glycoproteins was done. Application of ion exchange affinity and exclusion methods resulted in the isolation of two glycoproteins in pure form. The one with higher apparent molecular weight and more anionic character contains exclusively O-linked saccharide units, mainly tetra saccharide (NANA$_2$-Gal-GalNAc) with some trisaccharide (NANA-Gal-GalNAc) whereas the less anionic one has both O- and N-linked saccharide units (Fig. 1). Molecular weights are approximately 100,000, comparable to that observed for the B16 product. The synthesis of analogous glycoconjugates by control melanocytes could not be detected although very low levels (5 % or less of that present in the tumor cells) would not have been identified. Thus, the difference may be quantitative although a qualitative change remains a distinct possibility.

Studies with two human mammary carcinoma cell lines indicated that very similar glycoproteins are produced (7). Although there is a slightly different structure for the mammary tumor products (NANA-Gal-GlcNAc-Gal-GalNAc), key features such as residue clustering and affinity for WGA-Sepharose are present. Subsequent work has shown that human colon carcinoma and Morris hepatoma likewise produce glycoproteins with predominantly O-linked sugar units which in turn are responsible for interaction with WGA.

An important point to be noted is that those control cells that were available, (mouse or human melanocytes, normal human mammary cells) do produce a variety of glycoproteins, many of which are sialylated but do not appear to synthesize significant quantities of glycoproteins with the particular features noted above.

Increases of Sialoglycoproteins in Serum of Cancer Patients

Based on the above experiments, we undertook preliminary studies in patients aimed at defining the association of circulating sialic acid levels with malignant disease. A reasonable extrapolation might suggest that tumor-derived products are shed from the cell surface and appear in the circulation. The chemical properties of the glycoproteins described include features which improve the prospects for detection. Thus, estimated molecular weights in the 100,000 range make it unlikely that significant quantities would be excreted in the urine. The relatively high sialic acid content and failure to interact effectively with the galactose-binding lectin from *Ricinus communis* further suggests that few if any terminal galactosyl units are present. This chemical architecture should allow for greatly increased circulatory half-lives, thus permitting accumulation in the circulation even though a relatively small number of cells are functioning as a source. The initial screen was intended to ascertain if there was an increase in acid soluble circulating sialic acid which correlated with malignant disease and which was not observed to any significant degree in normal individuals. The data show significant differences in circulating acid soluble sialic acid between normal individuals and patients with metastatic disease (*13*). However, as might be expected, not all patients with metastatic disease show elevated sialic acid levels and some normal individuals do show elevated sialic acid levels. Patients who have localized disease also are elevated from normal but these elevations are not nearly as dramatic. Adjuvant and cured patients have levels that tend to return to normal but this is not true in all cases. The overall sialic acid data is impressive but needs further development for routine diagnostic use. One problem is that a number of inflammatory conditions—systemic infections, rheumatoid arthritis, and even pregnancy—can lead to a rise in the so-called acute phase circulating reactants, many of which are sialoglycoproteins. An examination of individual patient data taken on a serial basis indicates that for those patients where initial correlations with disease status were good, the correlations remain in that successful therapy leads to a reduction in sialic acid levels whereas spread of disease leads to continual increases, frequently prior to the development of overt clinical symptoms (*10*).

Based on the above data and on the physical and chemical properties of the sialoglycoproteins studied in cultured cell systems, patient material was examined for a component which would reflect those features already defined. The starting material for these experiments was plasma obtained by plasmapheresis of patients with disseminated cancer. Initial studies were carried out using plasma from patients with lung or mammary carcinoma; subsequent isolations have used material obtained from patients with melanoma, stomach cancer, and renal cancer. A glycoprotein was isolated, although in relatively low yield, with characteristic features: acid solubility, high content of sialic acid, and affinity for WGA-Sepharose which was dependent on sialic acid (*4*). This glycoprotein had an apparent molecular weight of 52,000 and could be differentiated from previously defined circulating glycoproteins on the basis of molecular weight, solubility properties or isoelectric point. Chemical similarity of this glycoprotein to one of the acute reactants, α-1 acid glycoprotein, was present but a difference in isoelectric point and a larger apparent molecular weight suggested that structural differences were present as well.

A polyclonal antibody has been raised in rabbits utilizing this glycoprotein as immunogen and a sensitive radioimmunoassay developed. The basis of the radioimmunoassay involves a standard competition protocol wherein radioiodinated antigen is mixed with an appropriate dilution of antibody and various dilutions of the perchloric acid-soluble fraction of patient serum are added. A standard curve is constructed by similar incubations containing known amounts of unlabeled antigen; detection levels are in the nanogram range. An examination of a number of patients with various types of malignant disease as well as a variety of control individuals for levels of this glycoprotein has given the general data summarized in Table I. The critical features are the following:

TABLE I. Mean Circulating Levels of TRG Determined by Radioimmunoassay

Patient status	Glycoprotein (ng)
Metastatic, pre-treatment	18.3 ± 3.4 (*p. vs.* normal, <0.00001)
Metastatic, on therapy	16.9 ± 3.1
Local disease, pre-treatment	15.9 ± 3.3 (*p. vs.* normal, <0.0001)
Cured (symptom free 5 years or more)	6.1 ± 2.8
Adjuvant, no evidence of disease	6.4 ± 3.4
Normal	4.8 ± 2.6

Statistically, the differentiation between levels in metastatic disease and normal levels is very good. The trend, as disease burden becomes less, is for the levels of circulating glycoprotein to be reduced while the levels for adjuvant and cured patients are not significantly different from those of normal individuals (*11, 12*).

These data suggest that following glycoprotein levels would be a suitable means for monitoring therapy and for early detection of recurrent disease; extensive data of this type is not yet available. A number of individuals in the non-malignant inpatient group showed elevated levels of glycoprotein probably reflecting the fact that the antibody as developed, although prepared with a pure antigen, crossreacts with one other circulating glycoprotein (α-1 acid glycoprotein). This crossreactivity reflects the chemical similarities noted above. Thus, what is being measured in the circulation is a composite of the levels of α-1 acid glycoprotein and the tumor related glycoprotein (TRG). In separate studies, immunoreactive material has been shown to be produced as a primary product by human tumor cells as well as by human tumors growing in athymic mice (*14*). A number of transient events can cause elevation in acute phase reactants which will lead to increased levels of circulating α-1 acid glycoprotein. What is more relevant is that individuals who are cured or have undergone successful therapy and are currently free of disease give normal glycoprotein levels. It is therefore realistic and feasible to carry out serial studies on individual patients, and to monitor for recurrent disease together with other para meters that would normally be followed such as carcinoembryonic antigen (CEA), or by tissue scans using radioimaging methods. It is not yet appropriate to apply this general screen to the population at large. Although normal individuals have a very low incidence of false positives, transient conditions can lead to changes which make interpretation difficult. An improvement of specificity while retaining sensitivity is the obvious next goal. We are preparing monoclonal antibodies which might allow a complete discrimination between normal circulating components and the glycoprotein of interest.

An interesting facet of these studies is the association of this class of macromolecule with a broad range of malignancy. Elevated values have been found for virtually all types of cancer with little distinction in terms of tissue localization. Thus, lung, mammary, gastrointestinal (GI), melanoma, renal, and prostate cancers all show positive correlations. A direct comparison with CEA in patients with GI malignancy has shown both sialic acid and glycoprotein levels to be somewhat better indicators of disease status than is CEA. Use of both (*i.e.*, CEA and glycoprotein) indicated some complementation but considerable overlap. Glycoproteins with similar or nearly identical properties to that originally isolated have been prepared from a variety of patient plasmas. It is premature to claim that this is a molecule universally associated with transformed or malignant cells. The physiologic role of this molecule and its production by tumor and normal tissues is currently under study. A summary of some patient data is given in Table II.

TABLE II. Glycoprotein Radioimmuoassay

Total sample	Negative	±[a]	Positive[b]
521 (normal)	488	18	15
140 (adjuvant)	123	6	11
36 (cured)	30	2	4

[a] Between one and 2 standard deviations above normal.
[b] Greater than 2 standard deviations above normal.

A rather different identification of approach to cell surface components has been followed. This is also based on the chemical structure of the mucin type glycoproteins identified in model systems. We were struck by the distinct similarity between the human melanoma glycoprotein and glycophorin, the major anionic glycoprotein of erythrocyte. Glycophorin carries the MN blood group determinants which reside in the first few amino acids from the amino terminus of the glycoprotein chain. This glycoprotein is not normally present in the circulation and has not routinely been associated with cell surfaces other than those of the erythrocyte. A key feature of glycophorin is the presence of clustered oligosaccharides which have a structure identical to those found in both the mouse and human melanoma glycoproteins. Further, the clustering of the sialyl oligosaccharides in glycophorin leads to a striking affinity for WGA-Sepharose which is mediated by sialic acid in a manner exactly analogous to that found for the tumor cell glycoproteins. Antibodies prepared to glycophorin have been raised in rabbits and by utilizing hybridomas derived from sensitized mouse spleen cells. In the latter case, we have specifically selected for those antibodies directed against the exterior portion of the glycophorin molecule by employing a complement mediated erythrocyte lysis assay. Preliminary results indicate that utilizing either the polyclonal or the monoclonal antibodies as initial reagents and then counterstaining the cells with an appropriate second antibody raised in goats which bears a fluorescent marker, the surfaces of a variety of tumor cells are sharply outlined (1). This technique has not yet been thoroughly tested but the general approach has promise as a means to examine frozen sections of tissue obtained at surgery which require evaluation for the presence or absence of tumor cells.

A number of laboratories are working in this area, focusing on tumor unique glycoproteins which can be identified using monoclonal antibody techniques. It has been shown that a glycoprotein from human melanoma cells is related to the circulating glycoprotein, transferrin (6). In a second case, a glycoprotein isolated from lung adenocarcinoma has been shown to cross-react with α-1 antichymotrypsin (9). Most of the procedures employed have used whole tumor cells or membranes obtained from such to raise monoclonal antibodies. These have then been employed to detect components on the surface of cells. The cross-reactivity of the monoclonal antibodies has generally not been thoroughly explored. It must be realized that the antibodies may be detecting conserved sites in these macromolecules which have structural features in common that allow them to function as antigenic determinants. It is usually assumed that a protein will have a number of antigenic determinants and that polyclonal antibodies will have different representatives capable of identifying discrete regions on the molecular surface. Monoclonal antibodies do not have this kind of diversity but may exhibit cross-reactivity where common determinants or common structural features exist.

The types of structural variability under study dictate approaches of this type in the hope that suitable macromolecules or antibody-producing clones will be found that will allow a clear discrimination between normal and abnormal structures. A derivative hope is that if specific cell surface recognition is achieved then a sophisticated means of toxic agent delivery can be employed. Model studies have been done whereby coupling of toxic agents to target directed molecules of high specificity allow selective cellular killing. However, it is not clear that either antibodies or other target directed reagents with the requisite degree of specificity exist. The generality of such an approach is made less likely by the very nature of the technique which allows for its success. Thus, each malignancy or the malignancy of any given patient probably represents a composite of common cell surface features from a particular organ but may represent unique features generated by the genetic diversity of the malignant process itself and the individual responses to it exhibited by the patient. Selection of a unique locus on the surface of one lung cancer cell does not hold out certainty that the same locus will be present on the cells of all such malignancies in spite of common tissue derivation. The prospects for targeted chemo- or immunotherapy exist but must be taken with considerable caution.

Acknowledgment

This work was supported in part by USPHS Grant CA 15483.

REFERENCES

1. Barsoum, A., Bhavanandan, V. P., and Davidson, E. A. "Sapporo Cancer Seminar, the 2nd Symposium on Membrane-Associated Alterations in Cancer: Biochemical Strategies against Cancer," July 14–17, Sapporo, Japan (1982) (abstr.).
2. Bhavanandan, V. P. and Davidson, E. A. *Biochem. Biophys. Res. Commun.*, **70**, 139–145 (1976).
3. Bhavanandan, V. P., Umemoto, J., Banks, J. R., and Davidson, E. A. *Biochemistry*, **16**, 4426–4437 (1977).
4. Bolmer, S. D. and Davidson, E. A. *Biochemistry*, **20**, 1047–1054 (1981).
5. Bhavanandan, V. P., Katlic, A. W., Banks, J., Kemper, J. G., and Davidson, E. A. *Biochemistry*, **20**, 5586–5594 (1981).
6. Brown, J. P., Woodbury, R. G., Hart, C. E., Hellstrom, I., and Hellstrom, K. E. *Proc. Natl. Acad. Sci. U.S.*, **78**(1), 539–543 (1981).
7. Chandrasekaran, E. V. and Davidson, E. A. *Biochemistry*, **18**, 5615–5620 (1979).
8. Codington, J. F. *In* "Glycoproteins and Glycolipids in Disease Processes," Am. Chem. Soc. Symp. Ser. 80, ed. E. F. Walborg, Jr., pp. 277–294 (1978). Am. Chem. Sci., Washington, D. C.
9. Gaffar, S. A., Princler, G. L., McIntire, K. R., and Braatz, J. A. *J. Biol. Chem.*, **255**(17), 8334–8339 (1980).
10. Harvey, H. A., Lipton, A., White, D., and Davidson, E. A. *Cancer*, **47**, 324–327 (1981).
11. Hatae, Y., Hatae, T., Bolmer, S. D., and Davidson, E. A. *Carbohydr. Res.*, in press.
12. Hatae, Y., Hatae, T., Lipton, A., Harvey, H., McCarthy, M., and Davidson, E. A. *Carbohydr. Res.*, in press.
13. Lipton, A., Harvey, H. A., Delong, S., Allegra, J., White, D., Allegra, M., and Davidson, E. A. *Cancer*, **43**, 1766–1771 (1979).
14. McCarthy, M. and Davidson, E. A. "The Synthesis of a Malignancy-related Glycoprotein by Colon Carcinomas," Soc. for Complex Carbohydr. Sept. 22–24, Hershey, PA (1982) (abstr.).

15. Satoh, C., Banks, J., Horst, P. Kreider, J. W., and Davidson, E. A. *Biochemistry*, **13**, 1233–1243 (1974).

16. Sheik Fareed, V., Bhavanandan, V. P., and Davidson, E. A. *Carbohydr. Res.*, **65**, 73–83 (1978).

17. Talmadge, J. E. and Fidler, I. J. *Nature*, **197**, 593–594 (1982).

18. Umemoto, J., Bhavanandan, V. P., and Davidson, E. A. *Biochim. Biophys. Acta*, **646**, 402–410 (1981).

19. Yogeeswaran, G. and Salk, P. L. *Science*, **212**, 1514–1516 (1981).

GANN Monograph on Cancer Research 29, 1983

ALTERATIONS OF GLYCOPROTEINS AND GLYCOSAMINOGLYCANS ASSOCIATED WITH MALIGNANT TRANSFORMATION

Ikuo Yamashina, Ikuo Funakoshi, Toshisuke Kawasaki, Akira Kurosaka, Masanori Sugiura, and Shigeyuki Fukui

Department of Biological Chemistry, Faculty of Pharmaceutical Sciences, Kyoto University*

An example was shown which indicated the considerable importance of glycosaminoglycans in controlling cell surface properties.

A mucin-type glycoprotein was isolated from plasma membranes of hepatoma cells and the structures of sugar units released by alkaline-borohydride treatment were determined using chemical and enzymatic procedures. Some of the structures are unique in that they are branched containing N-acetylglucosamine and are relatively short; hexasaccharide with sialic acid at the non-reducing end being the largest. From a mucin-type glycoprotein isolated from a human rectal adenocarcinoma, three oligosaccharides were isolated and their structures were determined. They are Galβ1 → 3 (Siaα2 → 6) GalNAc, GlcNAcβ1 → 3 (Siaα2 → 6) GalNAc, and GalNAc α1 → 3 (Siaα2 → 6) GalNAc. Based on the structures of the sugar units of these two mucin-type glycoproteins, the biosynthetic pathways of the mucin-type glycoproteins were discussed.

The enzyme involved in the initiation of biosynthesis of mucin-type glycoproteins, uridine diphosphate (UDP)-GalNAc: polypeptide N-acetylgalactosamine transferase, was purified to homogeneity from ascites hepatoma cells. The purified enzyme was capable of transferring N-acetylgalactosamine to various acceptors. However, the rate and amount of the transfer were much less than those found *in vivo* indicating that a special spatial arrangement must exist on a membrane which enables effective glycosylation of all available acceptor sites.

Membranes are composed mainly of proteins and lipids. However, some of the proteins are glycoproteins and some of the lipids are glycolipids although they are usually minor components. Their carbohydrate moieties account for less than 10% of the whole membrane (*3*). Proteoglycans are even more minor components of membranes. Their carbohydrate moieties, *i.e.*, glycosaminoglycans (GAG), comprise only about 10% of the total carbohydrates (glycoproteins and glycolipids). However, even such minor components may have a role to play in controlling the structure and function of plasma membranes, the surface structure of cells. In this paper, we will discuss the properties of mucin-type glycoproteins (mucins) and GAG on the surface of various types of cancer cells.

---

* Yoshida Shimoadachi-cho, Sakyo-ku, Kyoto 606, Japan (山科郁男, 船越育雄, 川崎敏祐, 黒坂 光, 杉浦正典, 福井成行).

An Example of Involvement of Mucins and GAG in Cell Surface Properties

Figure 1 shows the changes in cell surface architecture, determined by lectin-binding assays, caused by the enzymatic treatment of hepatoma cells (*8*). Ascites hepatoma cells such as AH 66 or AH 130 FN, possess on the surface, GAG (heparan sulfate on AH 66 and chondroitin sulfate A on AH 130 FN) and mucin in addition to asparagine-type glycoproteins (*6, 7*). Trypsin preferentially removed heparan sulfate from AH 66 cells (*9*). The binding capacity of AH 66 cells for concanavalin A (ConA) and *Ricinus communis* lectin (RCA) did not change remarkably. This indicates that binding sites of ConA and RCA on cell membranes are not covered by heparan sulfate. Tryptic treatment of AH 130 FN cells also resulted in very little change in binding capacities of the cells towards ConA and RCA. There was a slight decrease in the binding capacity towards ConA, due probably to release of some N-glycosidic glycopeptides that bind to ConA.

Marked changes occurred when AH 130 FN cells were treated with chondroitinase AC. The enzyme-dependent release of ³H radioactivity from the cells which had been labeled with ³H-glucosamine reached a plateau within 1 hr. After incubation for up to 2 hr more than 90% of the cells remained viable, as observed by trypan blue staining. The binding of RCA to the chondroitinase-treated cells increased several-fold, as shown

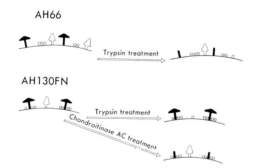

FIG. 1. Diagrammatic representation of the enzymatic release of glycopeptides and mucopolysaccharides (GAG) from cell surfaces of AH 66 and AH 130 FN cells. ⬆ proteoglycan; N-glycosidic glycoprotein; O-glycosidic glycoprotein.

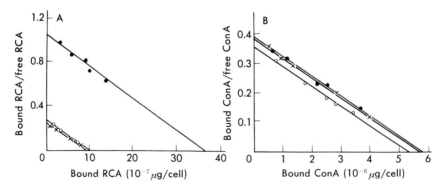

FIG. 2. Changes in lectin-binding capacities of AH 130 FN cells on treatment with chondroitinase AC. A, RCA binding; B, ConA binding. × freshly harvested intact cells; ○ cells incubated without chondroitinase AC; ● cells treated with chondroitinase AC.

in Fig. 2, without any change in the binding constant. In contrast, the capacities of the cells to bind ConA did not change after enzymatic treatment (Fig. 2). These results indicate that the RCA-binding sites which are composed mainly of O-glycosidically linked oligosaccharides are covered with chondroitin sulfate A. Unsaturated disaccharides derived from chondroitin sulfate A by digestion with chondroitinase AC were identified in the cell digest. On the other hand, the ConA-binding sites, which are mainly composed of N-glycosidically linked oligosaccharides are not covered by chondroitin sulfate A. Thus, it seems to be that GAG on the cell surface is not distributed uniformly, but is located at specific sites, interacting with other membrane components. Figure 1 is a diagrammatic representation of the enzymatic release of glycopeptides and GAG from the surfaces of AH 66 and AH 130 FN cells.

Comparison of Rat Liver and Hepatoma with Respect to Mucins and the Purification of Uridine Diphosphate (UDP)-GalNAc: Polypeptide GalNAc Transferase from Hepatoma

What are the differences in cell surface mucins between control and cancer cells? To approach this problem, we have compared the properties and structures of mucin-type glycoproteins and proteoglycans from plasma membranes of rat liver and hepatoma cells (*3, 6, 7*). It was found that the plasma membranes isolated from normal liver contained very little mucin-type glycoproteins. The low level of mucin in liver is consistent with the existing low level of the mucin-synthesizing enzyme activities, compared to hepatoma. In fact, the level of activity of the enzyme, UDP-GalNAc-polypeptide GalNAc transferase, that is the enzyme which is involved in the first step of the mucin biosynthesis, is much lower in liver than in hepatoma.

In order to know more about the mechanism of mucin biosynthesis, we purified the GalNAc transferase. This enzyme has been purified in the past with difficulty. We have purified the enzyme to homogeneity for the first time by various procedures including affinity chromatography on apomucin-Sepharose (*11*). Apomucin, deglycosylated bovine submaxillary mucin, was prepared by Smith degradation and used as the ligand for the affinity column and also as the acceptor for the enzyme assay. The purification by affinity

TABLE I.   Transfer of N-acetylgalactosamine UDP-GalNAc to Acceptors

Acceptor	Rate[a]	Amount[b] (%)	Amount[c] (%)
Al protein	0.216	5.02	
κ-Casein	0.082	11.4	
Apomucin (SD)	0.212	8.84	9.88
Apomucin (ET)	0.934	7.39	8.26
Apo-AFGP 8 (SD)	0.141	7.14	7.14
Apo-AFGP 8 (ET)	0.035	1.54	1.54
Apo-AFGP HMW (SD)	0.363	9.81	9.81
Apofetuin (ET)	0.005	0.56	8.99
Apofetuin (ET, endo D)	0.005	2.28	35.8

[a] Rate of transfer: μmol per min per mg of enzyme protein.
[b] Amount of transfer: mol per mol of total serine plus threonine.
[c] Amount of transfer: mol per mol of potential acceptor site.
SD, prepared by Smith degradation;   ET, prepared by enzymatic treatment;   AFGP, antifreeze glycoprotein;   HMW, high molecular weight;   ET, endo D, prepared by enzymatic treatments using exoglycosidases and endo-β-N-acetylglucosaminidase D.

chromatography was very effective, and was repeated three times. The final preparation was homogeneous on sodium dodecyl sulfate-polyacrylamide gel electrophoresis (SDS-PAGE) with a monomeric molecular weight of about 55,000. The enzyme was found to be different from those involved in the syntheses of blood group A active substances and Forssman glycolipid. The enzyme was capable of transferring GalNAc from UDP-GalNAc to various polypeptide acceptors without involvement of lipids or other cofactors except for Mn^{2+} ion. However, the rate of GalNAc transfer and the amount of GalNAc transferred varied greatly from one acceptor to another, as shown in Table I.

Apomucin and apoantifreeze-glycoprotein were good acceptors, followed by A1 protein and casein, as far as transfer acceptance is concerned. GalNAc is transferred to a very limited portion of the available serine and threonine residues. Only about 10% of the available sites could be glycosylated for most of the acceptors. These results can be interpreted as indicating that the GalNAc transferase requires a certain conformation of the acceptor polypeptides under *in vivo* conditions which cannot be mimicked *in vitro* with artificially prepared apoglycoproteins and a purified enzyme preparation.

Oligosaccharide Structure of the Major Mucin from Hepatoma

Most of the mucin-type oligosaccharides found in the plasma membranes of hepatoma cells could be isolated as components of the major glycoprotein of the membranes. We have isolated the major glycoprotein by a procedure similar to that used for the isolation of glycophorin from human erythrocytes (4). Chemical composition of this glycoprotein is shown in Table II. The carbohydrate composition, rich in glucosamine, galactosamine, galactose, and sialic acid, is similar to that of glycophorin. The glycoprotein was first digested with pronase, and the resulting glycopeptides were fractionated by gel filtration. Glycopeptides composed mainly of O-glycosidic types were obtained in the void volume fraction, and were then treated with alkaline-borohydride. The released sugar units with tritiated reducing ends were fractionated into neutral and acidic fractions by ion-exchange chromatography. Each group of sugar units was then fractionated further by gel filtration. Each oligosaccharide was purified to homogeneity by paper chromatography or by paper electrophoresis. One reduced monosaccharide, N-acetylgalactosaminitol, and three neutral and five acidic reduced oligosaccharides

TABLE II. Chemical Composition of the Major Glycoprotein
from AH 66 Plasma Membranes

Lysine	3.78	Methionine	1.28
Histidine	1.33	Isoleucine	2.86
Arginine	2.50	Leucine	5.20
Aspartic acid	7.14	Tyrosine	1.89
Threonine	6.94	Phenylalanine	2.40
Serine	6.89		
Glutamic acid	7.91	Glucosamine	6.73
Proline	4.69	Galactosamine	5.05
Glycine	5.35	Mannose	2.30
Alanine	4.59	Galactose	10.26
Half-cystine	1.17	Fucose	0.46
Valine	3.93	Sialic acid	5.26

Values are expressed as residues per 100 residues.

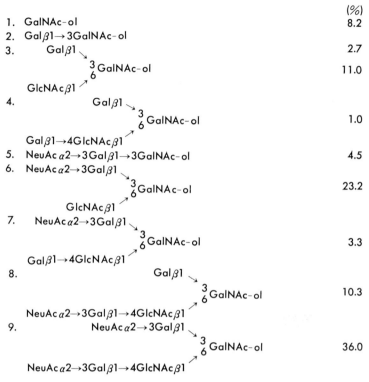

(%)

1. GalNAc-ol   8.2
2. Galβ1→3GalNAc-ol
3.   Galβ1   2.7
                    ³\₆ GalNAc-ol   11.0
      GlcNAcβ1
4.   Galβ1
                         ³\₆ GalNAc-ol   1.0
      Galβ1→4GlcNAcβ1
5. NeuAcα2→3Galβ1→3GalNAc-ol   4.5
6. NeuAcα2→3Galβ1
                         ³\₆ GalNAc-ol   23.2
         GlcNAcβ1
7.   NeuAcα2→3Galβ1
                         ³\₆ GalNAc-ol   3.3
      Galβ1→4GlcNAcβ1
8.   Galβ1
                              ³\₆ GalNAc-ol   10.3
      NeuAcα2→3Galβ1→4GlcNAcβ1
9.   NeuAcα2→3Galβ1
                              ³\₆ GalNAc-ol   36.0
      NeuAcα2→3Galβ1→4GlcNAcβ1

F IG. 3.   Structures of the O-glycosidically linked sugar units from plasma membranes of an ascites hepatoma, AH 66. In the right column, relative abundance (%
of total) of the oligosaccharides is indicated.

were isolated. The void volume fraction of the gel filtration was composed mainly of
undegraded O-glycosidic glycopeptides and some of the N-glycosidic glycopeptides.
This fraction could be degraded with a second alkaline-borohydride treatment after
acetylation of the amino group and esterification of the carboxyl group of the peptide
moieties, resulting in oligosaccharides similar to those obtained by the first degradation.
In Fig. 3, the structures of the isolated oligosaccharides are shown. These were determined on the basis of carbohydrate composition, mass spectra of permethylated oligosaccharides, methylation analysis, and exoglycosidase digestion (5).

The oligosaccharides are of relatively small size and characterized by most of them
having N-acetylglucosamine. As shown in Fig. 3, the glucosamine-containing sugar
units comprise more than 80% of the total. This structural pattern should reflect the
biosynthetic pathways. In Fig. 4, GalNAc is transferred to the polypeptide core in the
initiation of synthesis. Next step is the transfer of galactose and this is followed by the
GlcNAc transfer. As postulated by Schachter's group (12, 13), the GlcNAc transferase
requires a Gal-GalNAc structure as an acceptor. The reverse order, that is, the transfer
of GlcNAc followed by the transfer of Gal, is forbidden. Once the trisaccharide structure is formed, the sugar chain does not seem to be elongated, but rather terminated by
the transfer of sialic acid to either end or to both.

Glucosamine-containing mucin-type oligosaccharides have been reported to occur
in various mucins, but the sugar units in these mucins are larger in molecular size and

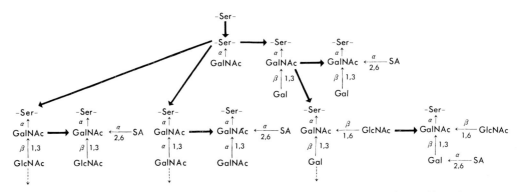

F IG . 4.   Biosynthetic pathways of mucin-type glycoproteins. Ser, serine residue of
the polypeptide core; SA, sialyl residue.

are devoid of sialic acid, as can be seen for example in the structure of oligosaccharides
with blood-group activities (2).

Based on the relative amounts of the sugar units, it may be possible to deduce
the relative activities of the transferases involved in the synthesis. As shown in Fig. 4,
sialyl transferase and GlcNAc-transferase which transfer these sugars directly to GalNAc
do not seem to operate. These reactions are forbidden. At the next step of the synthesis,
galactose is transferred to GalNAc, followed by the transfer of either GlcNAc to GalNAc
or sialic acid to galactose. The former, that is the GlcNAc transfer, seems to be greater
than the sialyl transfer. The GlcNAc-containing trisaccharide will either be directly
sialylated or lead to the formation of the fully sialylated hexasaccharide as the main final
product. This indicates that galactose transfer may be rate-limiting and sialylation,
even at one of the two non-reducing ends, is inhibitory to chain elongation.

Of the nine sugar units which we have studied (Fig. 3), 6, 7, 8, and 9 have not been
reported so far to occur in glycoproteins. These GlcNAc-containing, short oligosaccharides with sialic acid at the non-reducing ends might be characteristic of cancer
cell membranes. In fact, the presence of similar oligosaccharides on human mammary
cancer cells and on mouse mammary carcinoma cells has been reported (1, 14).

Oligosaccharide Structure of a Mucin from a Human Rectal Adenocarcinoma

We have recently discovered additional new oligosaccharide structures to occur in
a mucin from a human rectal adenocarcinoma. This mucin was obtained from the
metastatic masses of the greater omentum of a patient (10). The carcinoma weighted
approximately 400 g and the mucin content was at least 1% of the wet tissue weight.
The tumor tissue was extracted with an ethylenediamine tetraacetic acid (EDTA)-
containing buffer, and the extract was repeatedly fractionated by gel filtration. It was
difficult to assess the purity of the mucin, designated as rectal mucin-type glycoprotein
(RMG), since RMG has an extremely high molecular weight, like submaxillary mucin.
Purification was based on the increase in carbohydrate contents. In double diffusion
analysis using RMG and anti-RMG, one major and at least one minor precipitin line
was observed as is seen when submaxillary mucins are reacted with their antibodies in
agar gel. Anti-RMG did not react with carcinoembryonic antigen (CEA). A similar mucin
could be isolated from normal intestine with a much lower yield. In comparison with

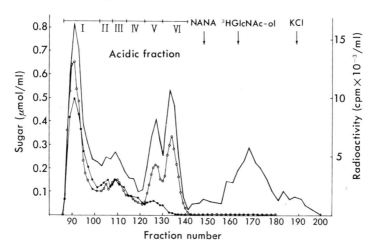

FIG. 5. Gel filtration on Sephadex G-25 of the acidic fraction (sialic acid-containing) prepared by alkaline-borohydride (^{3}H-NaBH$_4$) treatment of a glycoprotein from a human rectal adenocarcinoma. ○ sialic acid; ● hexose; —— radioactivity. NANA, N-acetylneuraminic acid.

RMG, the carbohydrate moiety of the normal mucin was much more heterogeneous. The carbohydrate composition of the purified mucin was: NeuAc, 92.6 mg/100 mg protein (1.19 in a molar ratio relative to GlcNAc); GlcNAc, 54.5 (1.00); GalNAc, 56,5 (1.04); Gal, 40.3 (0.91); Man, 3.2 (1.06); and Fuc, 2.4 (0.04). The mucin contained about 70% carbohydrate which consisted of nearly equal amounts of glucosamine, galactosamine, galactose, and sialic acid. The mucin was treated with alkaline-borohydride, and the products were fractionated by ion-exchange chromatography. Most of the oligosaccharides were obtained in the acidic fraction, that is the pyridine-acetic acid eluate, which is composed of sialic acid-containing sugar units. Some of the sugar units were recovered in the strongly acidic fraction, the 2 M NaCl eluate, which is composed of sulfate-containing saccharides of high molecular weight. The sialic acid-containing fraction was further fractionated by gel filtration, as shown in Fig. 5. Of the six discernible fractions, the void volume fraction has not yet been characterized and Fractions II–IV were minor fractions. Fraction VI was identified as Sialyl-GalNAc-ol. Fraction V was further fractionated by paper chromatography, and the structures of the isolated oligosaccharides were determined as follows: Galβ1→3(NeuAcα2→6)GalNAc-ol (1.0), GalNAcα1→3(NeuNAcα2→6)GalNAc-ol (1.5), GlcNAcβ1→3(NeuAcα2→6)GalNAc-ol (2.0 in a relative molar ratio) (unpublished results).

The total amount of trisaccharide units in Fraction V was about 20% of the total sugar units in RMG, and the relative amounts among these three were nearly equimolar. Of these three trisaccharides, GlcNAcβ1→3(NeuAcα2→6)GalNAc and GalNAcα1→3 (NeuAcα2→6)GalNAc have not been reported before. The last one contains the terminal structure of Forssman glycolipid, but neither RMG nor its desialated derivative reacted with anti-Forssman antibody.

The presence of these trisaccharide structures raise questions as to the biosynthetic routes of the mucin oligosaccharides. As shown in Fig. 4, it is now nearly definite that galactose is transferred to GalNAc, then either sialic acid or GlcNAc is transferred to the disaccharide, Gal-GalNAc. Once sialylated, chain elongation terminates. If the same rule is applied to the syntheses of the newly discovered trisaccharides, GlcNAc and GalNAc as well as galactose would be transferred to GalNAc prior to the sialylation. Since the direct transfer of GlcNAc to GalNAc was regarded as a forbidden reaction, the formation of GlcNAc-GalNAc or GalNAc-GalNAc structures might be permissible depending on the linkage position. In other words, β6-GlcNAc transfer to GalNAc prior to β3-Gal transfer to this GalNAc is forbidden, but β3-GlcNAc transfer to GalNAc might not be forbidden. Likewise, α3-GalNAc transfer to GalNAc, a new reaction, might not be forbidden either.

CONCLUSIONS

It was pointed out that mucin-type glycoproteins and GAG have considerable importance in determining the surface properties of cells. Cancer cells seem capable of producing sugar units of unique structure in cell surface mucins, at least in much larger amounts than do normal cells. Unique structures should be produced by unique sugar transferases. By characterizing these transferases, it may be possible to establish an effective cancer diagnosis.

Acknowledgment
    This work was supported in part by a Grant-in-Aid for Scientific Research from the Ministry of Education, Science and Culture of Japan.

REFERENCES

1. Chandrasekaran, E. V. and Davidson, E. A. *Biochemistry*, **18**, 5615–5620 (1979).
2. Feizi, T., Kabat, E. A., Vicari, G., Anderson, B., and March, W. L. *J. Immunol.*, **106**, 1578–1592 (1971).
3. Funakoshi, I., Nakada, H., and Yamashina, I. *J. Biochem.*, **76**, 319–333 (1974).
4. Funakoshi, I. and Yamashina, I. *J. Biochem.*, **80**, 1185–1193 (1976).
5. Funakoshi, I. and Yamashina, I. *J. Biol. Chem.*, **257**, 3782–3787 (1982).
6. Mutoh, S., Funakoshi, I., and Yamashina, I. *J. Biochem.*, **80**, 903–912 (1976).
7. Nakada, H., Funakoshi, I., and Yamashina, I. *J. Biochem.*, **78**, 863–872 (1975).
8. Nakada, H., Funakoshi, I., and Yamashina, I. *Biochem. Biophys. Res. Commun.*, **79**, 280–284 (1977).
9. Nakada, H. and Yamashina, I. *J. Biochem.*, **83**, 79–83 (1978).
10. Nakajima, H., Kurosaka, A., Fujisawa, A. (nee Sehara), Kawasaki, T., Funakoshi, I., Matsuyama, M., Nagayo, T., and Yamashina, I. *J. Biochem.*, **93**, 651–659 (1983).
11. Sugiura, M., Kawasaki, T., and Yamashina, I. *J. Biol. Chem.*, **257**, 9501–9507 (1982).
12. Williams, D., Longmore, G., Matta, K. L., and Schachter, H. *J. Biol. Chem.*, **255**, 11253–11261 (1980).
13. Williams, D. and Schachter, H. *J. Biol. Chem.*, **255**, 11247–11252 (1980).
14. Van den Eijnden, D. H., Evans, N. A., Codington, J. F., Reinfold, V., Silber, C., and Jeanloz, R. W. *J. Biol. Chem.*, **254**, 12153–12159 (1979).

GANN Monograph on Cancer Research 29, 1983

CARBOHYDRATE STRUCTURES EXPRESSED IN CERTAIN UNDIFFERENTIATED CELLS AND IN MALIGNANT CELLS

Takashi MURAMATSU

Department of Biochemistry, Kagoshima University School of Medicine*

Embryonal carcinoma (EC) cells, stem cells of teratocarcinoma express glycoprotein-bound large carbohydrates of molecular weight more than 7,500. The large carbohydrate chains were also detected in early mouse embryos. During differentiation of EC cells and the embryos, the large carbohydrates disappeared almost completely. The large carbohydrates carry several cell surface markers of early embryonic cells, including receptors for peanut agglutinin (PNA), *Dolichos biflorus* agglutinin (DBA), and fucose binding proteins of *Lotus* (FBP). Receptors for these lectins were differentially distributed in cell layers of teratocarcinomas and early embryos, indicating that non-reducing sugars of the large carbohydrates are altered according to the position of the cell in cell layers. Structural studies have shown that the building unit of the core portion of large glycan was $-4\text{GlcNAc}\beta1 \rightarrow 3\text{Gal}$. Branching occurred at C-6 of the galactosyl residues. Thus, the large carbohydrates appeared to be a highly complex form of lactosaminoglycan. The role of the complex glycan during embryogenesis will be an interesting subject for study. PNA and DBA are also useful in analyzing cell surface changes during differentiation in other systems. Moreover, antiserum raised against $\text{Fuc}\alpha1 \rightarrow 3\text{Gal}$ linkage reacted to human colon adenocarcinoma, but not to the normal mucosa of the colon.

Certain undifferentiated cells or malignant cells express unusual carbohydrate structures which are not commonly found in differentiated cells. Such carbohydrate structures can be used as markers to follow the process of cell differentiation. Cell surface recognition during the process of this differentiation is expected to be partially mediated by these structures. The carbohydrate structures might also be used in immunological diagnosis and even immunotherapy of human cancers. In this review, I would like to summarize the work we have performed along this line for the past several years.

Presence of High-molecular Weight Carbohydrates in Glycoproteins of Teratocarcinomas

Being interested in the possible role of glycoprotein-bound carbohydrates during the course of cell differentiation, I decided to study cell-surface glycoprotein of early embryonic cells of mammals. Although only a small amount of early embryos of mammals can be collected, there exists a suitable model system called teratocarcinomas *(19)*. Teratocarcinomas are tumors composed of cells of three germ layers plus the malignant

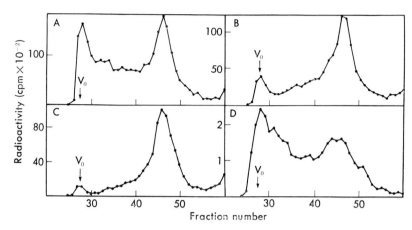

F<small>IG</small>. 1. Sephadex G-50 column chromatography of fucose-labeled glycopeptides from EC cells and early embryos. The elution positions of blue dextran and fucose were in fractions 36–38 and 88–91, respectively. A, undifferentiated EC cells (clone PCC3, 2 days after plating); B and C, differentiated EC cells (clone PCC3, 14 days and 28 days after plating, respectively); D, preimplantation embryos of mice (mainly morulae). (cited from Ref. 22)

stem cells called embryonal carcinoma (EC) cells. EC cells resemble multipotential cells of early embryos and yet can be propagated by standard cell culture techniques.

The first biochemical analysis of carbohydrates in EC cells was performed by fucose-labeling experiments when I visited the laboratory of Prof. F. Jacob. EC cells were grown in the presence of radioactive fucose, harvested, and extensively digested with pronase. The resulting glycopeptides were analyzed by Sephadex G-50 column chromatography (22). We found that a significant fraction of the fucosyl glycopeptides from EC cells was composed of large ones eluted in the excluded volume of the column (Fig. 1A).

The large fucosyl glycopeptides were found in all EC clones examined, which differed in origin and the ability to differentiate. Several experiments excluded the possibility that the large glycopeptides were products of incomplete pronase digestion, glycosaminoglycans or mucin-type glycopeptides of short oligosaccharide chains (22, 23). Thus, we concluded that EC cells contain a class of glycoprotein-bound large carbohydrate chains. It was a striking observation, since in a number of normal and malignant cells only a trace amount of fucosyl glycopeptides were eluted in these high-molecular-weight regions. It may be mentioned that erythroglycan, the high-molecular-weight carbohydrates of band III glycoprotein of erythrocytes, was not described at that time. In fact, the occurrence of the large carbohydrates in EC cells and of erythroglycan was published simultaneously in 1978 (11, 15, 22).

When PCC3, a clonal line of EC cells, was induced to differentiate by growing the cells at high density, the large fucosyl glycopeptides disappeared almost completely (22) (Fig. 1B, C). This phenomena was also observed during differentiation of another clonal line F9 by retinoic acid and di-butyryl cyclic AMP (29). In the latter case, the fucose content of the cell (amount of fucose/mg protein) also decreased as the result of differentiation.

In order to investigate whether the large glycopeptides are derived from the plasma membrane, we isolated the membrane fraction from F9 EC cells by ultracentrifugation in a discontinuous sucrose density gradient (23). Since EC cells have only a small amount of internal membranes, the isolated membranes can be considered to be relatively pure plasma membrane. Recovery of the non-dialyzable [³H]-fucose label in the membranes was about 44% and corresponded to the recovery of their cell surface antigens. The majority of the fucose-labeled glycopeptides from the plasma membrane fraction was found to be the large ones eluted in the excluded volume of a G-50 column (23).

The large glycopeptides were labeled not only by radioactive fucose but also by radioactive galactose and glucosamine. Autoradiographic experiments confirmed that more than half of the radioactive galactose incorporated into F9 EC cells was actually located in the plasma membrane (Kawamoto, Y. and Muramatsu, T. unpublished results). When F9 EC cells were externally labeled in their galactosyl residues by the galactose oxidase-NaB³H₄ method and extensively digested with pronase, most of the glycopeptides formed were again the large ones (38). All these results mentioned thus allowed us to conclude that the majority of the large glycopeptides were derived from the plasma membrane of EC cells.

Occurrence of the Large Carbohydrates in Murine Embryos

Preimplantation embryos of the mouse showed glycopeptide profiles very similar to those of EC cells (22) (Fig. 1D). A similar result was obtained for the embryonic part of 6-day-old embryos, which were dissected and cultured for 6 hr *in vitro* to incorporate [³H]-fucose (26). During the course of embryogenesis, the glycopeptide profile gradually changed as in the case of differentiating EC cells. In 10-day-old embryos, the profile was that of fully differentiated cells: only trace amounts of the large glycopeptides were detected. Brain cells of 10-day-old embryos and liver cells of 12-day-old embryos also displayed the glycopeptide profile of the differentiated cell type (26). Thus, the unusual large glycopeptides of EC cells are not peculiar to these malignant cells, but are properties common to and characteristic of an early embryonic phenotype. Furthermore, our studies were probably the first reliable biochemical studies on glycoproteins of mammalian early embryos. Although Pinsker and Mintz have analyzed "cell surface glycopeptides" of mouse embryos, their glycopeptide preparation was probably contaminated with monosaccharides and other low-molecular-weight substances and thus they apparently overlooked the large glycopeptides we detected (37).

Relationship of the Large Carbohydrates to Cell Surface Markers of EC Cells

When we found the large carbohydrates, EC cells were known to have three cell surface markers, which disappear from most of the cells segregated from EC cells after *in vitro* differentiation. The most thoroughly studied marker at that time was the F9 antigen defined by syngeneic antiserum against F9 EC cells (1). The F9 antigen was present not only on EC cells but also on early embryos and sperm, while it was reported to be absent in many differentiated cell types (1). Furthermore, serological experiments suggested the possibility that the F9 antigen was a wild type gene product of the T/t genetic region, which is located in the 17th chromosome of the mouse and apparently defines cell surface molecules required for embryogenesis (10). In addition, preliminary biochemical studies indicated that the molecular weight of the F9 antigen is around

44,000 (10), and thus is similar to that of the H-2 antigen. Since both H-2 and T/t genetic regions are located on the 17th chromosome, the above result even raised the hypothesis that the gene products of the T/t region are embryonic forms of H-2 antigen.

Other cell surface markers of EC cells in these days were receptors for two lectins, namely, peanut agglutinin (PNA), which binds to Galβ1→3GalNAc linkage (40) and fucose binding proteins of *Lotus* (FBP), which binds to certain α-L-fucose residues (6). The mode of disappearance of the three cell surface markers during *in vitro* differentiation of EC cells is similar to that of the large fucosyl glycopeptides. Thus, we investigated the possible correlation between the three cell surface markers and the large glycopeptides. EC cells cultured in the presence of radioactive monosaccharides were dissolved in detergent, and the cell surface markers were isolated by indirect immunoprecipitation (25). Approximately 5 to 10% of the fucose-label, galactose-label, and glucosamine-label were recovered in the immunoprecipitates, while scarcely any mannose-label was found. The isolated markers mainly migrated as glycoproteins of molecular weight around 44,000 upon sodium dodecylsulfate (SDS) gel electrophoresis. The glycopeptides obtained by extensive pronase digestion of the markers were found to be mostly the large ones excluded from a Sephadex G-50 column. Thus, the F9 antigen as well as receptors for the two lectins were revealed to be glycoproteins with large carbohydrate chains (25). These results correlated the carbohydrate alteration detected by biochemical methods with cell-surface changes detected by immunochemical methods. The finding that the F9 antigen belongs to glycoprotein(s) with unusual carbohydrate structures was rather unexpected at the time, and immediately yielded a new hypothesis that the T/t genetic region specifies glycosyl transferases.

Biochemical Properties of the Large Carbohydrates

The properties of the large glycopeptides from EC cells and also those from the isolated cell surface markers were at first studied by glycosidase digestion (23, 25). They were partially susceptible to endo-β-galactosidase of *Escherichia freundii* (4), which acts on substrates with GlcNAcβ1→3Gal sequence. Together with the observation that the large glycopeptides were efficiently labeled with fucose, galactose, and glucosamine but not with mannose, the susceptibility to the endoglycosidase indicated that the core portion of the glycan is formed by repeated and probably branched arrangements of galactose and N-acetylglucosamine. Furthermore, we observed that fucosyl residues of the large glycopeptides were susceptible to α-L-fucosidase I of almond emulsion (an enzyme specific for Fucα1→3,4GlcNAc), but not to that of *Bacillus fulminans* (an enzyme specific for Fucα1→2Gal). Subsequently, Feizi and co-workers have shown that I antigen is expressed on EC cells and early embryos (12) and that monoclonal antibody SSEA-1 reacting with EC cells recognizes the Fucα1→3GlcNAc linkage (7). It is most probable that both I and SSEA-1 antigenic determinants are on the large carbohydrates.

H. Muramatsu *et al.* have recently succeeded in clarifying the overall structural profiles of the large carbohydrates characteristic of early embryonic cells (33). The large glycopeptides from F9 cells grown *in vitro* and also *in vivo* as subcutaneous tumors were employed as the subject of structural studies. Compositional analysis revealed that galactose and N-acetylglucosamine were the major components of the glycan and were present in similar amounts (31, 33) (Table I). In addition, a small amount of fucose, N-acetylgalactosamine and mannose were present. No uronic acids nor sphingosine base

TABLE I. Sugar Composition of the Large Glycopeptides Isolated from F9 Cells

Monosaccharides	Glycopeptides from *in vitro* grown cells[a]	Glycopeptides from *in vivo* grown cells[b]
Galactose	1.0	1.0
Glucosamine	0.86	0.82
Galactosamine	0.15	0.12
Fucose	0.14	0.15
Mannose	0.08	0.07
Sialic acid	<0.05	<0.07

[a] Cited from Ref. *33*.
[b] Cited from Ref. *31*.

were detected. Amino acids were present only in small amount. Even assuming that the aspartic acid, threonine, and serine all are involved in the protein-carbohydrate linkage, the molecular weight of the glycan can be calculated to be 7,500, which is the minimum molecular weight of the large glycan. Furthermore, gel filtration of the glycopeptides treated with anhydrous hydrazine or with mild alkali in the presence of $NaBH_4$ to cleave the protein-carbohydrate linkage indicates that the major component of the glycan has a molecular weight around 25,000.

The structure of the glycan was studied by methylation analysis, [1]H-nuclear magnetic resonance (NMR) spectroscopy and alkaline thiophenol treatment followed by acid hydrolysis. From the result, the core portion of the glycan was concluded to have the structural unit, $-4GlcNAc\beta1 \rightarrow 3Gal\beta1 \rightarrow$, whose galactosyl residues served as branching points at C-6 (*33*).

Therefore, the building unit of the large glycan is very similar to that of erythroglycan, the high molecular weight glycan of band III glycoprotein of erythrocytes (*11, 15*) and to that of ABH blood group antigen of human ovarian cyst fluid (*16*). However, the large glycan from EC cells appear to be distinguished from erythroglycan and the ABH blood group antigen in the following two points. Firstly, the large glycan from EC cells did not have detectable amounts of ABH blood group antigens. Instead, they expressed non-reducing sugar sequences with restricted distribution, which served as lectin binding sites and antigenic determinants. Secondly, the estimated molecular weight of the major component of the large glycan is about 25,000, which is larger than that of erythroglycan (13,000–4,000) (*11, 15*) and that of the ABH blood group antigen (less than 20 monosaccharide units) (*16*). Glycans with repeating units of Gal-GlcNAc are now collectively called lactosaminoglycan (*8*). Our current view is that the large carbohydrates of early embryonic cells represent a highly complex form of lactosaminoglycan. We shall hereafter refer to the large carbohydrates as lactosaminoglycan of early embryonic cells or as "embryoglycan."

Problems under Current Investigation on Embryoglycan

Embryoglycan represents one of the major carbohydrate constituents of the surface of early embryonic cells. Non-reducing sugar sequences of restricted distribution are attached to its branched, complex core structure. Therefore, it is resonable to expect some specific function for embryoglycan during embryogenesis.

We have recently found that some of the non-reducing sugars in embryoglycan were differentially expressed in cell aggregates of teratocarcinoma and also in mouse embryos: FBP binding sites were preferentially expressed in the inner cell layer, namely the ecto-derm, *Dolichos biflorus* agglutinin (DBA) binding sites were preferentially expressed in the outer cell layer, or endoderm, and PNA binding sites were expressed in all cell layers including mesoderm (*9*). The gradual disappearance of embryoglycan from dif-ferentiating cells has been metioned before. Thus, biosynthesis of embryoglycan appears to be influenced both by time and space during embryogenesis. Expression of the specific sugar sequences in such an ordered manner is again consistent with the idea that they play essential roles during embryogenesis.

The specific function of embryoglycan can be related to cell adhesion and migration and also to the determination of the direction of differentiation. In connection with the latter possibility, it should be mentioned that cell surface molecules and chromosomes could be directly connected by cytoskeltons during mitosis; thereby asymmetrical cell surface interaction occurring only on one side of the cell could modify the chromosome structure only on this side.

Shur has recently provided evidence suggesting that cell surface glycosyl transferases play critical roles during embryogenesis and that the transferases interact with embryo-glycan on the surface of early embryonic cells (*41*). Studies on glycosyltransferases in-volved in the biosynthesis of embryoglycan will certainly be rewarding. In addition, we are also interested in protein moieties carrying embryoglycan and in endogeneous lectins recognizing embryoglycan. We expect that the function of embryoglycan will be ulti-mately clarified by a combination of such biochemical studies with cell biological and developmental biological approaches.

Embryoglycan is also interesting in clinical studies. Human teratocarcinoma cell lines invariably express embryoglycan, and the biochemical properties are very similar to those of the glycan from murine teratocarcinoma (*24*, *30*). Kawata *et al.* have recently found that sera from certain patients with ovarian germ cell tumors had antibodies against embryoglycan isolated from murine EC cells (*14*). Sera from normal human subjects and patients with other malignancies never showed the antibody activity. As above, embryoglycan may be used for diagnosis and classification of germ cell tumors.

Receptors for PNA

PNA is a lectin preferentially reacting with the $Gal\beta1 \rightarrow 3GalNAc$ linkage (*18*, *39*). Reisner, Sharon and others found that the lectin reacts with certain undifferentiated cells such as cortical thymocytes (*17*, *39*) and EC cells (*10*). Through the study of cell-surface glycoproteins of EC cells mentioned before, we learned the utility of PNA and attempted to exploit the lectin in certain specific problems of differentiation and malignancy.

First, we examined the distribution of PNA receptors in various tissues of adult mice (*44*, *45*) (Table II). Although the distribution of PNA receptors was rather broader than expected, we found two hitherto undescribed alterations of PNA receptors during cell differentiation. In squamous epithelium of esophagus, the receptors were expressed in undifferentiated cells in the basal layer, but disappeared from differentiated cells in the superficial layer. During the course of spermatogenesis, PNA receptors were absent in the stem cells, namely, spermatogonium, but came to be expressed at the spermatocyte stage.

PNA receptors were detected in more than half the established cell lines of human

TABLE II.   The Distribution of DBA Receptors and PNA Receptors in Mouse Organs

Organ	PNA	DBA	Organ	PNA	DBA
Esophagus			Stomach		
Epithelium;			Foveolar cells	±	±
Superficial layer	−	−	Parietal cells	−	+
Middle layer	+	−	Chief cells		
Basal layer	+	−	Upper half layer	±	±
Trachea			Lower half layer	−	−
Epithelium	−	−	Phloric gland	+	−
Cartilage	+	−	Samll intestine		
Lung			Brush border	+	+
Alveolar wall	+	−	Epithelial cells	−	+
Thymus			Goblet cells	+	±
Cortex	+	−	Paneth cells	−	+
Medulla	−	−	Testis		
Spleen			Spermatogonium	−	−
Lymphocytes	−	−	Spermatocytes	+	−
Liver			Sperm	+	+
Liver cells	−	−	Epididymis		
Bile duct	+	+	Epithelium	+	+
Pancreas			Sperm	+	+
Exocrine gland	+	+	Ovary		
Endocrine gland	−	−	Cytoplasm of oocyte	−	+
Pancreatic duct	+	+	Zona pellucidae	+	+
Kidney			Granular layer	+	−
Bowman's capsule	+	+	Basal lamina	+	−
Glomerulus	−	−	Fallopian tube		
Tubules;			Epithelium	+	±
Collecting tubules	+	+	Uterus		
Other tubules	+	−	Endometrium	−	−
Basement membrane	+	−	Brain		
Muscle			White matter	+	−
Fascia	+	−	Gray matter	−	−
Muscle fiber	−	−			

Cited from Refs. *44* and *45*. More precise descriptions will be found in these references.

malignant cells. Biochemical studies have been performed for the receptors from three different cell lines, namely, a Burkitt lymphoma line, Daudi, a lung squamous carcinoma QG-56, and a gastric signet ring carcinoma KATO-III (*21*). The isolated receptors from the three sources had similar properties and behaved as glycoproteins with apparent molecular weights of 160,000 to 280,000 upon SDS gel electrophoresis. However, they showed a molecular weight of about 70,000 upon gel filtration, suggesting that they contained large amounts of carbohydrates. The size of the carbohydrate chain was estimated to be in the range from 3,500 to less than 1,000 by gel filtration of oligosaccharides and glycopeptides released by mild alkaline treatment and pronase digestion (Fig. 2). Thus, carbohydrate moieties of PNA receptors from these malignant cells were not as large as those of PNA receptors from EC cells. Further biochemical studies on PNA receptors from malignant cells will be an interesting subject, since some PNA receptors from certain malignant cells appear to be tumor-associated transplantation antigens (Hamaoka, T. *et al.*; Adachi, M. *et al.*, unpublished results).

In the monkey retina, PNA receptors were specifically expressed in the membranes

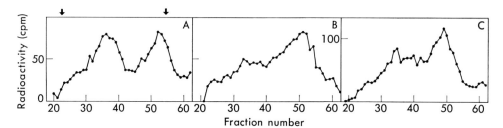

FIG. 2. Sephadex G-50 column chromatography of oligosaccharides and glycopeptides released from PNA receptors by mild alkaline treatment and pronase
digestion. Arrows indicate the elution position of blue dextran and galactose. A,
Daudi; B, QG-56; C, KATO-III. (cited from Ref *21*)

of cones (*43*). Thus, affinity chromatography using PNA may be helpful in isolating
cone-specific proteins which may participate in the recognition of color. Further, a
single glycoprotein of apparent molecular weight 65,000 has been isolated from human
nasal polyps by affinity chromatography on PNA-agarose (*5*).

Receptors for DBA

DBA is a lectin reacting with N-acetylgalactosamine residues (*2*). The lectin reacts
only with restricted areas in the organs of adult mice (*21, 45*) (Table II). In embryonic
mice tissues, the receptors are expressed in the following cells, with important characteristics. DBA receptors are expressed in preimplantation embryos until the early blastocyst stage (*3*). The intensity of staining with DBA labeled with a fluorescent dye was
found to decrease gradually, during the development of preimplantation embryos, and
the receptors disappeared in late blastocysts. The receptors reappeared in primitive
endoderm of 5-day-old embryos, and continued to be expressed in visceral endodermal
cells, parietal endodermal cells and embryonic gut cells (*34*). *In vitro* grown teratocarcinoma cells including certain EC cells express the receptors intensely. DBA receptors,
isolated from teratocarcinomas, were shown to be glycoproteins of molecular weights
more than 70,000 carrying the large carbohydrate chains, embryoglycan (*28*).

Most embryonic thymocytes of the 13th day of gestation were positive for DBA
receptors (*13*). The fraction of receptor-positive thymocytes gradually decrease during
embryogenesis, and thymocytes of newborn mice entirely lack them. GRSL leukemia
cells with the characteristics of pre-T leukemia cells also express DBA receptors, while
none of the lymphoid cells of the host express them (*27*). The receptors from GRSL
cells were shown to be glycoproteins of molecular weight around 100,000. Their carbohydrate moieties were only 4,000–1,000 in molecular weight and were smaller compared to those from teratocarcinomas (*27*).

Two new antigenic determinants were found in DBA receptors isolated from teratocarcinoma OTT6050. When the rabbit antiserum raised against the DBA receptors
was massively absorbed by a membrane fraction of liver, the antiserum reacted only
with visceral endoderm in early post-implantation embryos and with renal tubular brush
border of the adult (*35*). This antigen termed "brushin" was shown to be carried by
large glycoprotein(s) of molecular weight around 500,000 both in teratocarcinomas and
in the kidney. The antigenic marker will be helpful in following the differentiation

of visceral endoderm. Furthermore, the possible relationship of brushin with the nephrogenic antigen is of great interest.

By immunoaffinity chromatography on immobilized embryoglycan, anti-carbohydrate antibodies could be isolated from rabbit antiserum against DBA receptors from teratocarcinoma OTT6050. The antigen(s) defined by the antibodies was termed teratocarcinoma-derived carbohydrate (TC) antigen (36). In the mouse, the distribution of TC antigen was very similar to that of DBA receptors. Thus, the determinant of TC antigen appears to be the major DBA binding site in the mouse. It should be noted that TC antigen was not detected in human type A erythrocytes nor in sheep erythrocytes, although DBA reacts with these erythrocytes. The results with TC antigen thus appear to provide evidence that most of the DBA binding sites in the mouse are different from A antigen or Forssman antigen. The exact structure of the DBA binding site (TC antigen) in the mouse is under current investigation.

A New Fucosyl Antigen

Since EC cells express the unusual fucosyl carbohydrate, embryoglycan, we tried to detect the antigentic determinant by using synthetic carbohydrate haptens. A trisaccharide Fucα1→3Galβ1→4Glc, newly synthesized at the laboratory of Prof. S. Tejima was coupled to bovine serum albumin (BSA) by the p-isothiocyanate-phenethylamine (PIP) method (42). Rabbit antiserum raised against the synthetic antigen, 3'-fucosyllactose-PIP-BSA, reacted with the antigen, but not with 4'-fucosyllactose-IPI-BSA, 6'-fucosyllactose-PIP-BSA, lactose-PIP-BSA nor with BSA. This antiserum reacted only in a severely restricted area in mouse tissues, and from the reactivity it was confirmed that the antigen recognized by the antiserum was different from H antigen (Fucα1→2Gal) or from SSEA-1 (Fucα1→3GlcNAc). Thus, we proposed that the antiserum specifically recognized the Fucα1→3Gal linkage. The antigen recognized by the antiserum was termed "FG3 antigen" (20). FG3 antigen was detected in some EC cells, although the degree of its expression was rather weak. Unexpectedly, FG3 antigen was found to be intensely expressed in human colon adenocarcinoma. Out of 17 cancers examined, 12

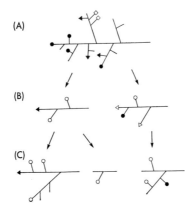

Fɪɢ. 3.   A model of carbohydrate alteration during differentiation. — core structure; ●, △, ○ non-reducing terminal. (cited from Ref 32) (A) early embryos; (B) late embryos; (C) adult.

were positive in the antigen. Normal colon tissue was negative in all cases (*20*). Many human tissues so far examined have also been negative.

CONCLUDING REMARKS

The alteration of cell surface carbohydrates during differentiation is a complex process and involves both the core structures and non-reducing terminal structures (Fig. 3). Further studies on the exact nature of these structural changes, on the mode of their genetic control and on the biological meaning of the structural changes will contribute to our basic understanding of the secret of cellular differentiation and its abnormalities in malignancy and other pathology.

Acknowledgments

I am grateful to many colleagues for collaboration in the work mentioned in this review. The expert secretarial assistance of Miss Kumiko Sato is greatly appreciated. Experiments performed in our laboratory were supported by grants from the Ministry of Education, Science and Culture, Japan (Grant-in-Aid for Cancer Research 56015061, 57015082, for Scientific Research 56480366, and for Special Project Research), the Ministry of Health and Welfare Japan (Grant-in-Aid for Cancer Research), the Otsuka Tokushima Institute and the Naito Foundation.

REFERENCES

1. Artzt, K., Dubois, P., Bennett, D., Condamine, H., Babinet, C., and Jacob, F. *Proc. Natl. Acad. Sci. U.S.*, **70**, 2988–2992 (1973).
2. Etzler, M. *Methods Enzymol.*, **28**, 340–344 (1972).
3. Fujimoto, H., Muramatsu, T., Urushihara, H., and Yanagisawa, K. O. *Differentiation*, **22**, 59–61 (1982).
4. Fukuda, M. N., Watanabe, K., and Hakomori, S. *J. Biol. Chem.*, **253**, 6814 6819 (1978).
5. Fukuda, K., Matsuyama, H., Fukami, K., Ozawa, M., Muramatsu, T., and Ohyama, M. *Acta Otol. Rhinol. Laryngol.*, in press.
6. Gachelin, G., Buc-Caron, M. H., Lis, H., and Sharon, N. *Biochim. Biophys. Acta*, **435**, 825–832 (1976).
7. Gooi, H. C., Feizi, T., Kapadia, A., Knowles, B. B., Solter, D., and Evans, M. J. *Nature*, **292**, 156–158 (1981).
8. Hakomori, S., Fukuda, M., and Nudelman, E. *In* "Teratocarcinoma and Embryonic Cell Interactions," ed. T. Muramatsu, G. Gachelin, A. A. Moscona, and Y. Ikawa, pp. 179–200 (1982). Japan Sci. Soc. Press, Tokyo / Academic Press, Tokyo and New York.
9. Hamada, H., Sato, M., Murata, F., and Muramatsu, T. *Exp. Cell Res.*, **144**, 489–495 (1983).
10. Jacob, F. *Immunol. Rev.*, **33**, 3–32 (1977).
11. Järnefelt, J., Rush, J., Li, Y.-T., and Laine, R. *J. Biol. Chem.*, **253**, 8006–8009 (1978).
12. Kapadia, A., Feizi, T., and Evans, M. J. *Exp. Cell Res.*, **131**, 185–195 (1981).
13. Kasai, M., Ochiai, Y., Habu, S., Muramatsu, T., Tokunaga, T., and Okumura, K. *Immunol. Lett.*, **2**, 157–158 (1980).
14. Kawata, M., Higaki, K., Sekiya, S., Takamizawa, Y., Muramatsu, T., and Okumura, K. *Clin. Exp. Immunol.*, **51** 401–406 (1983).
15. Krusius, T., Fiine, J., and Rauvala, H. *Eur. J. Biochem.*, **92**, 289 (1978).
16. Lloyd, K. O. and Kabat, E. A. *Proc. Natl. Acad. Sci. U.S.*, **61**, 1470–1477 (1968).
17. London, J., Berrih, S., and Bach, J.-F. *J. Immunol.*, **121**, 438 (1978).

18. Lotan, R. and Sharon, N. *Methods Enzymol.*, **50**, 361–367 (1978).
19. Martin, G. R. *Science*, **209**, 768–776 (1980).
20. Miyauchi, T., Yonezawa, S., Takamura, T., Chiba, T., Tejima, S., Ozawa, M., Sato, E., and Muramatsu, T. *Nature*, **299**, 168–169 (1982).
21. Miyauchi, T., Muramatsu, H., Ozawa, M., Mizuta, T., Suzuki, T., and Muramatsu, T. *Gann*, **73**, 581–587 (1982).
22. Muramatsu, T., Gachelin, G., Nicolas, J. F., Condamine, H., Jakob, H., and Jacob, F. *Proc. Natl. Acad. Sci. U.S.*, **75**, 2315–2319 (1978).
23. Muramatsu, T., Gachelin, G., and Jacob, F. *Biochim. Biophys. Acta*, **587**, 392–406 (1979).
24. Muramatsu, T., Avner, P., Fellous, M., Gachelin, G., and Jacob, F. *Somat. Cell Genet.*, **6**, 753–761 (1979).
25. Muramatsu, T., Gachelin, G., Damonneville, M., Delarbre, C., and Jacob, F. *Cell*, **18**, 183–191 (1979).
26. Muramatsu, T., Condamine, H., Gachelin, G., and Jacob, F. *J. Embryol. Exp. Morphol.*, **57**, 25–36 (1980).
27. Muramatsu, T., Muramatsu, H., Kasai, M., Habu, S., and Okumura, K. *Biochem. Biophys. Res. Commun.*, **96**, 1547–1553 (1980).
28. Muramatsu, T., Muramatsu, H., and Ozawa, M. *J. Biochem.*, **89**, 473–481 (1981).
29. Muramatsu, H. and Muramatsu, T. *Dev. Biol.*, **90**, 441–444 (1982).
30. Muramatsu, H., Muramatsu, T., and Avner, P. *Cancer Res.*, **42**, 1749–1752 (1982).
31. Muramatsu, T., Muramatsu, H., Gachelin, G., and Jacob, F. *In* "Teratocarcinoma and Embryonic Cell Interactions," ed. T. Muramatsu, G. Gachelin, A. A. Moscona, and Y. Ikawa, pp. 143–156 (1982). Japan Sci. Soc. Press, Tokyo/Academic Press, Tokyo and New York.
32. Muramatsu, T., Muramatsu, H., Ozawa, M., Hamada, H., Gachelin, G., and Tejima, S. *In* "Teratocarcinoma Stem Cells," ed. L. Silver, G. Martin, and S. Strickland, Cold Spring Harbor Press, Cold Spring Harbor, in press.
33. Muramatsu, H., Ishihara, H., Miyauchi, T., Gachelin, G., Fujisaki, T., Tejima, S., and Muramatsu, T. *J. Biochem.*, in press.
34. Noguchi, M., Noguchi, T., Watanabe, M., and Muramatsu, T. *J. Embryol. Exp. Morphol.*, **72**, 39–52 (1983).
35. Ozawa, M., Yonezawa, S., Sato, E., and Muramatsu, T. *Dev. Biol.*, **91**, 351–359 (1982).
36. Ozawa, M., Yonezawa, S., Miyauchi, T., Sato, E., and Muramatsu, T. *Biochem. Biophys. Res. Commun.*, **105**, 495–501 (1982).
37. Pinsker, M. C. and Mintz, B. *Proc. Natl. Acad. Sci. U.S.*, **70**, 1645–1648 (1973).
38. Prujanski-Jacobovits, A., Gachelin, G., Muramatsu, T., Sharon, N., and Jacob, F. *Biochem. Biophys. Res. Commun.*, **89**, 448–455 (1979).
39. Reisner, Y., Lenker-Israfli, M., and Sharon, N. *Cell Immunol.*, **25**, 129–134 (1976).
40. Reisner, Y., Gachelin, G., Dubois, P., Nicolas, J. F., Sharon, N., and Jacob, F. *Dev. Biol.*, **61**, 20–27 (1977).
41. Shur, B. D. *Dev. Biol.*, **91**, 149–162 (1982).
42. Smith, D. F., Zopf, D. A., and Ginsburg, V. *Methods Enzymol.*, **50**, 169–175 (1978).
43. Uehara, F., Sameshima, M., Muramatsu, T., and Ohba, N. *Exp. Eye Res.*, **36**, 113–123 (1983).
44. Watanabe, M., Muramatsu, T., Shirane, H., and Ugai, K. *J. Histochem. Cytochem.*, **29**, 779–790 (1981).
45. Watanabe, M., Takeda, Z., Urano, Y., and Muramatsu, T. *In* "Teratocarcinoma and Embryonic Cell Interactions," ed. T. Muramatsu, G. Gachelin, A. A. Moscona, and Y. Ikawa, pp. 217–228 (1982). Japan Sci. Soc. Press, Tokyo / Academic Press, Tokyo and New York.

GANN Monograph on Cancer Research 29, 1983

HUMAN GASTRIC CANCER-ASSOCIATED CHANGES IN GASTRIC GLYCOPROTEINS

Kyoko Hotta, Kazue Goso, Masao Kakei, Susumu Ohara, and Kazuhiko Ishihara

Department of Biochemistry, School of Medicine, Kitasato University*

Human gastric cancer-associated changes in gastric glycoproteins were investigated by organ culture technique using gastric biopsies and resection specimens. Radiolabeled glycoproteins were prepared by incorporation of [^{35}S]sulfate and [^{14}C] or [^{3}H]glucosamine into corpus and antral mucosa and separated by Bio-Gel A-1.5 m chromatography in void volume. Normal gastric mucosa synthesized sulfated glycoproteins in all age distribution. The sulfate incorporation increased in gastric mucosa obtained from specimens harboring gastric cancer whereas glucosamine uptake was almost unchanged. The increased ^{35}S-incorporation was mainly associated with sulfated glycoproteins and to lesser extent with glycosaminoglycan, and 70% of the sulfate was resistant with pronase digestion. The synthesized glycoproteins by non-cancer specimen were digestable with pronase treatment and characterized mainly as neutral glycoproteins.

Histochemical and biochemical studies indicate that neutral glycoproteins and acidic glycoproteins with or without sulfate are present in gastric mucosa, and that glycoproteins are the main carbohydrate-protein component of gastric mucus and cell membranes (*9*). Gastric mucus glycoproteins have well-defined features, distinct from polysaccharide-protein complexes of connective tissue origin and are high molecular weight compounds with large numbers of carbohydrate side chains attached to a protein core through an O-glycosidic linkage (*4, 9, 22*). Regional variations of the gastric glycoproteins exist qualitatively and quantitatively (*20*). While there is full agreement regarding the predominance of neutral mucins in the human gastric mucosa, the presence of sulfomucin is still a matter of debate (*15*). Although sulfated mucosubstances have been demonstrated in human gastric epithelium by autoradiography in *in vitro* ^{35}SO$_4$ uptake studies and by immunofluorescence, histochemical staining methods reveal traces only (*5*). Andre and Descos (*1*) could not detect sulfate in the gastric glycoprotein isolated from gastrectomy specimens. To test for the presence of sulfated glycoproteins in human gastric mucosa, we investigated sulfated glycoprotein biosynthesis in gastric mucosal biopsies assessed by incorporation of ^{35}S-sulfate and ^{14}C-glucosamine employing an organ culture, and the results suggest that normal gastric mucosa synthesizes sulfated glycoproteins although the synthetic rates are different in different stomach regions (*13*).

Histochemical observations show a significant association between sulfomucin secretion and intestinal metaplasia or gastric cancer (*12, 18*). Mucins secreted by gastric carcinomas frequently contain significant acid components (*9*). Moreover, it has been found that the synthetic levels of sulfated glycoproteins are elevated in gastric mucosa

---

* Kitasato 1-15-1, Sagamihara 228, Japan (堀田恭子, 五艘一恵, 筧　正雄, 小原　進, 石原和彦).

with gastric cancer induced by N-methyl-N′-nitro-N-nitrosoguanidine compared to that of normal rats (*19*).

We focus on trying to understand the qualitative and quantitative changes of gastric sulfated glycoproteins responsible for such gastric cancer.

Organ Culture of Human Gastric Mucosa by Biopsied Specimens and Gastric Mucus Glyco-proteins

In vitro organ culture of mucosa is a well-established technique in the studies of mucosal function and metabolism. The organ culture method was mainly used for label-ing of glycoproteins of intestinal mucosa, with isotopic precursors (*16, 17*). Since the method has proved useful for the investigation of gastric mucosal glycoprotein biosyn-thesis (*3, 11, 19, 21*), we examined its suitability using biopsied specimens obtained from human gastric mucosa (*13*). Biopsies of human gastric mucosa cultured for 8 hr main-tained an intact and morphologically near normal mucosa, and incorporated labeled precursors at a constant rate into gastric macromolecular glycoproteins. When individual biopsies from the same region of a single stomach were compared, reproducible results for the incorporation of labeled precursors into the glycoproteins were obtained. We therefore employed the cultured biopsies to investigate cancer-associated changes in gastric glycoprotein biosynthesis.

Gastric mucosa was obtained during routine endoscopy using biopsy forceps. Two biopsies were taken from the site of the lesser curvature of the pyloric antrum and two from the site of the greater curvature of the stomach body of normal volunteers or from patients with cancer, under direct vision. Specimens from patients were biopsied from the normal mucosal area apart from the mucosa covered with cancer tissue. The biosyn-

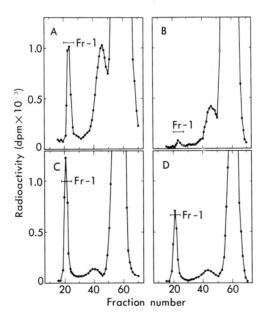

FIG. 1. Bio-Gel A-1.5 m column chromatography of the extract from healthy specimens incubated with [³⁵S]-sulfate (A and B) or [¹⁴C]-glucosamine (C and D). Solid bars indicate the fractions that were pooled as Fraction-1. A, C, antrum; B, D, corpus.

thesis of glycoproteins was assessed by incorporation of ^{35}S-sulfate and ^{14}C- or ^{3}H-glucosamine into the specimens. The glycoproteins were extracted from tissues with Tris buffer containing Triton X-100 followed by Bio-Gel A-1.5 m column chromatography. The first peak eluted with the excluded volume (Fr-1) corresponded to gastric mucus macromolecular neutral and acidic glycoproteins with or without sulfate as described previously (2). The elution pattern of one of the extracts from a healthy stomach on Bio-Gel A-1.5 m is shown in Fig. 1.

Biosynthesis of Glycoproteins by Gastric Healthy and Cancer Mucosa

There is histochemical evidence that sulfomucins are frequently found in gastric cancer (6, 12). It is necessary to investigate the evidence biochemically and to establish the relationship between this biochemical change and cancer. The biosynthetic rates of gastric sulfated glycoproteins have been found to differ markedly in patients with cancer compared to healthy subjects (7, 13, 14). The biopsied specimens were divided into three groups. Group I consists of healthy adults (7 males) aged 18 to 31 years, mean 22.0 years, and Group II (8 males and 3 females) aged 45 to 74 years, mean 58.6 years. Group III shown in Table I consists of patients with gastric cancer (5 males and 1 female) ranging from 52 to 72 years, mean 61.7 years. The mean values of incorporated ^{14}C-glucosamine into gastric mucus glycoproteins (Fr-1) remained at almost the same level among all the groups, I, II, and III (2,288–3,858 dpm/biopsy). Furthermore, there was no significant regional difference in the corpus and antral ^{14}C-labeled glycoproteins. The rate of incorporation of radioactive sulfate into the mucus glycoproteins (Fr-1) differed in the healthy and patient specimens, and in corpus and antral regions, shown in Fig. 2. Biopsies from patients with gastric cancer incorporated a significantly greater amount of ^{35}S-sulfate into the mucus glycoproteins than that obtained from healthy subjects. The highest mean value was found in antral glycoproteins of Group III (50,706 dpm/biopsy). Differences observed in ^{35}S-incorporation into healthy antral biopsies (Groups I and II) may be related to the age of specimens. There was a 10-fold increase in the mean value of the ^{35}S-incorporation into Group II glycoproteins (18,144 dpm/biopsy) than into those of Group I (1,698 dpm/biopsy). There was no age dependency in the corpus region. The ranges were limited in both Groups I (453 dpm/biopsy) and II (486 dpm/biopsy). The apparent and significant differences in the incorporation of ^{35}S-sulfate into corpus glycoproteins were present in healthy and cancer biopsies (Group III, 5,998 dpm/biopsy). By employing cultured biopsies, it is easily possible to obtain and measure sufficient numbers of normal subjects in a given age distribution. Although there are substantial differences of ^{35}S-incorporation between antral and corpus mucosa, the ^{14}C-incorporation rates are very similar in all cases. The increased ^{35}S-incorporation into antral mucosa observed

TABLE I. Summary of Patients with Gastric Cancer (Group III)

Case	Name	Age	Sex	Endoscopic diagnosis
1	T. O.	68	F	Borrman 3
2	M. K.	62	M	Borrman 2
3	H. S.	53	M	IIc
4	S. S.	52	M	IIc
5	S. U.	65	M	IIc+III like advanced
6	T. T.	70	M	Borrman 3

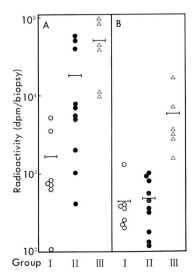

FIG. 2. Incorporation of [³⁵S]-sulfate into Fr-1 obtained from healthy volunteers
(○ Group I; ● Group II) and patients with gastric cancer (△ Group III). Solid
bars indicate the mean value of each group. A, antrum; B, corpus.

in Group II was seen in older individuals, that are at high risk for cancer. There is no
doubt that the biochemical change associated with gastric cancer might be detected prior
to the histochemically observable change. The increased ³⁵S-incorporation and unchanged ¹⁴C-incorporation into gastric mucus glycoproteins can be explained as follows:
1) The biosynthesis of sulfated glycoproteins is enhanced, while non-sulfated glycoprotein biosynthesis is inhibited, 2) part of the sulfate is transferred to the previously synthesized unlabeled glycoprotein, and/or 3) highly sulfated glycoproteins are synthesized.
Histochemical findings support the first possibility at present (6). However, there is in-
sufficient information to contradict the other possibilities.

Properties of Synthesized Sulfated Glycoproteins

Gastric sulfated glycoproteins have been studied with reference to their efficacy as
inhibitors of proteolysis by pepsin (23), the appearance of variants as detected by tumor
antigens (8) and as gastric juice components (10). Recently, aspects of the biosynthesis
of gastric sulfated glycoproteins *in vitro* have been reported (7, 13, 14, 19). To investigate
the quantitative differences between the synthesized sulfated glycoproteins by gastric
mucosa obtained from patients without cancer, with gastric cancer, or with gastric ulcer,
resected stomachs from patients were employed for organ culture experiments (7). The
³⁵S-sulfate and ³H-glucosamine labeled glycoproteins (Fr-1) of each specimen were
isolated with Bio-Gel A-1.5 m chromatography. Fr-1 obtained from corpus and antrum
regions of non-cancer specimens was completely resistant to chondroitinase ABC, chondroitinase AC, hyaluronidase, heparitinase, and keratanase digestion, whereas, Fr-1 from
the antral region of cancer specimens contained [³H]hyaluronic acid (7% ³H), [³H, ³⁵S]-
heparan sulfate (3% ³H, 10% ³⁵S) and [³H, ³⁵S] dermatan sulfate (3% ³H, 7% ³⁵S). The
increased ³⁵S-incorporation in the macromolecules of cancer specimens was mainly found
associated with sulfated glycoproteins and to a lesser extent with glycosaminoglycans.
Susceptibility to pronase digestion of Fr-1 was compared with elution patterns followed

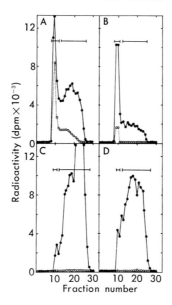

FIG. 3. Sepharose CL-4B column chromatography of pronase treated Fr-1. A and B were obtained from a patient with gastric cancer, and C and D were from gastric ulcer. Solid bars indicate the fractions which were pooled. A, C, antrum; B, D, corpus. ● ³H; ○ ³⁵S.

TABLE II. Specific Activity and Susceptibility to Pronase Digestion of Fr-1

		^{3}H		^{35}S	
		dpm[a]	%[b]	dpm[a]	%[b]
Cancer	Antrum	405.6		156.9	
	Undigested		41		67
	Digested		59		33
	Corpus	182.8		27.2	
	Undigested		50		69
	Digested		50		31
Ulcer	Antrum	331.4		4.6	
	Undigested		5		1
	Digested		95		99
	Corpus	277.3		0.7	
	Undigested		7		2
	Digested		93		98

[a] Expressed as dpm$\times 10^{-3}$ per mg protein of tissue homogenate.

[b] Expressed as percent distribution.

by Sepharose CL-4B chromatography of the digests (Fig. 3). The specific activity and distribution of radioactivities in each fraction separated by the Sepharose column are shown in Table II. Most of the glycoproteins synthesized by non-cancer specimens were digestible with the pronase treatment, and recovered as neutral glycoproteins with diethylaminoethyl (DEAE)-Sephacel. The presence of pronase-undigested material seems to reflect malignant or metaplastic change of gastric mucosa. The undigested fraction isolated from the antrum of cancer specimens consisted mainly of sulfated glycoproteins.

CONCLUDING COMMENT

It has been ascertained that normal gastric mucosa synthesizes sulfated glycoproteins in all ages and the synthetic rates of sulfated glycoproteins are elevated with gastric mucosa from specimens harboring gastric cancer. Present knowledge of the alterations of glycoproteins in gastric mucosa owes much to histochemistry. We believe that further biochemical investigations of this kind are necessary to lead to early cancer diagnosis.

Acknowledgment

This work was supported in part by Grants-in Aid from the Japanese Ministry of Education and the Ministry of Health and Welfare (Cancer 55–21).

REFERENCES

1. Andre, F. and Descos, E. *Biochim. Biophys. Acta*, **386**, 129–137 (1975).
2. Azuumi, Y., Ohara, S., Ishihara, K., Okabe, H., and Hotta, K. *Gut*, **21**, 533–536 (1980).
3. Browning, T. H. and Trier, J. S. *J. Clin. Invest.*, **48**, 1423 (1969).
4. Buddecke, E. *In* "Glycoproteins, A," Vol. 5, 2nd Ed., ed. A. Gottschalk, BBA library, pp. 535–545 (1972). Elsevier Publishing Co., Amsterdam.
5. Filipe, M. I. *Invest. Cell Pathol.*, **2**, 195–216 (1979).
6. God, A. *Br. J. Cancer*, **23**, 52–63 (1969).
7. Goso, K., Kakei, M., Ohara, S., Ishihara, K., and Hotta, K. *In* "Proc. 12th Int. Congr. Biochem.," Perth, 1982, Abstr. p. 344.
8. Häkkinen, I.P.T. *Transplant. Rev.*, **20**, 61–76 (1974).
9. Horowitz, M. I. *In* "The Glycoconjugates," Vol. 1, ed. M. I. Horowitz and W. Pigman, pp. 189–214 (1977). Academic Press, New York.
10. Hotta, K. and Goso, K. *Anal. Biochem.*, **110**, 338–341 (1981).
11. Ishihara, K., Ohara, S., Azuumi, Y., Hotta, K., Kakei, M., and Okabe, H. *Japan. J. Gastroenterol.*, **78**, 1896–1900 (1981) (in Japanese).
12. Jass, J. R. and Filipe, M. I. *Histopathology*, **3**, 191–199 (1979).
13. Kakei, M., Okabe, H., Ohara, S., Goso, K., Ishihara, K., and Hotta, K. *In* "Proc. 7th World Congr. of Gastroenterology," Stockholm, 1982, Abstr. p. 83.
14. Kakei, M., Ohara, S., Ishihara, K., Goso, K., Okabe, H., and Hotta, K. *Gut*, submitted for publication.
15. Lambert, R. and Andre, C. *Digestion*, **5**, 116–122 (1972).
16. LaMont, J. T. and Ventola, A. *Gastroenterology*, **72**, 82–86 (1977).
17. MacDermott, R. P., Donaldson, R. M., Jr., and Trier, J. S. *J. Clin. Invest.*, **54**, 545–554 (1974).
18. Matsukura, N., Suzuki, K., Kawachi, T., Aoyagi, M., Sugimura, T., Kitaoka, H., Numajiri, H., Shirota, A., Itabashi, M., and Hirota, T. *J. Natl. Cancer Inst.*, **65**, 231–240 (1980).
19. Ohara, S., Ishihara, K., Goso, K., and Hotta, K. *In* "Proc. VIth Int. Symp. Glycoconjugates," Tokyo, 1981, pp. 255–256.
20. Ohara, S., Ishihara, K., Kakei, M., Azuumi, Y., and Hotta, K. *Comp. Biochem. Physiol. B*, **72**, 309–311 (1982).
21. Ohara, S., Kakei, M., Ishihara, K., and Hotta, K. *Comp Biochem. Physiol. B*, submitted for publication.
22. Sheahan, D. G. and Jervis, H. R. *Am. J. Anat.*, **146**, 103–132 (1976).
23. Takagaki, Y. M. and Hotta, K. *Biochim. Biophys. Acta*, **584**, 288–297 (1979).

V. ENZYMES OF GLYCOCONJUGATE METABOLISM IN CANCER

ENZYMATIC CONTROL OF OLIGOSACCHARIDE BRANCHING DURING SYNTHESIS OF MEMBRANE GLYCOPROTEINS

Harry Schachter,[*1],[*2] Saroja Narasimhan,[*2] Paul Gleeson,[*2] and George Vella[*2]

*Department of Biochemistry, University of Toronto[*1] and Division of Biochemistry Research, Hospital for Sick Children[*2]*

Many mammalian and avian complex carbohydrates (glycoproteins and glycolipids) have highly branched oligosaccharides. Although the function of complex carbohydrates is not known, there is evidence to suggest that oligosaccharide branching may be an important factor in the process by which cells recognize one another and their environment. One of the most consistent biochemical correlations with malignant transformation is a relative increase in the release of high molecular weight glycopeptide from the cell surface by proteolytic cleavage. The increase in molecular weight on transformation is believed to be due to increased oligosaccharide branching. Asparagine-linked (N-glycosyl) oligosaccharides can be subdivided into at least 12 classes according to their branching patterns. It is presently believed that these classes all stem from a common precursor oligosaccharide containing 3 D-glucose, 9 D-mannose, and 2 N-acetyl-D-glucosamine residues. This precursor is incorporated into the protein backbone in the rough endoplasmic reticulum and is then processed within the endoplasmic reticulum and Golgi apparatus by a series of highly specific glycosidases and glycosyltransferases to yield the various classes of N-glycosyl oligosaccharides. The branches that occur in N-glycosyl oligosaccharides are usually initiated by the incorporation of a GlcNAc residue. Our laboratory has studied four of the N-acetylglucosaminyltransferases (GlcNAc-transferases) involved in this initiation process. We have defined various factors which determine the synthetic pathway. There are at least three types of control that are commonly found. (1) Tissues differ in the relative activities of the different glycosyltransferases and glycosidases and therefore competition between two or more enzymes for a common intermediate often determines the synthetic route. (2) The incorporation of a key glycosyl residue into an oligosaccharide may convert a non-substrate to a substrate for either a glycosyltransferase or a glycosidase. (3) Conversely, the incorporation of a key residue may convert a substrate into a non-substrate. Recent studies on the three-dimensional structures of N-glycosyl oligosaccharides have enabled us to explain certain features of glycosyltransferase substrate specificity on the basis of steric factors. It is hoped that similar three-dimensional studies on cell surface oligosaccharides may help to explain their role in normal cell-cell interactions and in pathological processes such as metastasis.

[*1],[*2] Toronto, Ontario, Canada M5G 1×8.

Although the function of most complex carbohydrates remains unknown, there is evidence to suggest that the branching of N-glycosyl oligosaccharides on the cell surface may play a role in cell-cell interactions. One of the most consistent biochemical correlations with malignant transformation is a relative increase in the release of high molecular weight sialic acid-rich glycopeptide material from the cell surface by proteolytic cleavage (40). This material is believed to contain highly branched asparagine (Asn)-linked oligosaccharides. For example, Takasaki et al. (35) found that transformation of baby hamster kidney cells with polyoma virus led to a reduction in bi-antennary oligosaccharides, an increase in tetra-antennary oligosaccharides and the appearance of novel penta- and hexa-antennary oligosaccharides.

Our laboratory has been concerned for many years with the enzymatic control of oligosaccharide branching in both N- and O-glycosyl oligosaccharides. Our studies have thus far been carried out only with normal tissues. It is clear, however, that important changes occur in cell surface oligosaccharide branching patterns during malignant disease and we are presently embarking on a study of enzyme changes in pathological tissues. The present review will, however, be limited to our studies on normal tissues, primarily mammalian liver and the hen oviduct.

Oligosaccharide Structure

Protein-bound oligosaccharides are classified according to the covalent linkage between amino acid and carbohydrate. The major linkages in avian and mammalian glycoproteins are the N-glycosidic linkage between Asn and GlcNAc and three types of O-glycosidic linkage, serine (threonine) [Ser (Thr)]-GalNAc, Ser-xylose and hydroxylysine-Gal (13). The synthesis of the Asn-GlcNAc linkage is presently believed to be carried out by an oligosaccharide transferase in the rough endoplasmic reticulum which catalyzes the transfer of oligosaccharide from dolichol pyrophosphate oligosaccharide to either nascent ribosome-bound peptide or to post-ribosomal peptide (30). In several tissues it has been shown that the initial peptide-bound oligosaccharide contains 3 D-glucose (Glc), 9 D-mannose(Man), and 2 N-acetyl-D-glucosamine (GlcNAc) residues but this structure has not been established for all tissues. The protein-bound oligosaccharide is believed to be the precursor of all N-glycosyl oligosaccharides. These oligosaccharides all share a common core containing 3 Man and 2 GlcNAc residues (Fig. 1).

The large protein-bound oligosaccharide undergoes a series of processing reactions to form the various N-glycosyl oligosaccharides shown in Fig. 2. The high mannose structures containing from 4 to 9 Man residues (Fig. 2) are the most primitive N-glycosyl oligosaccharides from an evolutionary point of view. More advanced organisms (birds

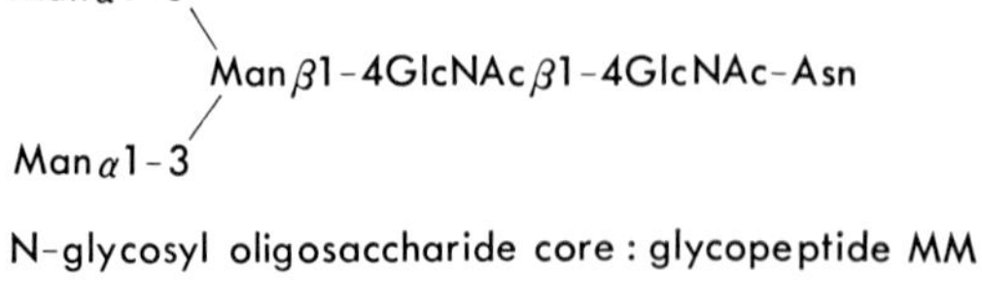

```
Manα1-6
         \
          Manβ1-4GlcNAcβ1-4GlcNAc-Asn
         /
Manα1-3
```

N-glycosyl oligosaccharide core : glycopeptide MM

FIG. 1. The structure of the core common to most N-glycosyl oligosaccharides. This structure is named MM to indicate that both arms are terminated in Man (M) residues.

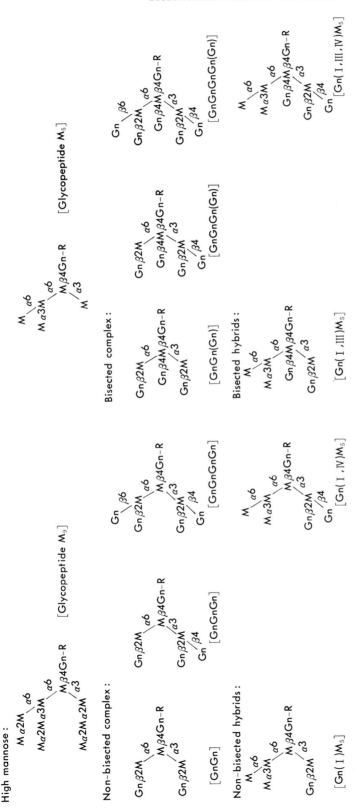

FIG. 2. N-glycosyl oligosaccharides can be classified into at least 12 types of structure. Examples of these types are shown in the figure. High mannose oligosaccharides are named according to the number of Man (M) residues, *e.g.*, M₅, M₉. Complex oligosaccharides are named according to the terminal sugars present on the arms (M, Man; Gn, GlcNAc; G, Gal; S, sialic acid; (Gn) represents a bisecting GlcNAc residue). The hybrids shown in the figure have only incomplete antennae (GlcNAc) and are named according to the positions of these GlcNAc residues using the code shown in Fig. 5.

and mammals) have retained these high mannose structures and have developed in addition a series of complex N-glycosyl oligosaccharides (Fig. 2).

Bi-, tri-, and tetra-antennary complex (also known as N-acetyllactosamine type) oligosaccharides carry 2, 3, or 4 branches or antennae attached to the common core (Fig. 2). A branch can be incomplete (either a single GlcNAc, or a Gal-GlcNAc disaccharide) or complete (a sialyl-Gal-GlcNAc trisaccharide). The linkage between Gal and GlcNAc is usually β1-4 (hence the name N-acetyllactosamine) but is occasionally β1-3. The linkage between sialic acid and Gal is either α2-3 or α2-6. Bisected complex oligosaccharides are similar except for an additional GlcNAc residue linked β1-4 to the β-linked Man residue of the core; this GlcNAc bisects the branches on the two arms of the core (Fig. 2), e.g., as in ovotransferrin (3). Hybrid oligosaccharides contain either 1 or 2 Man residues attached to the Man-α1-6 arm of the core and 1 or 2 complex-type branches (usually incomplete) on the Man-α1-3 arm of the core. The structure is thus a hybrid in the sense of having a high-mannose structure on one arm of the core and a complex structure on the other arm. Hybrid oligosaccharides are usually isolated as bisected structures, e.g., from ovalbumin (34). Non-bisected hybrid oligosaccharides have, however, been isolated from rhodopsin (6, 17). Poly-N-acetyllactosaminoglycan structures carrying i and I blood group antigenic determinants have also been found attached to the common N-glycosyl core in human erythrocyte band 3 (4, 5, 11), K-562 cells derived from human chronic myelogenous leukemia (38) and Chinese hamster ovary cell membranes (16).

Biosynthesis of High Mannose Oligosaccharides Precedes Synthesis of Complex Oligosaccharides

The synthetic process begins with the synthesis of dolichol pyrophosphate oligosaccharide (Fig. 3) and the transfer of oligosaccharide to polypeptide within the rough endoplasmic reticulum (Fig. 4). Processing (Fig. 4) of the protein-bound oligosaccharide (Glc)$_3$(Man)$_9$(GlcNAc)$_2$ begins with the removal of the 3 Glc residues by at least two

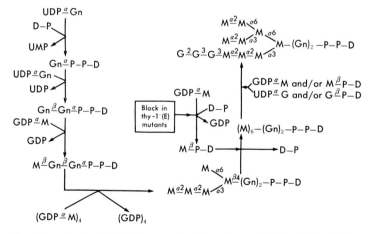

FIG. 3. Biosynthesis of dolichol pyrophosphate oligosaccharide. Abbreviations: D, dolichol; P, phosphate; UMP, uridine monophosphate; Gn, GlcNAc; M, Man; G, D-glucose. The final product is (Glc)$_3$ (Man)$_9$ (GlcNAc)$_2$ attached to dolichol by a pyrophosphate link.

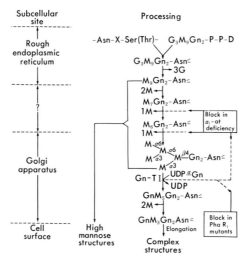

FIG. 4.   Oligosaccharide processing of protein-bound N-glycosyl oligosaccharides. Abbreviations: G, D-glucose; M, Man; Gn, GlcNAc; P, phosphate; D, dolichol; Gn-T I, UDP-GlcNAc: α-D-mannoside β1-2-GlcNAc-transferase I.

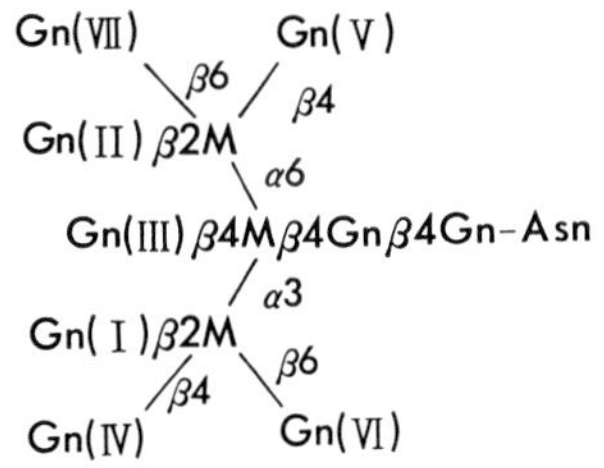

$$Gn(VII) \qquad Gn(V)$$
$$\begin{array}{cc} {}^{\beta 6} \searrow & / {}^{\beta 4} \\ & \end{array}$$
$$Gn(II)\,\beta 2M$$
$$\searrow {}^{\alpha 6}$$
$$Gn(III)\,\beta 4M\beta 4Gn\beta 4Gn-Asn$$
$$/ {}^{\alpha 3}$$
$$Gn(I)\,\beta 2M$$
$$/ {}^{\beta 4} \qquad \searrow {}^{\beta 6}$$
$$Gn(IV) \qquad Gn(VI)$$

FIG. 5.   A hypothetical structure showing all the possible GlcNAc residues that can be attached to the core. We have numbered these GlcNAc residues as indicated. This numbering system is used to name compounds (see hybrids in Fig. 2) and GlcNAc-transferases. Abbreviations as for Fig. 2.

α-glucosidases in the rough endoplasmic reticulum and 0 to 6 of the 9 Man residues are removed primarily in the Golgi apparatus (32). The number of Man residues removed varies from one oligosaccharide to the other. If 0 to 4 of the peripheral α2-linked Man residues are removed by α2-mannosidase(s) I, the result is a high-mannose type of oligosaccharide (Fig. 2). A sub-class of high mannose structure with mannose-6-phosphate residues has been found in some lysosomal hydrolases (14). Further oligosaccharide processing followed by a series of elongation reactions (discussed in detail in this review) lead the synthetic pathway from M_5 (the product of α2-mannosidase(s) I action, Fig. 2) towards at least 11 other classes of N-glycosyl oligosaccharides (Fig. 2; Ref. 2).

Some glycoproteins contain high-mannose oligosaccharides, others contain complex oligosaccharides and some glycoproteins contain both, e.g., calf thyroglobulin. The biosynthetic factors which determine whether an oligosaccharide remains high mannose or is processed further are not known but it is probable that the amino acid sequence near the glycosylation site is involved. The high mannose $(Man)_5(GlcNAc)_2$-Asn structure shown in Fig. 2 (M_5) is the starting point for the biosynthesis of all complex and hybrid N-glycosyl oligosaccharides. A series of Golgi apparatus-localized glycosyltransferases and α-mannosidases carry out these processing and elongation reactions.

Branches are usually initiated by the incorporation of a GlcNAc residue. In fact, branches can be initiated on the N-glycosyl core in at least seven different ways (Fig. 5) and if one assumes the one linkage-one enzyme hypothesis (27, 28), there should be at least 7 different initiating GlcNAc-transferases. This laboratory has described 4 of the 7 theoretically possible GlcNAc-transferases; these enzymes incorporate the GlcNAc residues labelled as I, II, III, and IV in Fig. 5 and the transferases are numbered accordingly. Evidence will be presented to show that these transferases play important roles in controlling the branching patterns commonly found in N-glycosyl oligosaccharides.

Uridine Diphosphate (UDP)-GlcNAc: α-D-Mannoside β1-2-GlcNAc-Transferase I

Johnston et al. (12) first reported the presence in goat colostrum of a GlcNAc-transferase acting on α_1-acid glycoprotein pre-treated with neuraminidase, β-galactosidase and β-N-acetylglucosaminidase. A similar enzyme has been found in many tissues (26, 28) of the rat, pig, guinea pig, and human and has been localized to the Golgi apparatus in rat liver (20). Studies on lectin-resistant mutants of Chinese hamster ovary cells (8, 22, 29) and baby hamster kidney cells (39) indicated that the high molecular weight acceptor detects at least two different GlcNAc-transferases. One of these enzymes, UDP-GlcNAc: α-D-mannoside β-1-2-GlcNAc-transferase I (GlcNAc-transferase I), attaches GlcNAc in β1-2 linkage to the Manα1-3- terminus of the tri-mannosyl core of glycopeptide M_5, as shown in Fig. 6. This enzyme has been purified from bovine colostrum (9), rabbit liver (24), pig liver, and pig tracheal mucosa (19, 25).

The substrate specificity of GlcNAc-transferase I is summarized in Table I. The enzyme appears to be specific for the terminal Manα1-3 residue of the core since it does not attack the other more peripheral terminal Manα1-3 residue of M_5 (Figs. 2 and 6).

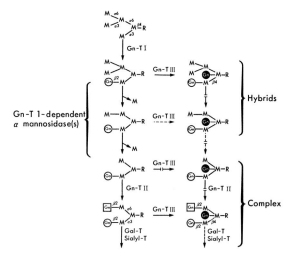

FIG. 6. Pathway showing the actions of GlcNAc-transferases I and II, GlcNAc-transferase I-dependent α3/6-mannosidase (mannosidase II) and the synthesis of hybrid oligosaccharides. M, Man; Gn, GlcNAc; T, transferase. Proven reactions are shown by solid arrows, unproven but likely reactions by discontinuous arrows and blocked reactions by blocked arrows.

TABLE I. Substrate Specificity of GlcNAc-transferases I and II

Substrate[a]	GlcNAc-transferase I K_m (mM)	GlcNAc-transferase II K_m (mM)
Mβ4Gn /α3 M M \α6	7.4	Not active
Mβ4Gn–R /α3 M Mα3M \α6	0.20	Not active
Mβ4Gn–R /α3 M M \α6 Mα3M \α6	Active	Not tested
Mβ4Gn–R /α3 M M \α6	0.12	Not active
Mβ4Gn–R /α3 Gnβ2M M \α6	10[b]	0.1
M \α6 Gnβ4Mβ4Gn–R /α3 Gnβ2M	Not active	Not active

[a] Abbreviations: M, Man; Gn, GlcNAc; R, (+/−Fucα6) Gn-Asn-.

[b] Oppenheimer and Hill (24) report that their highly purified GlcNAc-transferase I is totally inactive with this substrate.

The physiological substrate is probably the 5-mannose oligosaccharide M_5 since Chinese hamster ovary cell mutants lacking GlcNAc-transferase I accumulate glycoproteins with the M_5 structure (15, 33). However, Kornfeld (14) has pointed out that normal cells possess an alternate pathway involving the action of GlcNAc-transferase I on the 3-mannose structure MM shown in Fig. 1. This alternate pathway is usually a minor pathway in normal cells but becomes the major path under certain conditions in normal cells (e.g., glucose deprivation) or in cell mutants with an inability to make dolichol monophosphate mannose; the result is a truncated dolichol pyrophosphate oligosaccharide, containing 5 instead of 9 mannose residues, which on oligosaccharide processing leads to the MM structure (Fig. 1).

The fact that mutants lacking GlcNAc-transferase I accumulate the high mannose oligosaccharide M_5 (Fig. 2) and fail to make complex or hybrid structures indicates that the M_5 structure is the precursor of these oligosaccharides. Further, GlcNAc-transferase I action is essential for processing of M_5 to complex and hybrid structures.

GlcNAc-Transferase I-Dependent α3/6-Mannosidase(s) (Mannosidase II)

The product of GlcNAc-transferase I, Gn(I)M_5, sits at an important cross-roads

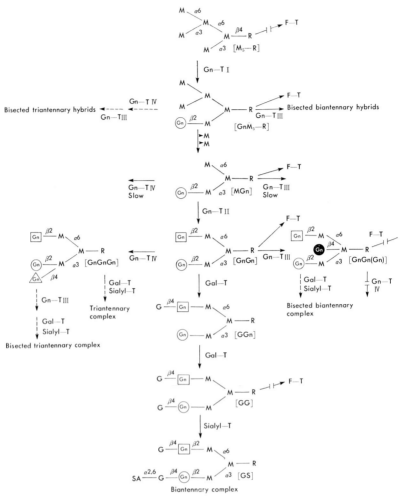

FIG. 7. Pathway showing the synthesis of complex oligosaccharides. Abbreviations: M, Man; Gn, GlcNAc; F, Fuc; T, transferase. Oligosaccharides are named according to the terminal sugars with the sugar on the Manα1-6- arm being named first. Proven reactions are shown by solid arrows, unproven but likely reactions by discontinuous arrows and blocked reactions by blocked arrows.

(top of Fig. 7) in that it can be acted on by at least three glycosyltransferases and one highly specific α-mannosidase. The glycosyltransferases lead towards the synthesis of hybrid oligosaccharides (discussed below). The 'main line' pathway *via* the α-mannosidase leads towards the various complex oligosaccharide structures shown in Fig. 2. These structures all have only 3 Man residues. The enzyme which removes 2 Man residues from Gn(I)M_5 is an α-mannosidase absolutely dependent on the prior action of GlcNAc-transferase I (*10, 31*); the enzyme will not work on M_5 but only on Gn(I)M_5 (Figs. 6, 7, and 8a). This GlcNAc-transferase I-dependent α3/6-mannosidase is the first committed step towards the synthesis of complex oligosaccharides. It appears to be the same enzyme as the α-mannosidase II purified from rat liver Golgi-rich membranes by Tulsiani *et al.* (*37*). The highly purified enzyme catalyzes the release of both the α3- and α6-Man residues from Gn(I)M_5. The formation of the 4-mannose intermediate

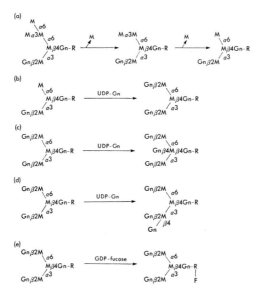

FIG. 8. Reactions catalyzed by five enzymes requiring the prior action of GlcNAc-transferase I which inserts GlcNAc(I) in β1-2 linkage into the Manα1-3- arm of the core. Abbreviations as for Fig. 7.

(Fig. 8a) is readily demonstrated but it is uncertain which Man residue is released preferentially (10). Tulsiani et al. (36) have recently shown that swainsonine causes the accumulation of high mannose intermediates by inhibiting the action of α-mannosidase II.

UDP-GlcNAc: α-D-Mannoside β1-2-GlcNAc-Transferase II

The study of lectin-resistant mutants of Chinese hamster ovary cells and baby hamster kidney cells deficient in GlcNAc-transferase I (see above) indicated the presence of a second UDP-GlcNAc: α-D-mannoside β1-2-GlcNAc-transferase designated GlcNAc-transferase II. The function of GlcNAc-transferase II is the initiation of the second antenna or branch by addition of GlcNAc in β1-2- linkage to the Manα1-6- terminus of glycopeptide MGn (Figs. 6, 7, and 8b). The enzyme has not been purified to homogeneity but partially purified preparations have been obtained from bovine colostrum (9), pig liver and pig trachea (25) and hen oviduct (G. Vella and H. Schachter, unpublished).

The only effective substrate for GlcNAc-transferase II is MGn (Table 1), the product of GlcNAc-transferase I-dependent α3/6-mannosidase. The enzyme does not act on MM (Fig. 1) indicating that GlcNAc-transferase I action must precede GlcNAc-transferase II. The product of GlcNAc-transferase II, GnGn (Fig. 2), is the major precursor for all complex oligosaccharides (see below).

UDP-GlcNAc: Glycopeptide GnGn β1-4-GlcNAc-Transferase III

GnGn, the product of GlcNAc-transferase II, sits at yet another cross-roads in the synthetic pathway. It is an excellent substrate for at least four glycosyltransferases

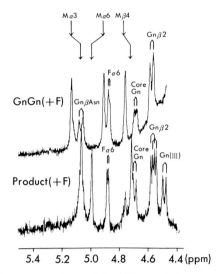

Fig. 9. Anomeric proton regions of the high resolution proton NMR spectra of glycopeptides GnGn (top) and GlcNAc-transferase III product (bottom). The identification of the signals is indicated. Gn(III) indicates the signal for the bisecting GlcNAc. This residue causes dramatic shifts (indicated at the top of the figure) in the signals of all three Man residues of the core.

TABLE II. Glycosyltransferase Substrate Specificities

Substrate[a]	Specific activity (µunits/mg)			
	Gn-T III pH 5.7	Gn-T III pH 7.0	Gn-T IV pH 7.0	Fuc-T pH 8.0
GnGn (+Fuc)	85	73	83	—[b]
GnGn (−Fuc)	—	75	95	1,800
MGn (+Fuc)	≤13	10	18	0
MGn (−Fuc)	—	—	—	3,100
MM (+Fuc)	≤7	≤16	≤16	0
MM (−Fuc)	—	—	—	0
GGn (+Fuc)	—	48	30	—
GnG (+Fuc)	—	≤5	≤5	—
GG (−Fuc)	—	≤8	≤8	0[c]
SS (−Fuc)	—	0	0	0
GnGn (Gn) (−Fuc)	—	—	≤3	0
MGn (Gn) (−Fuc)	—	—	—	0

Hen oviduct membranes were used for studies with GlcNAc-transferase III (Gn-T III) at pH 5.7 and 7.0, and GlcNAc-transferase IV (Gn-T IV) at pH 7.0. Golgi-enriched membranes from pig liver were used for the studies on GDP-Fuc: β-N-acetylglucosaminide (Fuc to Asn-linked GlcNAc) α1-6-fucosyltransferase (Fuc-T). These membranes are enriched 30-fold in Fuc-T relative to homogenate.

[a] Structures of glycopeptides GnGn, MGn, GGn, GG, and GnGn(Gn) are shown in Fig. 7. Glycopeptide MM is shown in Fig. 1. GnG is similar to GGn except that the Gal residue is on the Manα1-3-arm instead of the Manα1-6- arm. SS is fully sialylated bi-antennary complex glycopeptide with both sialyl residues linked α2-6-. The glycopeptides are named according to the terminal sugar residues with M, Man; Gn, GlcNAc; G, Gal; S, sialyl, and (Gn), bisecting GlcNAc. The sugar on the Manα1-6- arm is named first.

[b] Not done.

[c] Based on work with rat liver Golgi membranes (20) which lack fucosyltransferase activities towards Galβ1-4GlcNAc- terminated acceptors.

(Fig. 7): GlcNAc-transferases III and IV, β4-Gal-transferase and α6-fucosyltrans-ferase. GlcNAc-transferase III leads towards bisected bi-antennary complex oligosac-charides (Fig. 7). The enzyme has recently been reported in hen oviduct membranes (21). It attaches a bisecting GlcNAc residue to glycopeptide GnGn (see Figs. 7 and 8c for the reaction catalyzed). A similar reaction (discussed below) also occurs in hen ovi-duct membranes at the 5-Man, and possibly the 4-Man, stages (Fig. 6) but it is not yet known whether these various activities are catalyzed by one or more enzymes. GlcNAc-transferase III has been partially purified from hen oviduct (G. Vella and H. Schachter, unpublished data). The product of the reaction has been identified as GnGn (Gn) (Figs. 2 and 8c) by methylation analysis and high resolution proton nuclear magnetic resonance (NMR) spectrometry at 360 MHz (Fig. 9; Ref. 21).

The substrate specificity of GlcNAc-transferase III is shown in Table II. The ac-tivity of crude hen oviduct membranes towards glycopeptide GnGn is about 85 μunits/mg protein under standard assay conditions. GnGn preparations both with and without a Fucα1-6- residue attached to the Asn-linked GlcNAc give the same activity. Activities with MGn (Fig. 7) and MM (Fig. 1) relative to GnGn are less than 15% and 8%, re-spectively, at pH 5.7. Activity with glycopeptide GGn (Fig. 7) is about 60% of that with GnGn. However, the enzyme is essentially inactive with glycopeptide GnG (see Table II) and with the other glycopeptides tested.

UDP-GlcNAc: Glycopeptide GnGn β1-4-GlcNAc-Transferase IV

This enzyme has recently been described in hen oviduct membranes (7, 7a). It catalyzes the attachment of a GlcNAc residue in β1-4- linkage to the Manα1-3- arm of glycopeptide GnGn thereby initiating the third antenna or branch (see Figs. 7 and 8d for the reaction catalyzed). The enzyme therefore routes the synthetic pathway towards tri-antennary, bisected tri-antennary and tetra-antennary complex oligosaccharides. The enzyme has been partially purified from hen oviduct (G. Vella and H. Schachter, unpublished data).

The assay of both GlcNAc-transferases III and IV is complicated by the fact that they act on a common substrate, GnGn (Fig. 8c, d). It is therefore necessary to separate the products (GnGn(Gn) and GnGnGn, respectively) when crude enzyme sources con-taining both activities are being assayed. This can be accomplished by either concana-valin A (Con A)/Sepharose or pea lectin/agarose chromatography. Figure 10 shows a series of standard glycopeptides chromatographed on Con A/Sepharose; GnGn adheres to the column, GnGn(Gn) passes through in a retarded fashion and GnGnGn passes through unretarded. Figure 11 shows the Con A/Sepharose chromatogram of the prod-ucts of a standard enzyme incubation with crude hen oviduct membranes as enzyme source. GlcNAc-transferase III product is retarded on the column while GlcNAc-transferase IV product passes through unretarded. The latter product has been identi-fied as GnGnGn (Figs. 2 and 8d) by methylation analysis and high resolution proton NMR spectrometry at 360 MHz (Fig. 12) (7a).

The substrate specificity of GlcNAc-transferase IV is shown in Table II. Like GlcNAc-transferase III, the enzyme works on glycopeptide GnGn with or without a Fucα1-6- attached to the Asn-linked GlcNAc, works on glycopeptides MGn (Fig. 7) and GGn (Fig. 7) but at a lower rate than on GnGn, and works poorly or not at all on glycopeptide GnG (see Table II) and on the other glycopeptides tested. An interesting

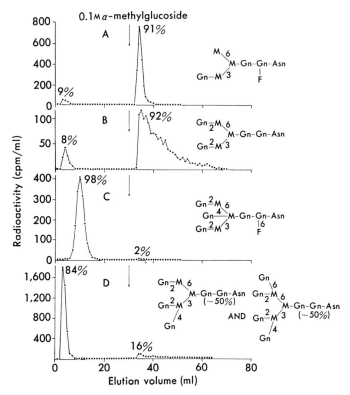

FIG. 10. N-[^{14}C]acetylated glycopeptide standards were chromatographed on Con A/Sepharose columns (0.6 × 9 cm) equilibrated and eluted at room temperature with 0.01 M Tris-HCl, pH 7.5, containing 0.1 M NaCl. At the arrow, 0.1 M methyl α-D-glucopyranoside was added to the buffer. Fraction size was 1.0 ml. (A) N-[^{14}C] acetyl glycopeptide MGn(+F). (B) N-[^{14}C]acetyl glycopeptide GnGn. (C) N-[^{14}C] acetyl glycopeptide GnGn(Gn)(+F). (D) A mixture of N-[^{14}C]acetyl tri- and tetra-antennary glycopeptides terminating in GlcNAc residues prepared from α_1-acid glycoprotein (18). Structural formulae are indicated in the figure using the abbreviations described in the legends to Figs. 2 and 7. The numbers over the peaks indicate the % recovery of radioactivity in that peak relative to the total radioactivity recovered from the column.

finding is that the presence of a bisecting GlcNAc on glycopeptide GnGn completely inhibits GlcNAc-transferase IV action (Table II). Thus, GlcNAc-transferase IV must act before GlcNAc-transferase III to form bisected tri-antennary complex oligosaccharides (Fig. 7) and this is probably true also for the synthesis of bisected tri-antennary hybrid oligosaccharides.

Substrate specificity studies on crude enzyme preparations (Table II) are often difficult and subject to artefacts. For example, not only is GnGn a substrate for both GlcNAc-transferases III and IV (discussed above) but the presence of β-N-acetylglucosaminidase in crude preparations can convert GnGn to MGn and MM, respective substrates for GlcNAc-transferases II and I (Fig. 13). This problem was approached in two ways. First, a β-N-acetylglucosaminidase inhibitor (e.g., GlcNAc) was always present in the incubation mixture. Second, the radioactive products of GlcNAc-transferases I and II (MGn and GnGn, respectively, Fig. 13) adhere to Con A/Sepharose and are

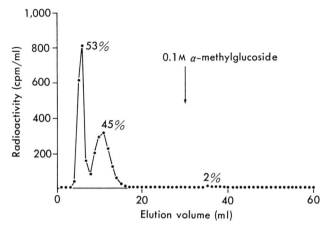

FIG. 11. Chromatography on Con A/Sepharose of the [¹⁴C]products from a standard GlcNAc-transferase IV incubation using hen oviduct membranes as enzyme source. Conditions of chromatography were as outlined in the legend to Fig. 10. The products were N-acetylated with non-radioactive acetic anhydride prior to chromatography. The % recoveries of radioactivity in the three peaks are indicated.

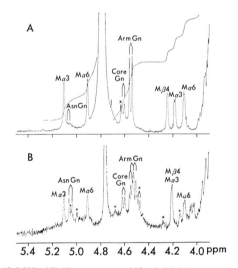

FIG. 12. The 360-MHz NMR spectra at 23° of GlcNAc-transferase IV substrate and product in the regions of anomeric hydrogen signals (4.4 to 5.5 ppm) and Man C-2 hydrogen signals (4.0 to 4.4 ppm). (A) Glycopeptide GnGn, the substrate for GlcNAc-transferase IV. (B) Enzyme product. The peak marked * has not been identified. The peaks marked with a star in Fig. 12B represent the signals from a minor enzymatic product which has been identified as bisected tri-antennary oligosaccharide formed by the sequential actions of GlcNAc-transferases IV and III (Fig. 7). The changes in the H-2 region are consistent with the addition of a GlcNAc in β1-4 linkage to the Manα1-3- arm of the core.

thus separated from the products of GlcNAc-transferases III and IV. Figure 11 shows that only 2% of the radioactive products from a standard hen oviduct incubation adhere to the lectin column. This is due to a relatively low rate of GnGn breakdown and to a relatively low level of GlcNAc-transferase I in hen oviduct membranes (G. Vella and

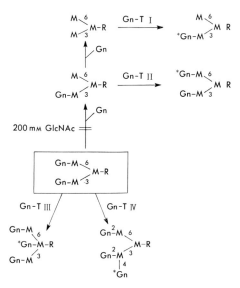

FIG. 13. Possible fates of glycopeptide GnGn in incubations with crude enzyme preparations. Abbreviations: M, Man; Gn, GlcNAc; star (*), radioactivity; T, transferase.

H. Schachter, unpublished). However, some tissues (*e.g.*, the monocyte fraction from normal human white cells) are very rich in glycosidases and the standard assay produces a very large radioactive peak adhering to Con A/Sepharose. This destruction of GnGn may interfere with the accurate assay of GlcNAc-transferases III and IV.

Both glycopeptides GnG and GGn were tested as substrates for GlcNAc-transferases III and IV (Table II). GGn is a good substrate for both transferases while GnG is a very poor substrate. Since we believe that the GlcNAcβ1-2Manα1-3- arm must be free for both transferases to act (see below), it is perhaps not surprising that substitution of the Manα1-3- arm by a Gal residue (such as in GnG) results in an inactive substrate whereas a Gal residue on the Manα1-6- arm (such as in GGn) has little effect. Recent data (M. Paquet, S. Narasimhan, H. Schachter, and M. A. Moscarello, unpublished) have shown that highly purified UDP-Gal: GlcNAc β4-Gal-transferase (from rat liver or bovine milk) prefers the GlcNAc on the Manα1-3- arm of the core to form GnG suggesting that, *in vivo*, the incorporation of even a single Gal residue into GnGn prevents further branching by either GlcNAc-transferase III or IV. Thus the action of the β4-Gal-transferase is the first committed step towards synthesis of non-bisected bi-antennary oligosaccharides. It is possible, however, that the relatively small amount of GGn that is formed provides an alternate but minor path towards bisected bi-antennary and highly branched oligosaccharides.

Guanosine Diphosphate (GDP)-Fuc: β-N-Acetylglucosaminide (Fuc to Asn-linked GlcNAc) α1-6-Fucosyltransferase

Fucose has been reported to occur linked α1-6- or α1-3- to the Asn-linked GlcNAc of N-glycosyl oligosaccharides (*1, 26, 28*). Fucose also occurs in a variety of antigenic determinants at the non-reducing termini of milk and urinary oligosaccharides, N- and O-linked protein-bound oligosaccharides and glycosphingolipids. Golgi apparatus-enriched membrane preparations from pig and rat liver and rat and mouse testis, crude extracts from HeLa cells, and human serum, can all transfer Fuc from GDP-Fuc to N-glycosyl oligosaccharides with terminal GlcNAc residues. The pork liver enzyme has been shown to catalyze the reaction shown in Fig. 8e (18). No product was detected with Fuc in α1-3 linkage to the Asn-linked GlcNAc.

The substrate specificity of the α1-6-fucosyltransferase is summarized in Table II. The enzyme will act on substrates with the structure GlcNAcβ1-2Manα1-3(R-Manα1-6)Manβ1-4GlcNAcβ1-4GlcNAc-Asn-X where R is H (glycopeptide MGn), GlcNAcβ1-2 (glycopeptide GnGn), or Manα1-6(Manα1-3) (glycopeptide Gn(I)M$_5$). The enzyme does not act on substrates which lack the GlcNAcβ1-2Manα1-3- sequence or on any substrate carrying a bisecting GlcNAc residue (GlcNAc attached β1-4- to the β-linked Man). Elongation of antennae by addition of Galβ1-4- or sialyl-Galβ1-4- sequences also prevents enzyme action. Glycopeptides with only a single Gal residue (GGn and GnG) have, however, not yet been tested as substrates for this enzyme. Some of these reactions are indicated in Fig. 7.

Hybrid Oligosaccharide Synthesis

Hybrid oligosaccharides can occur either in a bisected or non-bisected form (Fig. 2). It is not clear why a glycoprotein like rhodopsin has non-bisected hybrid structures; Fig. 6 suggests that there may be interference with either α-mannosidase II or GlcNAc-transferase II. Ovalbumin is rich in bisected hybrid oligosaccharides. We have observed that hen oviduct membranes are very rich in GlcNAc-transferase III and relatively deficient in GlcNAc-transferase I-dependent α3/6-mannosidase (mannosidase II). We have also observed (23) that GlcNAc-transferase III can incorporate a bisecting GlcNAc into Gn(I)M$_5$ (Fig. 6). Finally, it has been observed (10) that mannosidase II does not act if the substrate has a bisecting GlcNAc residue (Fig. 6). These observations suggest strongly that hen oviduct membranes shunt the synthetic pathway from Gn(I)M$_5$ to bisected bi- and tri-antennary hybrid structures (Fig. 6). Once GlcNAc-transferase III has acted, further Man removal cannot occur. The only available paths are further elongation by Gal- and sialyl-transferases. Since the presence of a bisecting GlcNAc prevents GlcNAc-transferase IV action (Table II), we also suggest that bisected bi-antennary hybrids result if GlcNAc-transferase III acts before GlcNAc-transferase IV and bisected tri-antennary hybrids result if transferase IV acts before transferase III. The existence of hybrids with only 4 Man residues suggests that GlcNAc-transferases III and IV can act at both the 5-Man and 4-Man stages but the 4-Man compound has not been tested as a substrate for these enzymes.

The α6-fucosyltransferase discussed above has been shown to act on Gn(I)M$_5$ (18; Fig. 7). This suggests that fucosylated hybrids are theoretically possible but such structures have not yet been described. Since prior GlcNAc-transferase I action is essential for α6-fucosyltransferase (Table II), it is not surprising that all high mannose oligosaccharides thus far described lack a core fucose residue.

Bisected Complex Oligosaccharide Synthesis

Bisected complex oligosaccharides are relatively uncommon but have been found in human immunoglobulins, hen ovotransferrin and ovomucoid, human erythrocyte glycophorin A and band 3, and in a few other glycoproteins (*21*). Such structures cannot be made by the action of GlcNAc-transferase III at either the 5-Man or 4-Man stages since mannosidase II cannot act if a bisecting GlcNAc is present (Fig. 6). A third point of entry at the 3-Man stage was therefore predicted by Harpaz and Schachter (*10*) and recently established by Narasimhan (*21*).

The substrate specificity studies shown in Table II indicate that GlcNAc-transferase III has a narrow window of action at the 3-Man stage (Fig. 7). MGn is a relatively poor substrate, GGn is probably not formed in large amounts *in vivo* (see above) and GnG, GG, and the sialylated compounds are not substrates. Thus GnGn is the major entry point for bisected bi-antennary complex oligosaccharides. GlcNAc-transferase IV has a similarly narrow window of action (Table II) and therefore GnGn is also the main point of entry for both bisected and non-bisected tri-antennary oligosaccharides (Fig. 7). The presence of a bisecting GlcNAc prevents GlcNAc-transferase IV action (Table II) and therefore GlcNAc-transferase IV action must precede GlcNAc-transferase III action.

Control Points and Key Residues

Polypeptides and nucleic acids are linear structures and are synthesized by a template mechanism. Oligosaccharides, being highly branched, cannot be assembled in this

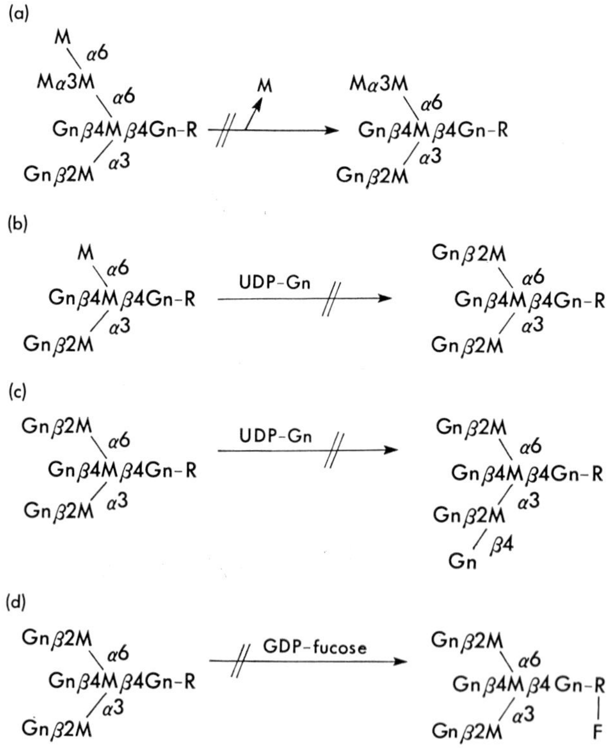

FIG. 14. Four enzymes which cannot act on oligosaccharide substrates containing a bisecting GlcNAc residue. (a) GlcNAc-transferase I-dependent α3/6 mannosidase (mannosidase II); (b) GlcNAc-transferase II; (c) GlcNAc-transferase IV; (d) GDP-Fuc: β-N-acetylglucosaminide (Fuc to Asn-linked GlcNAc) α1-6-fucosyltransferase.

manner. Although many factors such as compartmentation within the cell and the availability of various substrates and co-factors undoubtedly play important roles in the control of oligosaccharide synthesis, our studies suggest that enzyme availability and substrate specificities are primarily responsible for the routing of the synthetic pathway. Three types of control can be seen in the schemes shown in Figs. 6 and 7. First, there are several points at which two or more enzymes compete for a common intermediate, e.g., Gn(I)M$_5$, MGn, and GnGn are at especially critical cross-roads. Routing depends on the relative activities of the competing enzymes. For example, hen oviduct makes hybrid structures because GlcNAc-transferase III in this tissue is much more active than mannosidase II. In tissues with the reverse situation, complex oligosaccharides are favoured. Second, the addition of a key glycosyl residue to an oligosaccharide can convert it from a good substrate to a non-substrate. The bisecting GlcNAc is especially effective at this type of control since it prevents the action of at least four enzymes (Fig. 14). The bisecting GlcNAc thus serves to 'freeze' the synthetic pathway at hybrid structures (Fig. 6) or at bisected bi-antennary structures (Fig. 7). Galactose can also convert a substrate to a non-substrate, e.g., Gal serves this function for GlcNAc-transferases III and IV and for α6-fucosyltransferase (see above). Third, the insertion of a key glycosyl residue may convert a non-substrate to a substrate. The GlcNAc inserted by GlcNAc-transferase I is an excellent example of this type of control since it is essential for the action of at least five enzymes (Fig. 8).

The pathways in Figs. 6 and 7 are based on a series of assumptions and restrictions. It is assumed that all the GlcNAc residues are inserted before elongation by addition of Gal and sialic acid begins. All the reactions shown in Figs. 6 and 7 involving mannosidase II, GlcNAc-transferases I, II, III, and IV, Gal-transferase and sialyltransferase can involve both fucosylated and non-fucosylated structures; only the non-fucosylated paths are shown. The possible effects of the protein backbone on glycosyltransferase action cannot be assessed by our experiments since we use glycopeptides as transferase acceptors. It is also assumed that there are no restrictions due to intracellular compartmentation or lack of substrates and co-factors. Finally, the schemes shown pool data from different species and tissues. Differences do indeed occur between species and tissues involving availability of enzymes and substrate specificities and these differences will determine the routing of the synthetic path. It is hoped that oncogenic transformation will be shown to cause such changes in enzymatic control to account for the observed differences in cell surface complex carbohydrates.

Three-dimensional Oligosaccharide Structures

Recent studies have elucidated the three-dimensional structures of some of the oligosaccharides used as substrates in the above work. These studies have been useful in explaining some of our substrate specificity findings. We have shown that five different enzymes have an absolute requirement for the GlcNAcβ1-2Manα1-3Manβ1-4- sequence in N-glycosyl oligosaccharides (Fig. 8). Further, four of these enzymes cannot act if a bisecting GlcNAc is inserted into their substrates (Fig. 14). The three-dimensional analysis of these oligosaccharides shows that the GlcNAcβ1-2Manα1-3Manβ1-4- arm is sterically covered by a bisecting GlcNAc residue. Thus it is postulated that all five enzymes shown in Fig. 8 require this arm as a binding site and that binding is prevented by a bisecting GlcNAc residue.

Three-dimensional studies should prove important not only for elucidating the control of oligosaccharide synthesis but also in the study of cell surface oligosaccharides and their functions in cell-cell interactions.

Acknowledgment

This work was supported by the Medical Research Council of Canada and by NIH grant No. HD-07889.

REFERENCES

1. Beyer, T. A., Sadler, J. E., Rearick, J. I., Paulson, J. C., and Hill, R. L. *Adv. Enzymol.,* **52**, 23–175 (1981).
2. Carver, J. P. and Grey, A. A. *Biochemistry,* **20**, 6607–6616 (1981).
3. Dorland, L., Haverkamp, J., Vliegenthart, J.F.G., Spik, G., Fournet, B., and Montreuil, J. *Eur. J. Biochem.,* **100**, 569–574 (1979).
4. Fukuda, M., Fukuda, M. N., and Hakomori, S. *J. Biol. Chem.,* **254**, 3700–3703 (1979).
5. Fukuda, M. N., Fukuda, M., and Hakomori, S. *J. Biol. Chem.,* **254**, 5458–5465 (1979).
6. Fukuda, M. N., Papermaster, D. S., and Hargrave, P. A. *J. Biol. Chem.,* **254**, 8201–8207 (1979).
7. Gleeson, P., Vella, G., Narasimhan, S., and Schachter, H. *Fed. Proc.,* **41**, 1147 (1982).
7a. Gleeson, P. and Schachter, H. *J. Biol. Chem.,* in press.
8. Gottlieb, C., Baenziger, J., and Kornfeld, S. *J. Biol. Chem.,* **250**, 3303–3309 (1975).
9. Harpaz, N. and Schachter, H. *J. Biol. Chem.,* **255**, 4885–4893 (1980).
10. Harpaz, N. and Schachter, H. *J. Biol. Chem.,* **255**, 4894–4902 (1980).
11. Jarnefelt, J., Rush, J., Li, Y-T., and Laine, R. A. *J. Biol. Chem.,* **253**, 8006–8009 (1978).
12. Johnston, I. R., McGuire, E. J., Jourdian, G. W., and Roseman, S. *J. Biol. Chem.,* **241**, 5735–5737 (1966).
13. Kornfeld, R. and Kornfeld, S. *In* "The Biochemistry of Glycoproteins and Proteoglycans," ed. W. J. Lennarz, pp. 1–34 (1980). Plenum Press, New York.
14. Kornfeld, S. *In* "The Glycoconjugates," Vol. III, ed M. I. Horowitz, pp. 3–23 (1982). Academic Press, New York.
15. Li, E. and Kornfeld, S. *J. Biol. Chem.,* **253**, 6426–6431 (1978).
16. Li, E., Gibson, R., and Kornfeld, S. *Arch Biochem. Biophys.,* **199**, 393–399 (1980).
17. Liang, C-J., Yamashita, K., Muellenberg, C. G., Shichi, H., and Kobata, A. *J. Biol. Chem.,* **254**, 6414–6418 (1979).
18. Longmore, G. D. and Schachter, H. *Carbohydr. Res.,* **100**, 365–392 (1982).
19. Mendicino, J., Chandrasekaran, E. V., Anumula, K. R., and Davila, M. *Biochemistry,* **20**, 967–976 (1981).
20. Munro, J. R., Narasimhan, S., Wetmore, S., Riordan, J. R., and Schachter, H. *Arch. Biochem. Biophys.,* **169**, 269–277 (1975).
21. Narasimhan, S. *J. Biol. Chem.,* **257**, 10235–10242 (1982).
22. Narasimhan, S., Stanley, P., and Schachter, H. *J. Biol. Chem.,* **252**, 3926–3933 (1977).
23. Narasimhan, S., Tsai, D., and Schachter, H. *Fed. Proc.,* **40**, 1597 (1981).
24. Oppenheimer, C. L. and Hill, R. L. *J. Biol. Chem.,* **256**, 799–804 (1981).
25. Oppenheimer, C. L., Eckhardt, A. E., and Hill, R. L. *J. Biol. Chem.,* **256**, 11477–11482 (1981).
26. Schachter, H. *In* "The Glycoconjugates," Vol. II, ed. W. Pigman and M. I. Horowitz, pp. 87–181 (1978). Academic Press, New York.
27. Schachter, H. and Roden, L. *In* "Metabolic Conjugation and Metabolic Hydrolysis," Vol. III, ed. W. H. Fishman, pp. 1–149 (1973). Academic Press, New York.

28. Schachter, H. and Roseman, S. *In* "The Biochemistry of Glycoproteins and Proteoglycans," ed. W. J. Lennarz, pp. 85–160 (1980). Plenum Press, New York.

29. Stanley, P., Narasimhan, S., Siminovitch, L., and Schachter, H. *Proc. Natl. Acad. Sci. U.S.*, **72**, 3323–3327 (1975).

30. Struck, D. K. and Lennarz, W. J. *In* "The Biochemistry of Glycoproteins and Proteoglycans," ed. W. J. Lennarz, pp. 35–83 (1980). Plenum Press, New York.

31. Tabas, I. and Kornfeld, S. *J. Biol. Chem.*, **253**, 7779–7786 (1978).

32. Tabas, I. and Kornfeld, S. *Methods Enzymol.*, **83**, 416–429 (1982).

33. Tabas, I., Schlesinger, S., and Kornfeld, S. *J. Biol. Chem.*, **253**, 716–722 (1978).

34. Tai, T., Yamashita, K., Ito, S., and Kobata, A. *J. Biol. Chem.*, **252**, 6687–6694 (1977).

35. Takasaki, S., Ikehira, H., and Kobata, A. *Biochem. Biophys. Res. Commun.*, **92**, 735–742 (1980).

36. Tulsiani, D.R.P., Harris, T. M., and Touster, O. *J. Biol. Chem.*, **257**, 7936–7939 (1982).

37. Tulsiani, D.R.P., Hubbard, S. C., Robbins, P. W., and Touster, O. *J. Biol. Chem.*, **257**, 3660–3668 (1982).

38. Turco, S. J., Rush, J. S., and Laine, R. A. *J. Biol. Chem.*, **255**, 3266–3269 (1980).

39. Vischer, P. and Hughes, R. C. *Eur. J. Biochem.*, **117**, 257–284 (1981).

40. Warren, L., Buck, C. A., and Tuszynski, G. P. *Biochim. Biophys. Acta*, **516**, 97–127 (1978).

GANN Monograph on Cancer Research 29, 1983

NEOPLASTIC ALTERATIONS OF SIALYLTRANSFERASE AND ITS SIGNIFICANCE: STUDIES ON SIALYLTRANSFERASES OF RAT LIVER AND RAT HEPATOMAS

Shigeru Tsuiki and Taeko Miyagi

Biochemistry Laboratory, Research Institute for Tuberculosis and Cancer, Tohoku University*

Neoplastic alterations of sialyltransferase have been studied by comparing sialyltransferases of rat liver and rat hepatocellular carcinomas induced by feeding hepatocarcinogens. With asialofetuin as acceptor, rat liver was found to contain two forms of $Gal\beta1 \rightarrow 4GlcNAc$ $\alpha2 \rightarrow 6$ sialyltransferase, sialylated transferase I and unsialylated transferase II. Transferase II as well as desialylated transferase I could be sialylated autocatalytically. Though indistinguishable immunologically, transferase I has a lower molecular weight and a higher affinity for cytidine monophosphate-N-acetylneuraminic acid and desialylated rat liver plasma membrane than transferase II. Rat hepatomas, on the other hand, contain only a single form of $Gal\beta1 \rightarrow 4GlcNAc$ $\alpha2 \rightarrow 6$ sialyltransferase, which is identical to transferase I. Since transferase I is supposed to be more active than transferase II in sialylating membrane glycoproteins, the present data are consistent with the view that the sialylation of membrane glycoproteins is accelerated in cancer cells.

It has been suspected that the surface membrane of the cell is a primary site for malignant transformation. This idea has stemmed mainly from the consideration that the cell surface is important in cell-cell interaction, the recognition of regulatory signals and the control of cell division. That cancer cells have an altered surface membrane has been demonstrated by differences in the patterns of glycolipids and glycoproteins between cancer and control cells (*2, 16, 49*), but the reported differences are too diverse to draw any clear-cut conclusion from them.

The sialic acid residues of glycoproteins have been implicated in many biological processes (*21*). Possible involvement of the sialic acid in malignant transformation has been suggested from the observation that the membrane-associated glycoproteins of cancer cells are more highly sialylated than those of the normal counterparts (*13, 20, 47, 50, 52, 53*). Kobata and coworkers (*31, 43*), on the other hand, were able to show that the degree of branching in asparagine-linked oligosaccharides is also increased in cancer cells. The increased branching may result in an increase in the number of sialic acid-accepting site. Whether the higher degree of sialylation observed in cancer cells is due to increased substitution of the sialic acid-accepting site or simply a consequence of increased branching is an important question and may be answered, at least in part, by comparing sialyltransferase between cancer and control cells. Almost all previous

* Seiryo-machi 4-1, Sendai 980, Japan (立木　蔚，宮城妙子).

TABLE I.   Sialyltransferase Activity of Neoplastic and Virally Transformed Cells[a]

Tumors	Acceptors (acialo form)	Changes	Ref.
SV40-3T3	Fetuin	Decrease	
	Submaxillary mucin	Decrease	14
SV40(ts)-3T3	Fetuin	Increase	32
RSV-3T3, Py-3T3, MSV-3T3	Membrane glycopeptide	Increase	6
Py-BHK, RSV-BHK	Fetuin	No change	
	Submaxillary mucin	No change	
	"Group A" glycopeptide	Increase	50
Thyroid tumor (rat)	Fetuin	No change	
	Orosomucoid	No change	
	Thyroglobulin	Decrease	28
Ascites hepatomas (rat)	Submaxillary mucin	Decrease	
	Lactose	Decrease	38
Morris hepatomas (rat)	Fetuin	Decrease	19
	Orosomucoid	Decrease	4
Primary hepatomas (rat)	Fetuin	No change	26
	Submaxillary mucin	No change	24
Colonic tumor (human)	Orosomucoid	Decrease	
	Submaxillary mucin	Decrease	51
	Fetuin	Increase	7
Ovarian tumor (human)	Fetuin	Increase	8

[a] In the studies shown above, homogenates or particulate fractions of tumor cells were assayed for sialyltransferase using the asialo forms of glycoproteins indicated as acceptor. The results were expressed as changes from the values of the normal counterparts.
SV40, simian virus 40; RSV, Rous sarcoma virus; Py, polyoma virus; MSV, murine sarcoma virus.

TABLE II.   Types of Sialyltransferase that Participate in the Synthesis of Glycoproteins

A. Asparagine-linked oligosaccharides
   Type 1: $Gal\beta1 \rightarrow 4GlcNAc \ \alpha2 \rightarrow 6$ sialyltransferase
   Type 2: $Gal\beta1 \rightarrow 4GlcNAc \ \alpha2 \rightarrow 3$ sialyltransferase
   Type 3: $Gal\beta1 \rightarrow 3GlcNAc \ \alpha2 \rightarrow 3$ sialyltransferase
B. Threonine/serine-linked oligosaccharides
   Type 4: $Gal\beta1 \rightarrow 3GalNAc \ \alpha2 \rightarrow 3$ sialyltransferase
   Type 5: $GalNAc\alpha1-O \rightarrow$ threonine/serine $\alpha2 \rightarrow 6$ sialyltransferase

studies concerning neoplastic alterations of sialyltransferase, however, were quantitative and many of them indicated decrease rather than increase of the activity in cancer cells as compared to the normal counterparts (Table I). What seems clear is the necessity of qualitative comparison, but no work has ever been done, to our knowledge, along this line.

Sialyltransferase is the enzyme that transfers sialic acid from cytidine monophosphate-N-acetylneuraminic acid (CMP-NeuAc) to appropriate acceptors. The initial one enzyme-one linkage hypothesis for glycosyltransferases (15) has to be modified since their acceptor specificity extends beyond the non-reducing terminal sugar. At least three types of sialyltransferases are known to participate in the formation of asparagine-linked oligosaccharides (Table II). One, "β-galactoside $\alpha2 \rightarrow 6$ sialyltransferase," has been purified from bovine colostrum by Paulson et al. (33, 34) and shown to have strict specificity toward the terminal $Gal\beta1 \rightarrow 4GlcNAc$ sequence (type 1). A second sialyltransferase also sialylates the same terminal sequence but $\alpha2 \rightarrow 3$ glycosidically (type 2) (48). In addition,

Paulson *et al.* (*35*) quite recently reported the occurrence in rat liver Golgi apparatus of a sialyltransferase responsible for the formation of the sialyl linkage in the NeuAc α2 →3Galβ1→3GlcNAc sequence present in the asparagine-linked oligosaccharides of prothrombin (*27*) (type 3). Two other sialyltransferases listed in Table II, types 4 (*36*) and 5 (*37*), are involved in the formation of the NeuAcα2→3Galβ1→3GalNAc and NeuAcα2→6GalNAcβ1-O→threonine/serine sequences, respectively, of threonine/ serine-linked oligosaccharides.

It should also be noted that the polypeptide portion of glycoprotein acceptors influences recognition by glycosyltransferases. The best example for this is the two forms of α-mannoside β-N-acetylglucosaminyltransferase, designated transferases A and B, found in rat hepatomas (*25*). Although they recognize the same oligosaccharide sequence, transferase B has a preference for low-molecular-weight glycopeptides while transferase A prefers to act on high-molecular-weight glycoproteins (*25*). Interestingly, rat liver, unlike rat hepatomas, contains only transferase A (*25*). As for sialyltransferase, Aguanno *et al.* (*1*) demonstrated that the proteolytic digestion of α-1-antitrypsin significantly altered its acceptor efficiency in the reaction catalyzed by human liver sialyltransferase.

Prompted by all these considerations, we began to study the sialyltransferase of rat liver and rat hepatocellular carcinomas. The hepatomas were induced by feeding 3′-methyl-4-dimethylaminoazobenzene (3′-methyl-DAB) or diethylnitrosamine (DEN). Sialyltransferase was assayed by the transfer of [¹⁴C]sialic acid from CMP-[¹⁴C]NeuAc to asialofetuin, which contains both asparagine-linked and threonine/serine-linked oligosaccharides (*3, 30, 42*). Many of the experimental results shown in this review are described in detail elsewhere (*26*).

Molecular Forms

With asialofetuin as acceptor, the homogenates of rat liver and hepatomas exhibited similar sialyltransferase activities. These activities were particulate-bound but readily solubilized by 2% Triton X-100. The detergent extracts of rat liver and hepatomas were then chromatographed on phosphocellulose. While liver activity resolved into two peaks (Fig. 1A), designated transferases I and II in order of elution, the extract of hepatoma induced by 3′-methyl-DAB exhibited only a single peak, which was eluted at the same position as liver transferase I (Fig. 1B). Although hepatoma induced by 3′-methyl-DAB is known to be more poorly differentiated than that induced by DEN (*39*), the

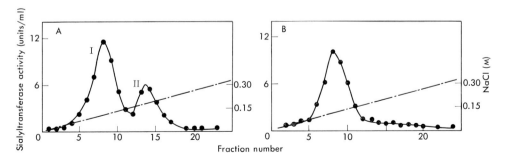

FIG. 1. Asialofetuin sialyltransferase of normal rat liver (A) and rat hepatoma induced by 3′-methyl-DAB (B) as chromatographed on phosphocellulose.

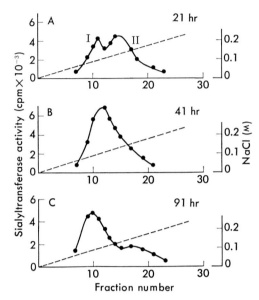

FIG. 2. Asialofetuin sialyltransferase of regenerating rat liver as chromatographed
on phosphocellulose.

activity level and molecular pattern of asialofetuin sialyltransferase were about the same
in the two hepatomas. The following experiments were therefore performed with 3′-
methyl-DAB-induced hepatoma.

To find a clue to the nature and significance of the deviation from the liver pattern
of the hepatoma pattern (Fig. 1), livers were removed from rats at various time intervals
following partial hepatectomy; detergent extracts were then made and they were chromatographed on phosphocellulose. The results obtained are illustrated in Fig. 2. Twenty-one
hr after the operation, liver still exhibited transferases I and II; transferase II then de-
clined and at 41 hr became undetectable. At 91 hr, however, the pattern almost reverted
to that seen before partial hepatectomy. It is therefore apparent that the lack of transferase II is not characteristic of neoplasia but should be associated with cell proliferation.

Neuraminidase   Treatment

In those enzymes containing asparagine- or serine/threonine-linked oligosaccharides,
chromatographic or electrophoretic multiplicity may arise from different degrees of
sialylation (9, 12, 20, 29). This prompted us to investigate the effect of neuraminidase
treatment on liver transferases I and II. When the enzymes were incubated with *Arthro-
bacter ureafaciens* neuraminidase (46) and then chromatographed on phosphocellulose,
the elution position of transferase I shifted toward transferase II while little change
occurred in transferase II. The behavior of hepatoma transferase in this respect was
similar to that of transferase I. Since the neuraminidase employed here is known to have
a broad substrate specificity (46), these observations suggest that liver transferase II is
unsialylated while all the transferase molecules in hepatoma are sialylated as is liver
transferase I.

Purification

In order to gain further insights into the nature of liver and hepatoma sialyltransferases, they were purified in the 8 step procedure, the details of which were described elsewhere (26). Purification was marked when the transferases were specifically eluted from a carboxymethyl-cellulose column by cytidine triphosphate, a potent inhibitor of sialyltransferase (5). The purified transferases I and II had specific activities approximately 3,000- and 2,700-fold greater, respectively, than those at the homogenates and were homogeneous as judged by sodium dodecyl sulfate gel electrophoresis. Hepatoma transferase was enriched 2,400-fold but had several minor bands besides the major transferase band on sodium dodecyl sulfate gel electrophoresis.

Specificity

Purified sialyltransferases described above transferred sialic acid to asialofetuin, asialotransferrin, and asialoorosomucoid at about the same rate and to lactose and oroso-N-octaose [(Galβ1→4GlcNAcβ1→2Man)$_2$ α1→3,6Manβ1→4GlcNAc] (22) with somewhat lower efficiencies. Asialo-bovine submaxillary mucin, its galactosylated product (25), asialo-mixed gangliosides and lacto-N-tetraose [Galβ1→3GlcNAcβ1→3Galβ1→4Glc], on the other hand, were totally inactive as acceptors. The results of periodate oxidation and treatment with Influenza virus neuraminidase of asialofetuin previously sialylated by these transferases revealed that sialylgalactoside linkage had been formed α2→6 glycosidically. Furthermore, with lactose as acceptor, these transferases formed α2→6 sialyllactose but not its α2→3 isomer. When all these results are considered together, they constitute strong evidence that the liver and hepatoma enzymes are type 1 (Table II), that is Galβ1→4GlcNAc α2→6 sialyltransferase.

Sialylation

When liver transferase I previously treated with *A. ureafaciens* neuraminidase was incubated with CMP-[^{14}C]NeuAc, its elution profile from phosphocellulose reverted to that seen before neuraminidase treatment. This reversion must be a consequence of resialylation of "desialylated" transferase I since the reverted enzyme contained ^{14}C readily releasable by neuraminidase. Liver transferase II was also incubated with CMP-[^{14}C]NeuAc. When subsequently chromatographed on phosphocellulose, the enzyme emerged at the same position as resialylated transferase I and contained ^{14}C. These observations make it clear that both transferases are capable of auto-sialylation and possess asparagine-linked oligosaccharide(s). It is also worth-noting that native transferase II possesses sialic acid-accepting site(s) even though it lacks sialic acid.

Immunological Study

Liver transferases I and II were studied using antibodies produced in rabbits against purified liver transferases I and II individually. The antibody to transferase I inhibited both transferases similarly. Exactly the same pattern of inhibition was obtained with the antibody to transferase II. The results suggest that the two transferases closely resemble each other or are identical in their polypeptide portion.

TABLE III. Molecular and Kinetic Properties of Rat Liver and Hepatoma Sialyltransferases

	Hepatoma	Liver I	Liver II
Molecular weight	37,000	37,000 (36,000)[a]	43,000
Inactivation after 20 min at 50° (%)	55	53	0
K_m for			
CMP-NeuAc (mM)	0.055	0.055	0.165 (0.165)[b]
Asialofetuin (mM)	0.44	0.44	0.44
Desialylated plasma membrane (μg/ml)		590	1,810

[a] The value for desialylated transferase I.
[b] The value for sialylated transferase II.

Molecular and Kinetic Properties

Even though indistinguishable immunologically, the supposition that transferases I and II are simply a sialo- and an asialo-form, respectively, of an otherwise identical glycoprotein may be incorrect as evidenced by the molecular and kinetic data summarized in Table III. The molecular weight values shown here are those calculated from Stokes' radius and the sedimentation constant (40). Transferase II is greater in molecular weight by about 6,000 than transferase I and this difference could not be eliminated by desialylation of transferase I. The two transferases also differ in stability: transferase I lost half its original activity after 20 min at 50° while transferase II was scarcely inactivated under the same conditions.

Kinetic studies reported here reveal that transferase I has a K_m for CMP-NeuAc 3 times lower than transferase II. This difference is not attributable to the sialic acid present in transferase I since sialylation of transferase II did not affect its K_m value. Furthermore, the K_m for desialylated rat liver plasma membrane of transferase I was also 3 times lower than that of transferase II.

Identification of Hepatoma Transferase as Transferase I

As already reported, rat hepatomas contain a single form of asialofetuin sialyl-transferase, whose chromatographic behavior and catalytic specificity are identical to liver transferase I. The enzyme purified from hepatoma was found to be indistinguishable immunologically from liver transferase. As shown in Table III, purified hepatoma transferase is identical to liver transferase I in all the molecular and kinetic properties that were examined. It is concluded that hepatomas contain transferase I but lacks transferase II.

DISCUSSION

1. Type of sialyltransferase

The structure of the oligosaccharide portion of fetuin is such that its asialo form (asialofetuin) should serve as acceptors for all the sialyltransferases in Table II except type 3 (3, 30, 42). Nevertheless, only Galβ1→4GlcNAc α2→6 sialyltransferase (type 1) has been purified from both rat liver and hepatoma. In a separate experiment, detergent extracts of rat liver and hepatoma were found to contain type 3 to 5 sialyltransferases, but their levels were lower than the level of type 1 transferase (23, 24). As to type 2 sialyl-transferase, we have recently found that both liver and hepatoma are totally devoid of this activity (23). There thus seem to be good grounds for accepting that type 1 sialyl-transferase is the major sialylating agent in rat liver and hepatoma.

2. Oligosaccharide portion of sialyltransferase

Since transferases I and II transfer sialic acid only to the terminal Galβ1→4GlcNAc sequence, the finding that both transferases are capable of autosialylation suggests that they are in nature a glycoprotein possessing asparagine-linked oligosaccharide(s) of the complex type. The desialylation-sialylation experiments shown above further suggest that the two transferases possess the same number of sialic acid-accepting sites, which are fully sialylated in transferase I and completely unsialylated in transferase II. In this respect, hepatomas differ from liver in that all the sialyltransferase molecules belong to fully sialylated transferase I. This finding is important as it certainly encourages the view that the higher degree of sialylation repeatedly observed in glycoproteins from cancer cells as compared to normal cells (9–13, 20, 29, 47, 50, 52) is due to increased substitution rather than to an increased number of sialic acid-accepting sites.

3. Polypeptide portion of sialyltransferase

In addition to the degree of sialylation, transferases I and II differ from each other in molecular weight, stability and kinetic properties. Either desialylation of transferase I or sialylation of transferase II failed to eliminate these differences. It is therefore suggested that the two transferases may in some manner differ in their polypeptide portion.

How transferases I and II differ structurally remains to be elucidated. They do not seem to be encoded by two distinct genes since they are close enough to be indistinguish-able immunologically. The two transferases may be products of mRNA splicing. It has been shown that μ chains of the membrane-bound and secreted forms of IgM are encoded by two species of mRNA (10). It seems, however, to be more reasonable that transferase I arises from transferase II by what appears to be cleavage of a 6,000-molecular weight fragment as hypothesized in Fig. 3. Lysosomal enzymes may undergo similar post-translational processing (18, 41, 45). To define the mechanisms underlying the emergence of the two distinct but closely related transferases in liver, the possibility of *in vitro*

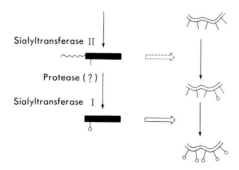

FIG. 3. Sialyltransferases I and II and sialylation of plasma membrane glycopro-teins (a hypothesis) | oligosaccharide side chain; ♭ sialylated oligosaccharide side chain; and ⌢ plasma membrane.

conversion of transferase II to transferase I is currently under investigation. Future studies will also be directed to the structural analysis of these transferases.

4.   Kinetic properties of sialyltransferase

Transferase I may be catalytically more active than transferase II *in vivo*. This idea has stemmed in part from the consideration that the K_m for CMP-NeuAc of transferase I (0.055 mM) but not that of II (0.165 mM) is low enough to utilize CMP-NeuAc, whose concentration in hepatocytes is not above 0.05 mM (*17*). This difference may be sufficient to explain why only transferase I is sialylated *in vivo* even though transferase II also possesses a sialic acid-accepting site. In addition to the K_m for CMP-NeuAc, the K_m for desialylated plasma membrane is also much lower in transferase I than in transferase II. The affinity for exogenously added asialofetuin, on the other hand, was the same between the two transferases. It therefore appears that transferase I is more easily accessible than transferase II to the sialic acid-accepting site of glycoproteins which is a part of the membranous structure.

5.   Neoplastic alterations of sialyltransferase

Increased membrane sialylation has often been considered as an essential feature of neoplasia (*13, 20, 47, 50, 52, 53*). Yet the results of the previous studies shown in Table I are such that the activities of asialofetuin or asialomucin sialyltransferases are slightly to greatly decreased in cancer cells. The studies presented above, however, demonstrate that although there is little change in the amount of Galβ1$\rightarrow$4GlcNAc α2$\rightarrow$6 sialyltransferase in hepatomas, the molecular pattern is altered so that transferase I predominates. If the hypothesis presented in Fig. 3 is correct, then the characteristic feature of cancer cells would be accelerated conversion of transferase II to transferase I. Since transferase I is more active than transferase II in sialylating membrane glycoproteins, it is entirely possible that the acceleration of transferase II to I conversion leads to an increase of membrane sialylation. One interesting finding to emerge from Table I is that in those cases where an increase in tumor sialyltransferase activity was observed, endogenous membrane proteins rather than asialofetuin or asialomucin were the acceptors (*6, 50*).

It should, however, be noted that the predominance of transferase I is by no means unique to neoplasia. Thus, regenerating liver exhibits this deviation at a specific time in the proliferative cycle (Fig. 2). It is therefore reasonable to assume that the accelerated conversion of transferase II to transferase I is associated more with cell growth than with neoplasia. Regenerating liver, however, differs from neoplastic liver in that chronological events soon result in a reversion to the normal liver pattern. Such a difference between neoplastic and regenerating liver probably arises from the occurrence in cancer cells of aberrant and misprogrammed gene expression (*44*).

Acknowledgment

This work was supported by Grants-in-aid for Cancer Research from the Ministry of Education, Culture and Science of Japan.

REFERENCES

1.   Aguanno, J. J., Roll, D. E., and Glew, R. H. *J. Biol. Chem.*, **253**, 6997–7004 (1978).

2. Atkinson, P. H. and Hakimi, J. *In* "The Biochemistry of Glycoproteins and Proteogly-cans," ed. W. J. Lennarz, pp. 191–239 (1980). Plenum Press, New York.

3. Baenziger, J. U. and Fiete, D. *J. Biol. Chem.*, **254**, 789–795 (1979).

4. Bauer, C. H., Vischer, P., Grunholz, H. J., and Reutter, W. *Cancer Res.*, **37**, 1513–1518 (1977).

5. Bernacki, R. J. *Eur. J. Biochem.*, **58**, 477–481 (1975).

6. Bosmann, H. B. *Biochem. Biophys. Res. Commun.*, **49**, 1256–1262 (1972).

7. Bosmann, H. B. and Hall, T. C. *Proc. Natl. Acad. Sci. U.S.*, **71**, 1833–1837 (1974).

8. Chatterjee, S. K., Bhattacharya, M., and Barlow, J. J. *Cancer Res.*, **39**, 1943–1951 (1979).

9. Dawson, J., Smith, G. D., Boak, J., and Peters, T. J. *Clin. Chim. Acta*, **96**, 37–42 (1979).

10. Early, P., Rogers, J., Davis, M., Calame, K., Bond, M., Wall, R., and Hood, L. *Cell*, **20**, 313–319 (1980).

11. Gasa, S., Makita, A., Kameta, T., Kodama, T., Koide, T., Tsumuraya, M., and Komai, T. *Eur. J. Biochem.*, **116**, 497–503 (1981).

12. Gerber, A. Ch., Kozdrowski, I., Wyss, S. R., and Berger, E. G. *Eur. J. Biochem.*, **93**, 453–460 (1979).

13. Glick, M. C. *Biochemistry*, **18**, 2525–2532 (1979).

14. Grimes, W. J. *Biochemistry*, **9**, 5083–5092 (1970).

15. Hagopian, A. and Eylar, E. H. *Arch. Biochem. Biophys.*, **129**, 422–433 (1968).

16. Hakomori, S. *Annu. Rev. Biochem.*, **50**, 733–764 (1981).

17. Harms, E., Kreisel, W., Morris, H. P., and Reutter, W. *Eur. J. Biochem.*, **32**, 254–262 (1973).

18. Hasilik, A. and Neufeld, E. F. *J. Biol. Chem.*, **255**, 4937–4945 (1980).

19. Hudgins, R. L., Murray, R., Pinteric, L., Morris, H. P., and Schachter, H. *Can. J. Biochem.*, **49**, 61–70 (1971).

20. Jaken, S. and Mason, M. *Proc. Natl. Acad. Sci. U.S.*, **75**, 1750–1753 (1978).

21. Jeanloz, R. W. and Codington, J. F. *In* "Biological Roles of Sialic Acid," ed. A. Rosenberg and C.-L. Schengrund, pp. 201–238 (1976). Plenum Press, New York.

22. Koseki, M. and Turumi, K. *Tohoku J. Exp. Med.*, **128**, 39–49 (1979).

23. Miyagi, T., Goto, T., and Tsuiki, S. *In* "Proc. Japan. Cancer Assoc. 41th Annu. Meet.," p. 281 (1982) (in Japanese).

24. Miyagi, T. and Tsuiki, S. *In* "Proc. Japan. Cancer Assoc. 38th Annu. Meet.," p. 247 (1980) (in Japanese).

25. Miyagi, T. and Tsuiki, S. *Biochim. Biophys. Acta*, **661**, 148–157 (1981).

26. Miyagi, T. and Tsuiki, S. *Eur. J. Biochem.*, **126**, 253–261 (1982).

27. Mizuochi, T., Yamashita, K., Fujikawa, K., Kisiel, W., and Kobata, A. *J. Biol. Chem.*, **254**, 6419–6425 (1979).

28. Monaco, F. and Robbins, J. *J. Biol. Chem.*, **248**, 2328–2336 (1973).

29. Niinobe, M., Tamura, Y., Arima, T., and Fujii, S. *Cancer Res.*, **39**, 4212–4217 (1979).

30. Nilsson, B., Norden, N. E., and Svensson, S. *J. Biol. Chem.*, **254**, 4545–4553 (1979).

31. Ogata, S., Muramatsu, T., and Kobata, A. *Nature*, **259**, 580–582 (1976).

32. Onodera, K., Yamaguchi, N., Kuchino, T., and Aoi, Y. *Proc. Natl. Acad. Sci. U.S.*, **73**, 4090–4094 (1976).

33. Paulson, J. C., Beranek, W. E., and Hill, R. L. *J. Biol. Chem.*, **252**, 2356–2362 (1977).

34. Paulson, J. C., Rearick, J. I., and Hill, R. L. *J. Biol. Chem.*, **252**, 2363–2371 (1977).

35. Paulson, J. C., Weinstein, J., and de Souza-e-Silva, U. *J. Biol. Chem.*, **257**, 4034–4037 (1982).

36. Rearick, J. I., Sadler, J. E., Paulson, J. C., and Hill, R. L. *J. Biol. Chem.*, **254**, 4444–4451 (1979).

37. Sadler, J. E., Rearick, J. I., and Hill, R. L. *J. Biol. Chem.*, **254**, 5934–5941 (1979).

38. Saito, M., Satoh, H., and Ukita, T. *Biochim. Biophys. Acta*, **362**, 549–557 (1974).
39. Sato, K., Takaya, S., Imai, F., Hatayama, I., and Ito, N. *Cancer Res.*, **38**, 3086–3093 (1978)
40. Siegel, L. M. and Monty, K. J. *Biochim. Biophys. Acta*, **112**, 346–362 (1966).
41. Skudlarek, M. D. and Swank, R. T. *J. Biol. Chem.*, **254**, 9939–9942 (1979).
42. Spiro, R. G. and Bhoyroo, V. D. *J. Biol. Chem.*, **249**, 5704–5717 (1974).
43. Takasaki, S., Ikehira, H., and Kobata, A. *Biochem. Biophys. Res. Commun.*, **92**, 735–742 (1980).
44. Tsuiki, S. *GANN Monogr. Cancer Res.*, **24**, 223–242, (1979).
45. Tulsiani, D.R.P., Six, H., and Touster, O. *Proc. Natl. Acad. Sci. U.S.*, **75**, 3080–3084 (1978).
46. Uchida, Y., Tsukada, Y., and Sugimori, T. *J. Biochem.*, **82**, 1425–1433 (1977).
47. Van Beek, W. P., Emmelot, P., and Homburg, C. *Br. J. Cancer*, **36**, 157–165 (1977).
48. Van den Eijnden, D. H. and Schiphorst, W.E.C.M. *J. Biol. Chem.*, **256**, 3159–3162 (1981).
49. Warren, L., Buck, C. A., and Tuszynski, G. P. *Biochim. Biophys. Acta*, **516**, 96–127 (1978).
50. Warren, L., Fuhrer, J. P., and Buck, C. A. *Proc. Natl. Acad. Sci. U.S.*, **69**, 1838–1842 (1972).
51. Whitehead, J. S., Fearney, F. J., and Kim, Y. S. *Cancer Res.*, **39**, 1259–1263 (1979).
52. Whyte, A. and Loke, Y. W. *Br. J. Cancer*, **37**, 689–700 (1978).
53. Yogeeswaran, G. and Tao, T.-W. *Biochem. Biophys. Res. Commun.*, **95**, 1452–1460 (1980).

GALACTOSYLTRANSFERASE:
BIOLOGY AND CLINICAL APPLICATIONS

Eric G. Berger,[*1] Jürgen Roth,[*2]
and Ger J.A.M. Strous[*3]

*Institute of Medical Chemistry, University of Bern,[*1] Biocenter,
Department of Electron Microscopy, University of Basle,[*2]
and Laboratory of Histology and Cell Biology,
Medical School, State University[*3]*

Galactosyltransferase (lactose synthetase A protein) is the best known representative of all glycosyltransferases and has drawn early attention for its interesting kinetics which consist in modification of specificity by binding of α-lactalbumin. Association of the enzyme with Golgi fractions led to its widespread acceptance as marker enzyme for this organelle.

Galactosyltransferase is an interesting enzyme also for the investigation of several types of protein heterogeneity as they may be observed in single polypeptide chains. It has been found that this enzyme exhibits size and unusual charge heterogeneity. Despite the availability of large scale purification procedures, no sequence information on its protein nor on its glycan part has been provided. However, considerable progress in understanding biosynthesis and cellular localization of galactosyltransferase has been achieved by the application of monospecific antibodies. Thus, presence of galactosyltransferase in Golgi membranes was confirmed and, in addition, heterogeneity of Golgi cisternae was disclosed as only trans (distal) cisternae exhibited presence of this enzyme. This approach permitted also detection of ecto-galactosyl-transferase on microvilli of enterocytes and gastric epithelial cells. Studies on biosynthesis and intracellular transport showed that the enzyme is formed at the rough endoplasmic reticulum, that it follows the secretory pathway but is retarded at the level of the trans Golgi cisternae and, in highly polarized cells, at the cell surface.

In growing cell cultures, galactosyltransferase is released into the supernatant and processed to a form smaller by 2 kilodaltons. Soluble galactosyltransferase is present in all body fluids, probably as a result of continuous shedding and/or secretion from cells. Thus, galactosyltransferase activity is found increased in sera and malignant effusions predominantly associated with ovarian and breast cancer. This finding may find some application in clinical chemistry and prove useful for patient monitoring.

Galactosyltransferase as reviewed in this article refers to a specific glycosyltransferase which catalyses the formation of a Galβ1$\rightarrow$4GlcNAc linkage (EC 2. 4. 1. 22). This

---

[*1] CH-3000 Bern 9, Switzerland.
[*2] CH-4056 Basle, Switzerland.
[*3] 3511 HG, Utrecht, The Netherlands.

enzyme has received much attention for its kinetic properties as it is able to synthesize lactose in the presence of α-lactalbumin; these aspects as well as purification procedures and principles of its assay have been reviewed by Ebner (*16*) and Hill and Brew (*26*).

The present review deals with biological aspects of galactosyltransferase enzymology which have been investigated in this laboratory and in collaboration with others during the past 6 years. Interest in this enzyme was mainly inspired by its potential use as tumor marker in clinical chemistry (*10, 48*), its classical use as Golgi marker enzyme in fractionation methodology (*14*) and its possible hormonal induction during lactation (*12*).

Assay Methodology

The assay for galactosyltransferase activity routinely used in our laboratory is based on the incorporation of ^{3}H or ^{14}C labeled galactose into an acceptor protein which exposes solely GlcNAc as acceptor site (ovalbumin) followed by acid precipitation of protein and counting of incorporated galactose by liquid scintillation counting. The assay is described in detail in Ref *6*; it is imperative, however, that products are rigorously identified whenever a crude enzyme source is used. In serum, for instance, two different galactosyltransferase (GT) activities have been distinguished by several criteria including analysis of the linkage type catalyzed: GT-A produced a $Gal\beta1 \rightarrow 3GalNAc$-protein linkage using asialo-ovine submaxillary mucin, GT-B a $Gal\beta1 \rightarrow 4GlcNAc$ linkage using free GlcNAc as acceptor substrate. Separation of both enzyme activities was possible using affinity chromatography on GlcNAc-agarose. The GT-B enzyme preparation, however, still catalysed transfer of galactose to asialomucin. This activity could be ascribed to contamination with GT-A or, alternatively, could represent an unknown specificity of GT-B. Careful analysis of the products formed by GT-B on asialomucin, however, led to the identification of otherwise undetectable amounts of terminal GlcNAc residues in ovine submaxillary mucin (*60*). This finding illustrates and strengthens the concept of "one glycosyltransferase—one glycosidic linkage" and demonstrates that in a given assay system, either the specificity of the enzyme or the accepting carbohydrates must be characterized. If this has not been done, the nature of the observed sugar transferase remains ill defined.

Purification

The purification procedure of soluble human galactosyltransferase routinely used in our laboratory was devised basically according to Barker *et al.* (*3*) and Andrews (*1*). After defattening of breast milk by centrifugation and removal of casein by acid precipitation, the resulting whey is passed over a GlcNAc-agarose column. An easy synthesis of this affinity ligand was described by Bloch and Burger (*11*) and found suitable for purification of soluble galactosyltransferases from various sources (*4*). As the construction of this ligand involves only reduction of *p*-nitrophenyl-N-acetylglucosamine to its *p*-amino derivative which can easily be coupled to CNBr-activated Sepharose (*11*), synthesis of large volumes (1–2 liters) of this ligand can be achieved within a few days. Adsorption and specific elution of the enzyme was carried out according to Barker (*3*) with only slight modifications. The second purification involves use of a bovine or human α-lactalbumin-agarose column according to Andrews (*1*). A single passage through this column is sufficient if a prepurified preparation of galactosyltransferase eluted from the

TABLE I. Purification Scheme of Human Milk Galactosyltransferase

Step	Volume (ml)	Protein concentration[a] (mg/ml)	Specific activity (U/mg)[b]	Total activity (U)	Purification factor	Recovery of activity (%)
Whey	4,400	10.9	0.59×10^{-3}	28.3	1	100
Dialysis	6,000	8.4	0.78×10^{-3}	39.3	1.3	144
Removal of casein by centrifugation	5,800	4.8	1.34×10^{-3}	37.3	23	131
Affinity chromatography on GlcNAc-agarose	950	0.050	0.41	19.3	689	68
Affinity chromatography on α-lactalbumin-agarose and concentration on PM10	16.5	0.675	1.6	17.8	2,712	63

[a] Determined according to Lowry (36) using bovine serum albumin as standard.
[b] 1 U: 1 μmol/min.

GlcNAc-Sepharose is applied. The resulting enzyme preparation appears electrophoretically pure. A typical purification scheme as shown in Table I is routinely used in our laboratory.

If the resulting preparation is injected into rabbits in order to raise an antiserum, the rabbit may form an antiserum directed also against human IgG. In the purified galactosyltransferase preparation obtained from human milk, contaminating IgG is not detectable except by its immunogenicity in the rabbit. If galactosyltransferase is purified from other sources such as malignant effusions, after the two affinity chromatographies on GlcNAc-sepharose and α-lactalbumin-sepharose, respectively, half of the protein still represents IgG (66). The phenomenon of copurification of IgG and galactosyltransferase over two affinity chromatographies specifically designed for galactosyltransferase is intriguing but cannot yet reasonably be explained. In any event, this finding made it necessary to remove contaminating IgG from the galactosyltransferase preparation either by protein A-Sepharose (9) or anti-IgG-Sepharose (66).

Heterogeneity

Different molecular forms of galactosyltransferase may be classified according to the following criteria: a) membrane-bound *versus* soluble enzyme forms; b) heterogeneity by size; c) heterogeneity by charge.

1. Membrane-bound versus soluble enzyme forms

It has long been recognized that galactosyltransferase copurifies with Golgi membranes upon fractionation (19, 41, 55). This finding, in fact, led to the increasing application of galactosyltransferase measurements to monitor Golgi fractions (14, 17). This membrane-associated activity was shown to be activated by detergents (13), whereas soluble galactosyltransferases tend to be inhibited by high detergent concentrations. Thirty percent of the maximum activity of membrane-bound galactosyltransferase is still measurable without detergents using high molecular weight acceptor substrates and 50% using free GlcNAc as acceptor. This detergent-independent activity of the membrane-associated enzyme may indicate a relatively free accessibility of substrates to the substrate binding sites as one would expect in the case of a glycosyltransferase specific for small molecular weight acceptors (lactose synthetase). In contrast, an erythrocyte membrane $\beta 1 \rightarrow 3$GalNAc galactosyltransferase is virtually unmeasurable in the absence of detergents whether assayed in right-side out or inside out membrane vesicles (25).

It has been assumed that soluble galactosyltransferase derives from an intracellular enzyme by "shedding" (26, 50, 56). Direct evidence in support of this assumption was relatively poor. A difference of 15 kilodaltons (kD) between the sizes of the intracellular precursor and the soluble enzyme forms was found by Smith and Brew (56). It was, however, unclear to what extent Triton X-100 contributed to the estimation of the molecular size of membrane-bound galactosyltransferase by gel filtration. In a recent study, we have confirmed work by LaMont et al. (35) by demonstrating release of galactosyltransferase enzyme protein from growing cell cultures. Using a protocol involving metabolic labeling of galactosyltransferase, immunoprecipitation and analysis by sodium dodecylsulphate/polyacrylamide gel electrophoresis/fluorography (SDS/PAGE/FG), it was found that the released form differs only by 2 kD from the intracellular mature form of 54 kD (57). As a working hypothesis, based on these findings, we assume that the intracellular Golgi associated form is processed to a soluble form by cleavage of a stretch of amino acids accounting for approximately 20 amino acids which may represent the hydrophobic anchoring peptide (54).

2. Heterogeneity by size of soluble galactosyltransferase

Using the purification protocol indicated above, single enzyme species are obtained from different sources as judged by SDS/PAGE/FG (Fig. 1) (22). Occasionally proteolytic degradation products may be detected in human milk which are still enzymatically active (51) or inactive (9); in this latter case they are detectable by the immune replica technique (59). In bovine milk, proteolytic degradation by plasmin has been extensively studied by Ebner et al. (38, 39). Interestingly, the presence of approximately dimeric

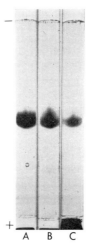

FIG. 1. SDS/PAGE of galactosyltransferase isolated from (A) human milk, (B) malignant ascites, and (C) amniotic fluid. Electrophoresis was carried out according to Fairbanks (18). A typical purification scheme for the human milk enzyme is shown in Table 1. From Gerber et al. (22).

galactosyltransferase has been reported by Khatra *et al.* (*30*) and recently in our laboratory using an enzyme linked immunosorbent assay for specific detection of galactosyltransferase antigen (*8, 9*). It is, however, unclear, how these findings are related.

It may be noted that prepurified serum galactosyltransferase reveals a broad band by the immune replica technique which moves slightly faster than the milk enzyme corresponding to approximately 50 kD (*9*), a mobility also found by Fujita-Yamaguchi and Yoshida (*21*); this higher mobility may reflect absence of O-glycosylation as suggested by these authors.

Another type of high molecular weight galactosyltransferase which appeared to be associated with cancer was reported by Podolsky and Weiser (*48*). This putative isoenzyme, termed GT-II, was detected as a slowly migrating enzyme activity peak eluted from PAGE gel slices run under nondenaturing conditions. This finding is discussed in more detail below (see Sect. entitled "*Clinical Use*")

3. Heterogeneity by size of membrane-bound galactosyltransferase

In HeLa cells galactosyltransferase immunoreactive protein can be identified after metabolic labeling using ^{35}S-methionine (*57*). The size of the molecular forms which are detectable by SDS/PAGE/FG depends on the pulse/chase protocol applied. After a 10 min pulse, two forms of immunoreactive galactosyltransferase are identified having molecular weights of 47 and 45 kD, respectively. These forms are sensitive to endo-N-acetylglucosaminidase H (Endo H) treatment which converts them to 44 and 42 kD forms; these are also detected after preincubation of cells with 5 μg/ml tunicamycin for 16 hr. Upon fractionation these precursor forms are found in dense fractions. After

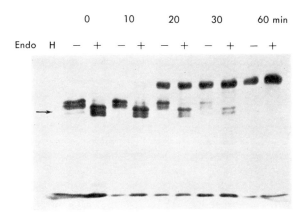

Fɪɢ. 2.   Treatment of metabolically ^{35}S-methionine labeled galactosyltransferase from HeLa cells with endo-N-acetylglucosaminidase H (Endo H). HeLa cells were grown on a 6 cm plate, labeled for 10 min with ^{35}S-methionine and chased with unlabeled methionine for the time indicated on the figure. The cells were lysed and subjected to immunoprecipitation with monospecific anti-galactosyltransferase antibody according to a method described by Zilberstein *et al.* (*67*) in a SDS-denatured, reduced and alkylated protein mixture derived from immunoprecipitates. Analysis of the treated enzyme was carried out by electrophoresis according to Laemmli (*34*) in 10% polyacrylamide and developed by fluorography. Endo H treatment is designated with (+), controls with omission of Endo H (−). The arrow points to the position of actin which often contaminates the immunoprecipitation after short chase periods. From Strous and Berger (*57*).

212   E. G. BERGER ET AL.

20 to 30 min chase, they disappear and a 54 kD species emerges, which is Endo H resistant (Fig. 2) and appears in light fractions upon cell fractionation which contain detectable galactosyltransferase activity. In the presence of tunicamycin, a 52 kD could be
identified after a 60 min chase. During release from the cell, the 54 kD form is converted
to a 52 kD soluble form.

From these metabolic studies, it is apparent that during maturation of galactosyltransferase, several transient forms of galactosyltransferase can be identified depending
on the degree of maturation. The general pattern of maturation resembles the one described for secretory glycoproteins (43). Several questions remain to be answered: Does
heterogeneity of precursor forms reflect heterogeneity in mRNA coding for the enzyme
or fast conversion of the 47 kD to the 45 kD form? Does the increase in molecular weight
observed between the precursor and mature form correspond to O-glycosylation? At
which stage of exocytocis is the intracellular membrane-bound form processed to the
soluble form and how does this phenomenon relate to "shedding"?

Intracellular, membrane-bound galactosyltransferase has also been purified from
sheep mammary gland (56) and from rat liver (20). In the first case, a molecular weight
of 69 kD was found whereas in the second case, after correction for detergent binding,
a 48.2 kD form was found. Our evidence from metabolic studies points to a small difference in molecular weight between intra- and extracellular forms which does not
exceed 2 kD or approximately the 15–20 amino acids, which is compatible with the size
of a hydrophobic anchoring peptide (54).

4. Heterogeneity by charge of soluble galactosyltransferase

The enzyme species purified from human milk which appears to migrate as a single
band on SDS/PAGE (*cf.* Fig. 1) resolves into 7 to 13 different forms by isoelectric
focusing (Fig. 3). This considerable charge heterogeneity is very consistently observed
(22, 53); a structural basis other than 3 to 4 different amino acids found at the amino
terminus has not been established. The facts, however, that (i) charge heterogeneity of
native galactosyltransferase assayed by its activity in serum or milk (5) is similar to the

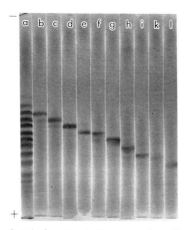

FIG. 3.   Analytical isoelectric focusing in 8 M urea of purified human milk galactosyltransferase. Purified enzyme was resolved on polyacrylamide gels in a pH gradient
3.5–10 (gel a). A similar gel was cut in slices which were placed individually on top
of other gels and refocused under similar conditions (gels b–l). From Gerber *et al.*
(22).

heterogeneity of purified enzyme, (ii) the single heteromorphs after refocusing retain their original respective isoelectric points (Fig. 3), (iii) presence of urea does not simplify the pattern, and (iv) each heteromorph exhibits enzymatic activity (22) and crossreacts with antibody (53) tend to exclude arte-factual resolution of galactosyltransferase by isoelectric focusing. Cleavage of sialic acid by neuraminidase shifts the isoelectric points to the cathodic part of the pH gradient and reduces the heterogeneity of the native enzyme to approximately six isoproteins. This treatment appears also to abolish charge differences observed between galactosyltransferase purified from milk and other sources such as ascitic or amniotic fluid (22). At the present time, it cannot be decided whether the observed charge heterogeneity reflects genetic or posttranslational (or both) modifications. The recently published example of the interferon gene family (42), which produces a similar degree of charge heterogeneity as the one identified for galactosyltransferase sets an interesting precedent for the genetic origin of this phenomenon. Alternatively, sulphation has recently been reported to produce a similar degree of charge heterogeneity in the case of the vesicular stomatitis virus (VSV)-G protein (27). In contrast to other serum glycosyltransferase activities (23, 29), resolution of galactosyltransferase into charge heteromorphs has not found any application in clinical chemistry.

5. *Heterogeneity by charge of membrane-bound galactosyltransferase*
    No data are yet available on this topic.

Localization

An important aspect of glycosyltransferase enzymology relates to intracellular localization of glycosyltransferases. In the late sixties, it was discovered on the basis of fractionation studies that galactosyltransferase activity is enriched in putative Golgi fractions (19, 41, 55). These findings have been amply confirmed (14, 17, 26) and led to the classical use of galactosyltransferase activity measurements to define Golgi membranes in fractionation studies. It was, however, not clear to what extent and in which cells galactosyltransferase would be exposed at the cell surface where they were attributed a role in recognition and adhesion (52). Biochemical evidence for the existence of cell surface or "ecto-galactosyltransferase" has been summarized in a recent review by Pierce et al. (47). Evidence is based mainly on activity measurements using intact cells as enzyme source and impermeant substrates such as beaded acceptors (61) or glycoproteins (47). Despite many precautions, biochemical methodology to determine ecto-glycosyltransferase activity has been criticized (28). Most recently, immunohistochemical evidence for the existence of both Golgi and cell surface association of galactosyltransferase has been provided in our laboratory: It has been found that galactosyltransferase serves as an excellent marker for the Golgi apparatus in HeLa cells and fibroblasts (7) as no evidence for cell surface localization was found in these cells at the level of the light microscope (Fig. 4). Moreover, an immunocytochemical study in HeLa cells permitted the unique localization of galactosyltransferase in the 2 to 3 trans cisternae of the Golgi apparatus where it is codistributed with thiamine pyrophosphatase (TPPase) activity (53) (Fig. 5). Codistribution of both enzymes supports a model of concerted action of both enzymes in chain elongation: uridine diphosphate (UDP) which is generated by galactosyltransferase reaction and which kinetically inhibits the reaction is split by TPPase to uridine monophosphate (UMP) and P, both freely diffusible through Golgi

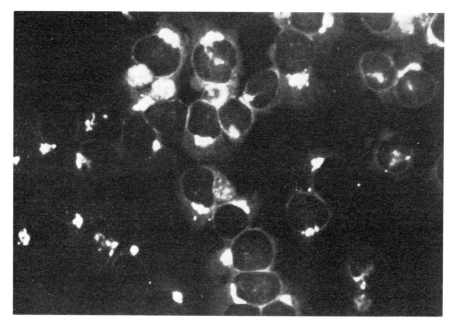

FIG. 4. Immunohistochemical staining of galactosyltransferase in HeLa cells. Sub-
confluent HeLa cells grown on Cooke microprint stock slides were fixed and per-
meabilized in chilled acetone, washed with phosphate-buffered saline and incubated
with approximately 10 μg of affinity purified rabbit anti-human galactosyltransferase antibody. Swine anti-rabbit Ig-fluorescein-isothiocyanate (FITC) was used
to detect presence of rabbit antibodies. ×2,080. From Berger *et al.* (*7*).

membranes (*33*). In contrast to cells in culture in which the Golgi apparatus tends to
adopt a crescent shaped juxtanuclear position (*40*), in polarized cells such as intestinal
epithelial cells, the membranes facing the intestinal lumen (brush borders) were also
heavily labeled (Fig. 6), whereas basolateral membranes exhibited only faint staining
at the light microscope level. In addition, in enterocytes located halfway along the crypt-
villus differentiation gradient (*63*), heavy labeling was also found adjacent to the brush
border in the region of the terminal web. More closely to the villus tips, some individual
cells exhibit labeling at the brush borders whereas adjacent cells remain entirely negative;
at the villus tips, however, most cells are intensely labeled over the brush borders (*46*).
Several conclusions can be drawn from these findings: galactosyltransferase being a good
marker for the trans Golgi membranes in cultured cells appears to mark for cytoplasmic
vesicles and plasma membranes in other systems as well. This finding has to be taken
into account whenever attempts are made to separate Golgi from plasma membranes
by fractionation of cells which exhibit cell surface galactosyltransferase (*65*). Interestingly,
also in enterocytes distribution of galactosyltransferase appears to mimic TPPase (*45*),
including expression at the cell surface.

Biosynthesis, Intracellular Transport, and Release of Galactosyltransferase

The absence of detectable galactosyltransferase antigen at the level of the endoplasmic reticulum and cis Golgi membranes raises questions on the site of biosynthesis and
intracellular transport of the enzyme. In HeLa cells, we have found by metabolic labeling

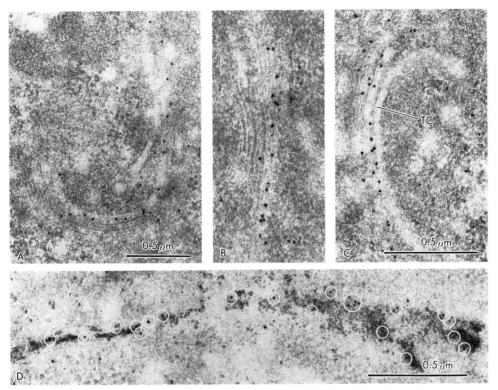

FIG. 5. Immunoelectron microscopic localization of galactosyltransferase immunoreactive sites. Confluent HeLa cells were fixed in glutaraldehyde and embedded in Lowicryl K4M resin at low temperature. Thin sections were cut and incubated with monospecific anti-galactosyltransferase antibodies and, subsequently, with protein A-gold complexes. For technical details see Ref. *53*. In perpendicularly cut (along the *cis-trans* axis) Golgi apparatus, galactosyltransferase immunoreactive sites are present in 2 to 3 trans cisternae (A–C) but absent from the transmost cisterna (TC in C). In D, double staining for TPPase activity (revealed by preembedding enzyme cytochemistry) and galactosyltransferase immunoreactivity (postembedding staining of thin sections with the protein A-gold technique on the same material) is shown. An obliquely sectioned trans cisterna contains amorphous reaction product for TPPase and, at the same time, is labeled with gold particles (white circles) indicative of galactosyltransferase immunoreactivity. ×48,000 (A); ×66,000 (B, C); ×73,000 (D). From Roth and Berger (*53*).

of the enzyme that early forms which are detectable by immunoprecipitation after a 10 min pulse with ³⁵S-methionine cosediment with dense fractions, whereas mature forms which appear after 20 min of chase cosediment with light fractions in a sucrose density gradient. Enzyme activity is measurable in these light fractions only. Thus, intracellular transport of galactosyltransferase appears to follow the general pathway of secretory proteins in being synthesized at the rough endoplasmic reticulum, transported to the trans Golgi cisternae and finally released (*57*). The observations that the enzyme is only detectable by activity and by cytochemistry in light fractions and trans Golgi cisternae, respectively, imply a mechanism which retards intracellular galactosyltransferase at this site. Absence of detection of galactosyltransferase in endoplasmic reticulum and cis Golgi membranes probably reflects rapid passage at these sites which prevents accumulation of the enzyme to a detectable level. This finding also argues against the

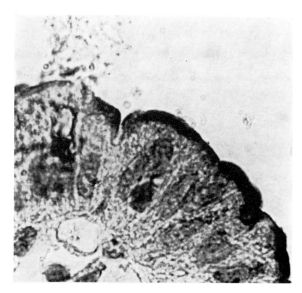

FIG. 6. Immunohistochemical staining of galactosyltransferase in a villus tip of human jejunal mucosa. The procedure included isotonic formaldehyde fixation of postmortem tissue, paraffin embedding and cutting of 5 μm sections which were mounted on slides. After deparaffinization the sections were briefly trypsinized, first treated with anti-galactosyltransferase antibody and thereafter with protein A-peroxidase. Staining was with 3,3′-diaminobenzidine, counterstaining with hematoxylin. On the left side, a goblet cell after discharge of mucus containing a well developed Golgi apparatus is readily identified. Other cells are enterocytes which show intense staining of brush borders and juxtanuclear staining for Golgi cisternae. ×1,000. From Pestalozzi *et al.* (*46*).

concept of cisternal progression of Golgi membranes as recently discussed by Tartakoff (*58*).

In tissue culture supernatants galactosyltransferase activity accumulates during cellular growth (*35*). This interesting finding led to the assumption that the enzyme is being released from the cells by a mechanism which converts the intracellular membrane-bound to the extracellular soluble (non sedimentable) form (*26, 50, 56*). Our recent studies support this assumption (*35*) since the soluble form recovered from the tissue culture supernatant by immunoprecipitation was smaller by 2 kD. However, it appears very difficult to detect cell surface galactosyltransferase in HeLa cells as fractionation studies (*24*) and immunocytochemistry (*53*) did not allow detection by activity nor by specific antibodies, respectively, at this site. In other cells, such as enterocytes, galactosyltransferase is expressed at the cell surface, predominantly on brush borders (Fig. 6). Thus, at the present time, two main alternatives of the destiny of this trans-Golgi membrane protein emerge: Either the enzyme is rapidly shed or it is expressed at the cell surface for a defined period of time. Further investigations will tell whether endocytosis and recycling of galactosyltransferase are a third possibility.

Intracellular transport, expression at the cell surface and release as discussed above are aspects of the same general mechanism of cell membrane biogenesis and renewal. It is, at present, not clear whether galactosyltransferase can be used as a reliable marker for these phenomena as the possibility of endocytosis and recycling in specialised cell types needs careful evaluation. The data related to release (shedding) and processing, however, form a rationale for activity measurements in body fluids for clinical purposes.

Clinical Use

Galactosyltransferase activity is readily measured in normal human serum (*32, 62*), which contains, on the basis of its activity, approximately 0.2 U/l or 125 μg/l enzyme protein. Increased levels of activity have been reported in patients suffering from ovarian (*10*) and breast cancer (*44*), whereas cancers of other organs as investigated in Ref. *64* are not correlated with significantly increased activity levels.

Preliminary results obtained in this laboratory in collaboration with the Bern Branch of the Ludwig Institute for Cancer Research confirm these findings and indicate a correlation with total sialic acid in serum (*37*). It is, however, important to note that activity increases related to ovarian and breast cancer usually remain within the same order of magnitude. The fact that these differences do not reliably discriminate between normal and pathological populations prevents the application of enzyme measurements for screening. As serum galactosyltransferase activity closely relates to tumor mass (*15, 62*), its use in clinical chemistry will mainly be restricted to patient monitoring and evaluation of therapeutic efficiency. Podolsky and Weiser reported a cancer associated "isoenzyme" of galactosyltransferase (GT-II), a hitherto unconfirmed observation (*48*). As their data are based on electrophoretic separation of a usually slow moving enzyme activity eluted from polyacrylamide gels, it is not clear whether the difference in electrophoretic mobility relates to higher molecular size or lower charge density or both. We have shown in this laboratory (*22*) that in neuraminidase treated serum, migration of galactosyltransferase activity in a similar system as the one described by Podolsky is considerably retarded. It is, therefore, conceivable that GT-II represents an incompletely glycosylated form of galactosyltransferase. In this case, the generally low serum level of GT-II may be the consequence of rapid removal from the circulation by receptors specific for terminal galactose, N-acetylglucosamine or mannose as recently reviewed by Ashwell and Harford (*2*). A probably unrelated species of enzyme present in malignant pleural exudates was described by Kim *et al.* (*31*). As sialic acid-galactose free fetuin was used as acceptor substrate in this work, it is not possible to ascertain that this cancer-related species belongs to galactosyltransferases specific for GlcNAc residues, the more as the enzyme was assayed apparently in the presence of free GlcNAc. GT-II could also represent a variant of galactosyltransferase of higher molecular weight as suggested by Podolsky and Weiser (*49*). Unfortunately, the enzyme preparations of GT-I and GT-II used for structural analysis appear to be contaminated by substantial amounts of immunoglobulins (*66*). Higher molecular weight variants of galactosyltransferase activity have been described (see Sec. on "*Heterogeneity*"). Since newly formed enzyme proteins recovered by immunoprecipitation from heavy HeLa cell fractions have molecular weights between 45 and 47 kD, high molecular weight forms of this enzyme most likely represent postsynthetically formed homo- or heteropolymers. Evidence for the occurrence of such enzyme forms in milk has been presented (*8, 9*). It is also possible that "isoenzyme II" represents one of these enzyme forms. Convincing evidence for a distinct gene coding for "isoenzyme II" (as the term "isoenzyme" implies) has not been presented.

Perspectives

Since glycosyltransferases appear to confer fundamental properties in terms of adhesion and recognition to cell surface glycoproteins and glycolipids, factors governing expression of glycosyltransferase activity are of crucial importance for the "social behavior" of cells. It appears promising, therefore, to investigate regulation of genetic expression of these enzymes as this approach may give insight into phenomena in which the social behavior is severely disturbed, as in malignant transformation and metastasis. Current efforts in this laboratory are aimed at the study of enzyme forms synthesized in cell free systems, at the construction and cloning of the cDNA in order to establish the structure of its gene(s) and, as a consequence, its putative amino acid sequence(s). Knowledge of the structure of galactosyltransferase may reveal some specific requirements which eventually could explain the intriguing finding that the enzyme is only detectable in trans cisternae of the Golgi apparatus. This approach may also pave the way for the study of factors governing expression of galactosyltransferase at the genetic level.

REFERENCES

1. Andrews, P. *FEBS Lett.*, **9**, 297–300 (1970).
2. Ashwell, G. and Harford, J. *Annu. Rev. Biochem.*, **51**, 531–544 (1982).
3. Barker, R., Olsen, K. W., Shaper, J. H., and Hill, R. L. *J. Biol. Chem.*, **247**, 7135–7147 (1972).
4. Berger, E. G., Weiser, M. M., and Isselbacher, K. J. *Experientia*, **32**, 690–691 (1976).
5. Berger, E. G., Weiser, M. M., Alpert, E., and Isselbacher, K. J. *Fed. Proc.*, **35** (1976) (Abstr.)
6. Berger, E. G., Kozdrowski, I., Weiser, M. M., van den Eijnden, D. H., and Schiphorst, W.E.C.M. *Eur. J. Biochem.*, **90**, 213–222 (1978).
7. Berger, E. G., Mandel, Th., and Schilt, U. *J. Histochem. Cytochem.*, **29**, 364–370 (1981).
8. Berger E. G., Verdon, B., and Roth, J. *In* "Glycoconjugates," ed. T. Yamakawa, T. Osawa, and S. Handa, pp. 299–300 (1981). Japan Sci. Soc. Press, Tokyo.
9. Berger, E. G., Verdon, B., Mandel, T., Fey, H., and Strous, G. *Enzyme*, **29**, 175–182 (1983).
10. Bhattacharya, M., Chatterjee, S. K., and Barlow, J. J. *Cancer Res.*, **36**, 2096–2101 (1976).
11. Bloch, R. and Burger, M. M. *FEBS Lett.*, **44**, 286–289 (1974).
12. Bolander, F. F., Jr. and Topper, Y. J. *Endocrinology*, **108**, 1594–1596 (1981).
13. Bretz, R. and Stäubli, W. *Eur. J. Biochem.*, **77**, 181–192 (1977).
14. Bretz, R., Bretz, H., and Palade, G. E. *J. Cell Biol.*, **84**, 87–101 (1980).
15. Chatterjee, S. K., Bhattacharya, M., and Barlow, J. J. *Cancer Lett.*, **5**, 239–244 (1978).
16. Ebner, K. E. *In* "Enzymes," Vol. IX, ed. P. D. Boyer, pp. 363–377 (1973). Academic Press, New York.
17. Ehrenreich, J. H., Bergeron, J.J.M., Siekevitz, P., and Palade, G. E. *J. Cell Biol.*, **59**, 45–72 (1973).
18. Fairbanks, G., Steck, Th.L., and Wallach, D.H.F. *Biochemistry*, **10**, 2606–2617 (1971).
19. Fleischer, B. and Fleischer, S. *Biochim. Biophys. Acta*, **219**, 301–319 (1970).
20. Fleischer, B. and Smigel, M. *J. Biol. Chem.*, **253**, 1632–1638 (1978).
21. Fujita-Yamaguchi, Y. and Yoshida, A. *J. Biol. Chem.*, **256**, 2701–2706 (1981).
22. Gerber, A. Ch., Kozdrowski, I., Wyss, S. R., and Berger, E. G. *Eur. J. Biochem.*, **93**, 453–460 (1979).

23. Griffiths, J. and Reynolds, S. *Clin. Biochem.*, **15**, 46–48 (1982).
24. Hagopian, A., Bosmann, B. H., and Eylar, E. H. *Arch. Biochem. Biophys.*, **128**, 387–396 (1968).
25. Hesford, F. J. and Berger, E. G. *Biochim. Biophys. Acta*, **649**, 709–716 (1981).
26. Hill, R. L. and Brew, K. *Adv. Enzymol.*, **43**, 411–490 (1975).
27. Hsu, Ch.-H. and Kingsbury, D. W. *J. Biol. Chem.*, **257**, 9035–9038 (1982).
28. Keenan, T. W. and Morré, D. J. *FEBS Lett.*, **55**, 8–13 (1975).
29. Kessel, D., Shah-Reddy, O., Mirchandani, I., Khilanani, P., and Chou, T.-H. *Cancer Res.*, **40**, 3576–3578 (1980).
30. Khatra, B. S., Herries, D. G., and Brew, K. *Eur. J. Biochem.*, **44**, 537–560 (1974).
31. Kim, Y. D., Weber, G. F., Tomita, J. T., and Hirata, A. A. *Clin. Chem.*, **28**, 1133–1136 (1982).
32. Kim, Y. S., Perdomo, J., and Whitehead, J. S. *J. Clin. Invest.*, **51**, 2024–2032 (1972).
33. Kuhn, N. J. and White, A. *Biochem. J.*, **168**, 423–433 (1977).
34. Laemmli, U. K. *Nature*, **227**, 680–685 (1970).
35. LaMont, J. T., Gammon, M. Th., and Isselbacher K. J. *Proc. Natl. Acad. Sci. U.S.*, **74**, 1086–1090 (1977).
36. Lowry, O. H., Rosebrough, N. J., Farr, A. L., and Randall, R. J. *J. Biol. Chem.*, **193**, 265–275 (1951).
37. Luder, A., Goldhirsch, A., and Berger, E. G. Unpublished results.
38. Magee, S. C., Mawai, R., and Ebner, K. E. *J. Biol. Chem.*, **248**, 7565–7569 (1973).
39. Magee, S. C., Green, C. R., and Ebner, K. E. *Biochim. Biophys. Acta*, **420**, 187–194 (1976).
40. Louvard, D., Reggio, H., and Warren, G. *J. Cell Biol.*, **92**, 92–107 1(982).
41. Morré, D. J., Merlin, L. M., and Keenan, T. W. *Biochim. Biophys. Res. Commun.*, **37**, 813–819 (1969).
42. Nagata, S., Mantei, N., and Weissmann C. *Nature*, **287**, 401–408 (1980).
43. Palade, G. *Science*, **189**, 347–358 (1975).
44. Paone, J. F., Waalkes, T. P., Baker, R. R., and Shaper, J. H. *J. Surg. Oncol.*, **15**, 59–66 (1980).
45. Pavelka, M. and Ellinger, A. *Eur. J. Cell Biol.*, **24**, 53–61 (1981).
46. Pestalozzi, D. M., Hess, M., and Berger, E. G. *J. Histochem. Cytochem.*, **30**, 1146–1152 (1982).
47. Pierce, M., Turley, E. A., and Roth, S. *Int. Rev. Cytol.*, **65**, 1–47 (1980).
48. Podolsky, D. K. and Weiser, M. M. *Biochim. Biophys. Res. Commun.*, **65**, 545–551 (1975).
49. Podolsky, D. K. and Weiser, M. M. *J. Biol. Chem.*, **254**, 3983–3990 (1979).
50. Powell, J. T., Jaerlfors, U., and Brew, K. *J. Cell Biol.*, **72**, 617–627 (1977).
51. Prieels, J.-P., Maes, E., Dolmans, M., and Leonis, J. *Eur. J. Biochem.*, **60**, 525–531 (1975).
52. Roseman, S. *Chem. Phys. Lipids*, **5**, 270 (1970).
53. Roth, J. and Berger, E. G. *J. Cell Biol.*, **92**, 223–229 (1982).
54. Sabatini, D. D., Kreibich, G., Morimoto, T., and Adesnik, M. *J. Cell Biol.*, **92**, 1–22 (1982).
55. Schachter, H., Jabbal, I., Hudgin, R. L., Pinteric, L., McGuire, E. J., and Roseman, S. *J. Biol. Chem.*, **245**, 1090–1100 (1970).
56. Smith, Ch. A. and Brew, K. *J. Biol. Chem.*, **252**, 7294–7299 (1977).
57. Strous, G.J.A.M. and Berger, E. G. *J. Biol. Chem.*, **257**, 7623–7628 (1982).
58. Tartakoff, A. M. *Trends Biochem. Sci.*, **7**, 174–176 (1982).
59. Towbin, H., Staehelin, T., and Gordon, J. *Proc. Natl. Acad. Sci U.S.*, **76**, 4350–4354 (1979).
60. van den Eijnden, D. H., Schiphorst, W.E.C.M., and Berger, E. G. *Biochim. Biophys. Acta*, **755**, 32–39 (1983).

61. Verbert, A., Cacan, R., and Montreuil, J. *Eur. J. Biochem.*, **70**, 49–54 (1976).
62. Verdon, B. and Berger, E. G. *In* "Methods of Enzymatic Analysis," Vol. III, ed. H. U. Bergmeyer. Verlag Chemie, Weinheim, in press.
63. Weiser, M. M. *J. Biol. Chem.*, **248**, 2536–2541 (1973).
64. Weiser, M. M., Podolsky, D. K., and Isselbacher, K. J. *Proc. Natl. Acad. Sci. U.S.*, **73**, 1319–1322 (1976).
65. Weiser, M. M. Neumeier, M. M., Quaroni, A., and Kirsch, K. *J. Cell Biol.*, **77**, 722–734 (1978).
66. Wilson, J. R., Weiser, M. M., Albini, B., Schenck, J. R., Rittenhouse, H. G., Hirata, A. A., and Berger, E. G. *Biochem. Biophys. Res. Commun.*, **105**, 737–744 (1982).
67. Zilberstein, A., Snider, M. D., Forster, M., and Lodish, H. F. *Cell*, **21**, 417–428 (1980).

GANN Monograph on Cancer Research 29, 1983

GLYCOSYLTRANSFERASES OF THE GOLGI COMPLEX IN RELATION TO CELL SURFACE CHANGES IN RAT HEPATOMA

Yukio Ikehara[*1] and Keikichi Takahashi[*2]

*Department of Biochemistry, Fukuoka University School of Medicine[*1] and Cancer Research Institute, Kyushu University School of Medicine[*2]*

Highly purified Golgi fractions were obtained from normal rat liver and ascites hepatoma AH-130 cells. Some properties of glycosyltransferases in the two Golgi fractions were compared using various purified glycoproteins as acceptors. A remarkable decrease of sialyltransferase activity was observed in the hepatoma Golgi fraction, while there was no significant difference in galactosyltransferase activity. Glycosyltransferases in the hepatoma and liver Golgi fractions were then assayed with plasma membranes from both sources as exogenous acceptors. Hepatoma sialyltransferase activity was also much lower (1/2 to 1/4) than that of the normal liver. Acceptor plasma membranes which had been glycosylated *in vitro* by each Golgi enzyme were separated into protein and lipid fractions, and the latter fraction was further analyzed by thin layer chromatography. The results demonstrated that the hepatoma Golgi had much lower levels of glycoprotein: sialyltransferase and asialo-GM_1: sialyltransferase, but had an increased activity of asialo-GM_3: sialyltransferase. It is suggested that the decrease of sialyltransferase level is related to the decreased sialylation of plasma membrane marker enzymes in the hepatoma cells.

Much interest has focused on the cell surface glycoproteins and glycolipids of normal and malignant cells. This is due to the fact that changes in the composition of these components are known to accompany malignant transformation. Transformed cells exhibit a reduction in complexity of glycolipids (*5, 21*) and an overall decrease in the number of membrane glycoproteins (*7, 19, 24, 33*). Some studies, however, have demonstrated an increased glycosylation of membrane glycoproteins in the transformed cells (*3, 32*). These alterations in the carbohydrate chains are suggested to be associated with changes in glycosyltransferases (*20*) and/or of glycosidases (*2*) which are localized on the cell surface.

On the other hand, the current concept of "membrane transformation," that the exoplasmic membranes are differentiated from the endoplasmic membranes (*15*), suggests that the Golgi complex plays an important role in the biogenesis of the plasma membrane and its modification (Fig. 1). Involvement of the Golgi complex is especially emphasized in the terminal glycosylation of glycoproteins and glycolipids of the plasma membrane, as shown in the case of secretory proteins (*25*). This concept is supported by considerable evidence (*15*), a part of which is based on the findings that glycolipid-glycosyltransferases

---

[*1] Nanakuma 34, Jonan-ku, Fukuoka 814-01, Japan (池原征夫).
[*2] Maidashi 3-1-1, Higashi-ku, Fukuoka 812, Japan (高橋慶吉).

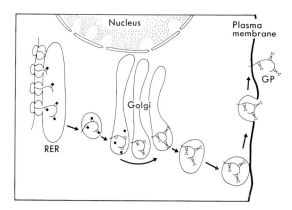

Fɪɢ. 1.   A diagram summarizing the structural and functional relationships among endoplasmic reticulum, Golgi complex, and the plasma membrane. The diagramed concept of the Golgi complex function involves the input of new membrane material from endoplasmic reticulum and its progressive transformation and utilization in the elaboration of membranes of secretory vesicles which are plasma membrane-like and ultimately capable of fusing with plasma membrane. RER, rough endoplasmic reticulum; GP, glycoprotein; □, ■, ×, △ components of sugar chains.

as well as glycoprotein: glycosyltransferases are almost exclusively localized in the Golgi complex (*12, 25*), and that the highest acceptor activities for galactose and sialic acid are found in the Golgi membranes (*8*). Thus, it is likely that the structural changes in glycoconjugates at the cell surface which accompany malignant transformation are provoked by alterations of glycosyltransferases in the Golgi complex. In the present study, rat ascites hepatoma AH-130 cells were used as the malignant cells for the following reasons. First, the rapid growth of ascites hepatoma cells readily provided a large enough number of cells for subcellular fractionation. Second, since the isolation of rat hepatic Golgi complex has been established, we can easily compare results obtained from the hepatoma cells with those from the normal liver.

Isolation of Golgi Fractions

As pointed out by Morré (*14*), the first homogenization step is most important for preparation of the Golgi complex with good yield and purity. The liver Golgi fraction was isolated by using the isotonic solution for homogenization, followed by a combination of differential and discontinuous sucrose gradient centrifugations (*16, 31*). The same homogenization conditions were not effective for the hepatoma cells which were free cells different from the liver tissues. After various trials, the homogenization conditions used for the plasma membrane preparations from the same hepatoma cells (*9*) were found to be most useful to obtain the Golgi complex in good yield and purity (*28*). An electron microscopic view of the typical Golgi fraction isolated from the ascites hepatoma AH-130 cells showed that it consisted primarily of cisternae, vesicles, and tubular elements which were similar to those structures of the Golgi fraction isolated from rat liver (*16, 31*).

Galactosyl- and sialyl-transferases were concentrated about 55- and 75-fold, respectively, in this fraction compared with the homogenate, indicating that these enzymes are useful markers for the Golgi complex of rat ascites hepatoma AH-130 cells, as they are for those of normal tissues (*16, 25, 31*). Further biochemical analyses including assays of various marker enzymes for other organelles, DNA, and RNA revealed that the isolated Golgi fraction had the purity of at least 80–90%, which is comparable to that of the Golgi fraction from normal liver (*16, 31*).

Comparison of Activity Levels of Glycosyltransferases in Hepatoma AH-130 Cells and Normal Liver

Two marker enzymes for the Golgi complex, sialyl- and galactosyltransferases, were determined in both homogenates and Golgi fractions isolated from AH-130 cells and normal liver using various acceptors (*29*) (Table I). In both the homogenate and Golgi fraction, the specific activity of the hepatoma sialyltransferase was markedly lower than that of the normal liver. Decrease of the enzyme activity varied with the acceptors used: the hepatoma Golgi fraction had activity levels of 21–22% with asialo-fetuin or asialo-orosomucoid and 41% with asialo-mucin, as compared with those of the liver Golgi fraction with the same acceptors. On the other hand, the specific activity of galactosyltransferase in the hepatoma was similar to that of normal liver both in the homogenate and Golgi fraction.

Similar results have been observed in solid hepatomas (*6*) and another ascites hepatoma (*23*). Hudgin *et al.* (*6*) showed that sialyltransferase activity of Morris hepatoma 7777 and 7800 was decreased to one-third of that of normal liver, while the hepatoma N-acetylglucosaminyltransferase activity was not significantly different from that of the liver. The reduction in sialyltransferase activity was also observed in the rat ascites hepatoma AH-108 AF by Saito *et al.* (*23*), although they did not give any data on other glycosyltransferases.

We also compared the activity levels of glycosyltransferases in plasma membranes prepared from both sources. Both plasma membranes had trace levels of the activities and showed no significant difference from each other: sialyltransferase activity with asialo-fetuin was 13.3 nmol/hr/mg protein and 14.0 for the hepatoma and liver, respectively; galactosyltransferase activity with GlcNAc was 48.8 nmol/hr/mg protein and 43.3 for the hepatoma and liver, respectively. Thus, it is likely that the much lower level of sialyltransferase activity observed in the hepatoma homogenate is primarily attributable to its decrease in the Golgi complex, not in the plasma membrane.

TABLE I. Comparison of Specific Activities of Glycosyltransferases in the Homogenates and Golgi Fractions from Hepatoma and Normal Liver[a] (*29*)

Acceptor	Hepatoma AH-130		Normal liver	
	Homogenate	Golgi	Homogenate	Golgi
Sialyltransferase				
Asialo-fetuin	8.2	648.2	27.6	3,047.2
Asialo-orosomucoid	16.2	923.1	64.0	4,094.6
Asialo-mucin	n.d.	123.5	n.d.	297.2
Galactosyltransferase				
N-acetylglucosamine	26.5	1,453.4	14.7	1,541.6
Asialo-agalacto-fetuin	28.0	2,178.3	26.8	2,533.3
Asialo-mucin	28.6	2,105.3	27.5	2,384.6

[a] Values are expressed as nmol/hr/mg protein, the mean of at least five different experiments.
n. d., not determined.

Comparison of Kinetic Properties of Glycosyltransferases between the Hepatoma and Liver

Sialyltransferase in both Golgi fractions showed similar pH activity curves with optimum pH between 6 and 7, with either asialo-fetuin or asialo-mucin as the acceptor. Similarly, no significant difference was observed in the pH activity curve of galactosyl-transferase between the two Golgi fractions (*29*).

Sialyltransferase of both Golgi fractions was activated by Triton X-100, and slightly inhibited by β-mercaptoethanol. Requirements for galactosyltransferase were essentially the same for both Golgi fractions: it absolutely required Mn^{2+} and Triton X-100 for the maximum activity. K_m values for both donor (substrate) and acceptors for each enzyme were found to be similar in both the hepatoma and normal liver. These results suggest that the kinetic properties of sialyltransferase as well as galactosyltransferase are very similar in the hepatoma and liver, although sialyltransferase is markedly decreased in quantity in the hepatoma Golgi as compared with that in the normal liver fraction.

Comparison of Glycosyltransferase Activities Using Plasma Membranes as Acceptors

Plasma membranes isolated from the hepatoma cells and liver were used as acceptors for the determination of glycosyltransferase activities. Figure 2 shows the transfer of [^{14}C]sialic acid from cytidine monophosphate (CMP)-[^{14}C]sialic acid to the denatured plasma membranes which was catalyzed by each Golgi fraction. As compared with the normal Golgi fraction, the hepatoma Golgi fraction had much less transfer activity of [^{14}C]sialic acid to plasma membrane preparations from both the hepatoma cells (Fig. 2A) and normal liver (Fig. 2B). The transfer of [^{14}C]galactose from uridine diphosphate (UDP)-[^{14}C]galactose to plasma membranes was also determined. As opposed to the results shown in Fig. 2, the hepatoma Golgi fraction exhibited a slightly higher transfer activity either with the hepatoma plasma membrane or with the liver membrane (*29*).

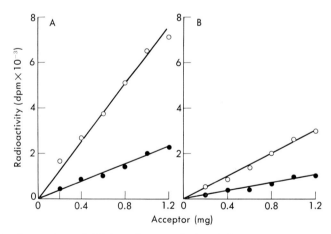

FIG. 2. Comparison of sialyltransferase activities of the hepatoma and liver Golgi fractions. Plasma membranes prepared from the hepatoma (A) and normal liver (B) were used as acceptors, and the Golgi fractions (50 μg) of the hepatoma ($\bullet$) and normal liver ($\bigcirc$) were used as enzyme sources. Activities are expressed as the radioactivity of [^{14}C]sialic acid incorporated from CMP-[^{14}C]sialic acid into the acceptor used (*29*).

These results also clearly demonstrate the difference between the two plasma membranes with respect to the acceptor activity for sialic acid and galactose: the hepatoma plasma membrane (Fig. 2A) showed higher acceptor activity than the liver membrane (Fig. 2B), irrespective of the enzyme sources used.

The deficiency of sialyltransferase in the hepatoma Golgi complex might result in incompleteness of sugar chains of the plasma membrane glycoconjugates, which in turn might exert an increased acceptor capacity (8, 29). It is reasonable that this acceptor capacity was expressed more effectively by the liver Golgi with higher specific activity of sialyltransferase. On the other hand, the increased acceptor capacity for galactose could not be explained on the same basis as above, since the hepatoma Golgi fraction had similar galactosyltransferase activity as that of the liver Golgi. It is noteworthy, however, that galactose is also transferred to the N-acetylgalactosamine residue of mucin-type oligosaccharide chains (1). Thus, it is possible that the increased acceptor activity for galactose in the hepatoma plasma membrane may be due to the presence of incomplete mucin-type sugar chains resulting from lack of terminal sialic acid residues.

The Golgi complex is also known to contain glycolipid: glycosyltransferses (12). Consequently the plasma membranes used for *in vitro* glycosylation may have served as glycolipid acceptors in addition to glycoprotein acceptors. To discriminate these two types of glycosylation, we subfractionated the plasma membranes into lipid and protein fractions after the membranes had been glycosylated *in vitro* by each Golgi fraction (Table II). Most of the [^{14}C]sialic acid transferred to each plasma membranes was found in its protein fraction, to which the hepatoma Golgi fraction exhibited much less transfer activity than the liver Golgi fraction: 41% with the hepatoma plasma membrane and 35% with liver membrane. To the lipid fraction (though the transfer was much less than to the protein fraction), the liver Golgi fraction had an increased transfer activity with the liver plasma membrane as the acceptor, but a decreased activity with hepatoma acceptor. On the other hand, glycoprotein:galactosyltransferase activity was slightly higher in the liver Golgi fraction than in the hepatoma Golgi with either of the two plasma membranes. A remarkable increase of glycolipid-galactosyltransferase activity, however,

TABLE II. Comparison of Glycosyltransferase Activities in the Golgi Fractions from Hepatoma and Normal Liver Using Plasma Membranes as Exogenous Acceptors (29)

Acceptor[a] (plasma membrane)	Enzyme source[b] (Golgi fraction)	Amounts of sugar transferred to acceptor[c]	
		Protein fraction	Lipid fraction
Sialyltransferase:			
Hepatoma	Hepatoma	160.2	26.7
	Liver	391.0	18.8
Liver	Hepatoma	47.9	28.5
	Liver	137.9	47.3
Galactosyltransferase:			
Hepatoma	Hepatoma	470.7	326.5
	Liver	580.6	23.0
Liver	Hepatoma	324.9	268.2
	Liver	375.0	14.7

[a] 1 mg of plasma membranes.

[b] 50 μg of Golgi fractions.

[c] Values are expressed as pmol/hr/mg of Golgi proteins which were obtained from four experiments.

was found in the hepatoma Golgi fraction. The specific activity of the hepatoma Golgi fraction was 14- to 19-fold greater than that of the liver Golgi.

Glycolipid Patterns of Plasma Membranes In Vitro Glycosylated with [^{14}C]Sialic Acid and [^{14}C]Galactose

In order to identify differences of glycolipid:glycosyltransferases between the hepatoma and normal liver, we analyzed the glycolipid fractions of plasma membranes glycosylated *in vitro* as above. The analysis was carried out by radioscanning thin layer chromatograms of lipid extracts to which [^{14}C]sialic acid was transferred from CMP-[^{14}C]sialic acid (29). The major product of both membrane glycolipids glycosylated by the hepatoma Golgi fraction was GM_3, although GM_1 and GM_2 were also found as minor components. In contrast, the liver Golgi fraction glycosylated both membrane-lipids to form GM_1 as the major component and GM_3 as a minor one. In addition, individual major peaks obtained with each enzyme preparation showed different heights, namely, different extents of sialylation. These results suggest two important points. One is that the hepatoma Golgi fraction contained an increased activity of asialo-GM_3: sialyltransferase but a decreased activity of asialo-GM_1: sialyltransferase, as compared with the liver Golgi fraction. The other is that there was a quantitative difference in each available acceptor (asialo-glycolipids) between the two plasma membranes.

Many reports have stated that changes in glycolipid: sialyltransferase activity occur at the cell surface as a function of tumorigenesis, resulting in a simplified ganglioside composition (5, 26). However, it may be reasonable to assume that the alteration of enzymes occurs at the Golgi apparatus, because enzymes for ganglioside synthesis are also concentrated in this organelle in the normal (12) and malignant tissues (21).

Glycolipids labeled with [^{14}C]galactose were also analyzed by thin layer chromatography (29). Irrespective of the plasma membrane used as the acceptor, the major glycolipids glycosylated by the hepatoma Golgi fraction were di- and tri-hexosylceramides (CDH and CTH, respectively), and GM_1 was also found as a minor component. When glycosylated by the liver Golgi fraction, both plasma membranes gave only GM_1 as the labeled glycolipid in an amount similar to that obtained with hepatoma Golgi fraction. It has been demonstrated that enzymes for the formation of lactosylceramide are located in the endoplasmic reticulum (13, 27). Chandrabose et al. (4) have indicated that the activities of two galactosyltransferases catalyzing the formation of CDH and CTH are found in the endoplasmic reticulum in NIL-2 hamster cells. Thus, our results suggest that considerable changes of glycolipid: glycosyltransferases occur in the hepatoma cells with respect to their activity and subcellular localization.

Comparison of Plasma Membrane Marker Enzymes between the Hepatoma and Normal Liver

To know the possible relationships between the decrease of sialyltransferase and structural changes in cell surface glycoproteins, we analyzed plasma membrane marker enzymes which are glycoproteins. Table III shows a comparison of activity levels of some marker enzymes between the hepatoma and liver plasma membranes, indicating a great contrast between the two membranes depending upon the marker enzymes. Activities of 5′-nucleotidase and dipeptidyl peptidase IV were much higher in the liver

TABLE III. Comparison of Activity Levels of Plasma Membrane Marker
Enzymes between Liver and Hepatoma AH-130 Cells

Marker enzyme	Specific activity[a]		Ratio (AH-130/liver)
	Liver	AH-130	
5'-Nucleotidase	850	67	0.08
Dipeptidyl peptidase IV	580	250	0.43
Alkaline phosphatase	53	2,200	41.5
γ-Glutamyl transpeptidase	15	1,400	93.3

[a] Mean values obtained from at least ten preparations of plasma membranes (nmol/min/mg protein).

TABLE IV. Comparison of Carbohydrate Compositions of Alkaline Phosphatases
Isolated from Rat Liver and Hepatoma

	Hepatoma AH-130		Liver	
	Weight (%)	mol/mol[a]	Weight (%)	mol/mol[a]
Mannose	5.28	40	5.40	41
Galactose	3.42	26	3.55	27
Fucose	0.96	8	0.84	7
Glucosamine	5.72	44	5.85	45
Galactosamine	1.04	8	0.58	4
Sialic acid	5.03	22	5.91	26
	21.45		22.13	

[a] Molecular weight of alkaline phosphatase = 136,000.

plasma membrane, while those of alkaline phosphatase and γ-glutamyl transpeptidase
were much higher in the hepatoma plasma membrane.

The hepatoma alkaline phosphatase was found to be electrophoretically different
from the liver enzyme in standard gels at pH 8.6 (9). To determine whether their difference is in the polypeptide chain or in the carbohydrate chain, we purified the enzyme
from plasma membranes of the hepatoma and liver (10, 11). The purified two enzymes
were identical in immunological properties and in amino acid composition, but different
in carbohydrate composition. As shown in Table IV, both enzymes contained 21 to 22%
carbohydrate by weight. Significant differences were observed in the contents of sialic
acid and galactosamine. The hepatoma alkaline phosphatase contained less sialic acid
and more galactosamine than the liver enzyme. When the two purified enzymes were
compared by standard gel electrophoresis before and after neuraminidase treatment,
different mobilities observed for the intact samples could no longer be detected after
treatment (11). The results clearly indicate that the difference of negative charge in the
two forms is due to the different contents of sialic acid. Similar results were obtained
in preliminary experiments with dipeptidyl peptidase IV, 5'-nucleotidase and γ-glutamyl
transpeptidase; these enzymes were also less sialylated in the hepatoma than in the
liver. In addition, we have demonstrated that the Golgi complex was involved in the
intracellular transport of newly synthesized alkaline phosphatase to the plasma membrane (17). Taken together, these results suggest that the decrease in sialyltransferase
activity of the hepatoma Golgi was actually reflected in less sialylation of carbohydrate
chains of the glycoproteins, alkaline phosphatase and other marker enzymes, of the
plasma membrane.

As the Golgi complex has now been established as the site of synthesis of complex carbohydrates, including their processing (22, 30), cell surface functions mediated by glycoproteins and glycolipids might be in some way regulated by Golgi function. Therefore, Richardson *et al.* (21) have proposed that the Golgi apparatus plays an important role in tumorigenesis. The alterations in glycosyltransferase activities of the hepatoma Golgi complex observed in the present study are consistent with their proposal. Nevertheless, the possibility should also be kept in mind that these differences between the two Golgi fractions simply reflect altered metabolism in these cells, because the hepatoma AH-130 cells grow rapidly in ascites as free cells (18) and lack many cellular functions, particularly synthesis and secretion of plasma proteins including glycoproteins.

Acknowledgments

We wish to thank Dr. K. Kato, Faculty of Pharmaceutical Sciences, Kyushu University, where part of this work was carried out, for his encouragement, and Dr. A. Makita (Hokkaido University School of Medicine) for useful suggestions and for providing us with authentic glycolipids. This work was supported in part by grants from the Ministry of Education, Science and Culture of Japan.

REFERENCES

1. Andersson, G. N. and Eriksson, L. C. *J. Biol. Chem.*, **256**, 9633–9639 (1981).
2. Bosmann, H. B. *Biochim. Biophys. Acta*, **264**, 339–343 (1972).
3. Buck, C. A., Glick, M. C., and Warren, L. *Biochemistry*, **9**, 4567–4576 (1970).
4. Chandrabose, K. A., Graham, J. M., and Macpherson, I. A. *Biochim. Biophys. Acta*, **426**, 112–122 (1976).
5. Hakomori, S. *Biochim. Biophys. Acta*, **417**, 55–89 (1975).
6. Hudgin, R. L., Murray, R. K., Pinteric, L., Morris, H. P., and Schachter, H. *Can. J. Biochem.*, **49**, 61–70 (1971).
7. Hynes, R. O. *Biochim. Biophys. Acta*, **458**, 73–107 (1976).
8. Ikehara, Y., Oda, K., and Kato, K. *J. Biochem.*, **81**, 349–354 (1977).
9. Ikehara, Y., Takahashi, K., Mansho, K., Eto, S., and Kato, K. *Biochim. Biophys. Acta*, **470**, 202–211 (1977).
10. Ikehara, Y., Mansho, K., Takahashi, K., and Kato, K. *J. Biochem.*, **83**, 1471–1483 (1978).
11. Kawahara, S., Ogata, S., and Ikehara, Y. *J. Biochem.*, **91**, 201–210 (1982).
12. Keenan, T. W., Morré, D. J., and Basu, S. *J. Biol. Chem.*, **249**, 310–315 (1974).
13. Mårtensson, E., Ohman, R., Graves, M., and Svennerholm, L. *J. Biol. Chem.*, **249**, 4132–4137 (1974).
14. Morré, D. J. *Methods Enzymol.*, **22**, 130–148 (1971).
15. Morré, D. J. *In* "The Synthesis, Assembly and Turnover of Cell Surface Components," ed. G. Poste and G. L. Nicolson, pp. 1–83 (1977). North-Holland, Amsterdam, New York, and Oxford.
16. Oda, K., Ikehara, Y., Ishikawa, T., and Kato, K. *Biochim. Biophys. Acta*, **552**, 212–224 (1979).
17. Oda, K. and Ikehara, Y. *Biochim. Biophys. Acta*, **640**, 398–408 (1981).
18. Odashima, S. *Natl. Cancer Inst. Monogr.*, **16**, 51–87 (1964).
19. Ohta, N., Pardee, A. B., MacAuslan, B. R., and Burger, M. M. *Biochim. Biophys. Acta*, **158**, 98–102 (1968).
20. Patt, L. M. and Grimes, W. J. *J. Biol. Chem.*, **249**, 4157–4165 (1974).
21. Richardson, C. L., Baber, S. R., Morré, D. J., and Keenan, T. W. *Biochim. Biophys. Acta*, **417**, 175–186 (1975).

22. Rothman, J. E. *Science*, **213**, 1212–1219 (1981).

23. Saito, M., Satoh, H., and Ukita, T. *Biochem. Biphys. Acta*, **362**, 549–557 (1974).

24. Sakiyama, H. and Burge, B. W. *Biochemistry*, **11**, 1366–1377 (1972).

25. Schachter, H., Jabbal, I., Hudgin, R. L., Pinteric, L., McGuire, E. J., and Roseman, S. *J. Biol. Chem.*, **245**, 1090–1100 (1970).

26. Shur, B. D. and Roth, S. *Biochim. Biophys. Acta*, **415**, 473–512 (1975).

27. Stoffyn, R., Stoffyn, A., and Hauser, G. *J. Biol. Chem.*, **248**, 1920–1923 (1973).

28. Takahashi, K., Ikehara, Y., and Kato, K. *J. Biochem.*, **92**, 725–736 (1982).

29. Takahashi, K., Ikehara, Y., Ogawa, M., and Kato, K. *J. Biochem.*, **92**, 737–748 (1982).

30. Tartakoff, A. M. *Int. Rev. Exp. Pathol.*, **22**, 227–251 (1980).

31. Tsuji, H., Hattori, N., Yamamoto, T., and Kato, K. *J. Biochem.*, **82**, 619–636 (1978).

32. Warren, L., Fuhrer, J. P., and Buck, C. A. *Proc. Natl. Acad. Sci. U.S.*, **69**, 1838–1842 (1972).

33. Wu, H. C., Meezan, E., Black, P. H., and Robbins, P. W. *Biochemistry*, **8**, 2509–2517 (1969).

ALTERATIONS OF LYSOSOMAL HYDROLASES IN HUMAN LUNG CANCER

Akira Makita, Shinsei Gasa, Masaki Narita,
Michiyasu Fujita, and Naoyuki Taniguchi

*Biochemistry Laboratory, Cancer Institute, Hokkaido
University School of Medicine**

Lysosomal hydrolases from human lung cancers of various histological types were examined for their activity levels and properties. The levels of β-hexosaminidases A and B, β-glucuronidase, and arylsulfatases A and B were significantly elevated in the tumors of almost all types as compared to those of uninvolved tissue. Arylsulfatase B, β-glucuronidase and β-hexosaminidase B purified from tumors demonstrated considerable charge-heterogeneity with their anionic variant forms. The anionic property of the variants was examined by treatment with exogenous enzymes. By exogenous phosphatase treatment, most anionic forms of arylsulfatase B and β-glucuronidase were converted to less anionic forms, and by endo-β-N-acetylglucosaminidase H treatment the variants were converted to the respective enzyme forms which are predominant in normal lung. Thus, the heterogeneity of the tumor enzymes is due to modification by the phosphate groups which are bound to the carbohydrate moieties of the hydrolases, though an arylsulfatase B variant was suggested to be modified by sialylation in addition. Arylsulfatase B variant was found to be phosphorylated both on the carbohydrate and protein moieties by ^{32}P-phosphorylation experiments with *in vivo* labeling and the *in vitro* protein kinase reaction. Mannose-6-phosphate, phosphoserine, and phosphothreonine were identified in the hydrolyzates of the labeled enzyme. On the other hand, the β-hexosaminidase B variant was modified at its sulfhydryl group by the possible formation of a mixed disulfide, based on the results of isoelectric focusing and titration of the sulfhydryl group before and after treatment with dithiothreitol.

Neoplastic transformation of cells is accompanied by alterations of carbohydrates in cell membrane glycolipids (*16*) and glycoproteins (*38*). Direct cause of such alterations can be sought in quantitative as well as qualitative changes of the synthetic and catabolic enzymes involved in glycoconjugate metabolism.

In a series of biochemical studies on enzymes involved in glycoconjugate synthesis and degradation in human lung cancer, we have demonstrated that the activity levels of transferases in the tumor (*10, 22, 35, 40*) can be correlated with the histological type of lung cancer. Since many lysosomal hydrolases which catalyze degradation of glycoconjugates can be readily prepared in purified form, it is feasible to investigate whether or not the hydrolases themselves from lung cancer undergo alterations of their properties. In this article, we show that three lysosomal hydrolases from human lung cancer are not

---

* Kita 15, Nishi 7, Kita-ku, Sapporo 060, Japan (牧田　章, 賀佐伸省, 成田真幸, 藤田充康, 谷口直之).

only elevated in their activity, but also exhibit changes of their protein and/or carbo-hydrate components.

Arylsulfatases

Lysosomal arylsulfatases A and B catalyze the desulfation of 3-sulfo-galactosylcera-mide (cerebroside sulfate) and 4-sulfo-N-acetylgalactosamine present in glycosamino-glycans, respectively. They can be distinguished from one another by their enzymatic properties (reviewed in Ref. 31).

1. Activity

The accumulation of glycosaminoglycans in lung carcinomas of three histological types (18, 19, 21), and of cerebroside sulfate in lung adenocarcinoma (39), could be ex-plained by the diminished activities of arylsulfatases. However, significantly higher activities of these sulfatases were observed in almost all the primary lung carcinomas as compared to corresponding uninvolved tissues (11). These observations imply that the increment of sulfated glycoconjugates in lung carcinoma is not due to diminished aryl-sulfatase activities. Rather, an increased activity of cerebroside sulfotransferase in human lung adenocarcinoma is probably responsible for the accumulation of cerebroside sulfate in the tumor (10). However, elevation of these enzyme activities is not common to all organ carcinomas; rather the activities appear to be either elevated or depressed in an organ-specific manner (7, 26). On the other hand, the levels in human lung tumors transplanted into nude mice were considerably higher (2 to 4-fold) than those of the tumor tissues obtained at surgery (12). Histological examination has revealed that the amount of interstitial tissue in the tumor is decreased when a surgical tumor is trans-planted into nude mice. Therefore, transplanted tumor tissue which is "enriched" in tumor cells may express more clearly biochemical phenotypic characteristics of these cells that may be attributable to the enhancement of various enzyme activities.

2. Properties of arylsulfatases A and B in surgical and transplanted tumors

Arylsulfatases of normal human lung were separated into two components (peaks B and A) (Fig. 1a) by diethylaminoethyl (DEAE) chromatography. The carcinoma tissue obtained at surgery had an additional minor component designated peak B_1 (Fig. 1b). This minor component consistently appeared also in other lung cancer types. In trans-planted tumors, peak B_1 enzyme was a predominant form with arylsulfatase B activity in

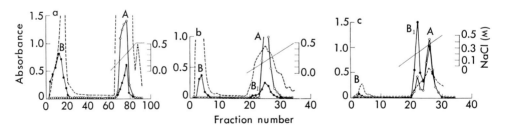

FIG. 1. DEAE chromatograms of human lung arylsulfatase (11, 12). a, normal lung; b, squamous cell carcinoma at surgery; c, transplanted squamous cell carcinoma. --- protein amount; ○ and ● "specific" arylsulfatase A and B activities, respectively.

squamous cell carcinoma (Fig. 1c) and adenocarcinoma types. The amount of peak B_1 was nearly equal with that of peak B in the large cell type of carcinoma.

The properties of peak A enzyme of normal lung and surgical and transplanted tumors were essentially identical in terms of pH optimum, K_m value, time course profile, heat stability, molecular weight, pI, and substrate specificity (11, 12), but were clearly distinguishable from those of arylsulfatase B. The properties of peak B_1 enzyme from surgical and transplanted tumors were similar to those of peak B enzyme from normal lung and tumors, and of the established arylsulfatase B (31), differing only in pI; pI 9.1 to 9.7 for B enzyme and pI 6.9 to 7.6 for B_1 enzyme (11, 12). The B and B_1 enzymes also had identical antigenicity. Thus, the assignment of arylsulfatase A to peak A enzyme, and of arylsulfatase B to peak B and B_1 enzymes was made.

To determine the nature of the negative charge in the anionic arylsulfatase B variant (B_1 enzyme), the B_1 enzyme preparation was treated with sialidase and phosphatase followed by gel isoelectric focusing (12). Treatment with either phosphatase or sialidase resulted in a shift of the B_1 enzyme to an alkaline range. Since treatment of B_1 enzyme with both the hydrolases gave the same pI value with that of B enzyme, the negative charge of B_1 enzyme can be ascribed to both sialic acid and phosphate groups linked to arylsulfatase B enzyme. The B_1 enzyme was also increased in human myelogenous leukemic cells, and decreased in response to chemotherapy (36).

3. *Evidence for phosphorylation of tumor arylsulfatase B_1 in its protein and carbohydrate moieties*

In order to examine the site of phosphorylation, human lung tumor transplanted into a nude mouse was radiolabeled *in vivo* with ^{32}P-phosphate (13). Arylsulfatases from the ^{32}P-labeled tumor were clearly separated into three enzyme-active components (A, B, B_1). Labeled B_1 enzyme was further purified by immunoprecipitation using anti-arylsulfatase B antiserum. The isolated B enzyme was only slightly labeled. The labeled B_1 enzyme was homogeneous for ^{32}P-activity, and the mobility of the radioactive peak coincided with the protein band of human liver B enzyme with a molecular weight (Mr)

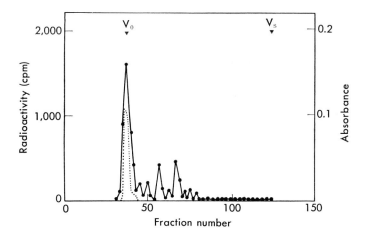

FIG. 2. Gel filtration of the enzymatic hydrolyzate of ^{32}P-labeled B_1 enzyme. ● ^{32}P activity; --- protein; V_s, elution volume of *p*-nitrocatechol sulfate which is used for assay of arylsulfatase activity as a substrate.

60×10^3, as shown by a polyacrylamide gel electrophoresis in the presence of sodium dodecyl sulfate. The immune complex was hydrolyzed by endo-β-N-acetylglucosaminidase H (endoglycosidase H), which cleaves a chitobiose unit on high mannose-type sugar chains, followed by gel filtration using a Bio-gel column. ^{32}P-label was found both in the excluded region together with the protein and in the included region with heterogenous components (Fig. 2). The labeled carbohydrate fractions in the included region were pooled, hydrolyzed and subjected to two-dimensional separation on a thin layer plate. Fluorography of the plate demonstrated two radioactive spots: One of them was identified as mannose-6-phosphate (M6P), and the other compound which migrates more than M6P has not yet been characterized. On the other hand, the excluded material from the column was subjected to a restricted hydrolysis followed by two-dimensional separation on a thin layer plate. An autoradiogram of the hydrolyzate clearly demonstrated phosphoserine and phosphothreonine in a ratio of 4:5. Thus, the lung tumor B variant (B_1) proved to be phosphorylated on both the sugar and peptide moieties (13).

4. Arylsulfatase B is a substrate for protein kinase

From the above results, it is probable that B enzyme and/or its anionic variant B_1 enzyme may serve as substrates for a protein kinase. This possibility was examined by two in vitro experiments using γ-^{32}P-ATP and endogenous or exogenous protein kinase. After the tumor homogenate containing an appreciable arylsulfatase B activity was incubated with ^{32}P-ATP, the isolated B_1 enzyme was labeled to a significant extent, whereas the B enzyme was barely labeled. When the B and B_1 enzymes were presented as substrates for exogenous protein kinase of beef heart, the B enzyme was phosphorylated 35 times more than was the B_1 enzyme. Considerable phosphorylation of the B enzyme over the B_1 enzyme by exogenous protein kinase implies that the sites available for phosphorylation on the protein moiety of the B_1 enzyme are almost saturated.

Concerning phosphorylation, the evidence presented above raises the following problems: How does protein phosphorylation correlate with phosphorylation on the carbohydrate moiety which occurs during a post-translational processing of lysosomal hydrolases? Is protein phosphorylation a truly cancer-associated alteration, possibly through an elevated protein kinase activity in neoplastic cells? Are other lysosomal hydrolases of neoplasms phosphorylated on their protein component?

β-Glucuronidase

β-Glucuronidase hydrolyzes the β-glucuronide bond at the non-reducing terminals of glycosaminoglycans. The enzyme is a glycoprotein containing high mannose-type oligosaccharide chains (25, 29).

We observed that the degree of elevation of β-glucuronidase activity in human lung cancers was different among the histologically separable types. Furthermore, some properties of the enzyme isolated from lung cancer were found to differ from those of normal lung (9).

1. Activity

β-Glucuronidase activities in the individual specimens of lung carcinomas were elevated in almost all cases as compared to that in their corresponding univolved tissue. A statistical analysis revealed that in the lung adenocarcinoma (1.25 ± 0.04 munits/mg protein; $n=29$) and squamous cell carcinoma (0.713 ± 0.029; $n=18$) the enzyme activity was increased significantly ($p<0.01$) as compared to that in the adjacent normal tissue. Moreover, the activity in adenocarcinoma was significantly ($p<0.01$) higher than that in the squamous cell carcinoma. The elevation of β-glucuronidase activity was demonstrated in several human neoplastic tissues such as bladder (27), skin (37), ovary (20), and other tissues (8). However, there was no statistical difference in the activity between human lung tumor and uninvolved tissue when the activity was expressed by tissue wet weight basis (24). Thus, increased specific activity expressed on a protein basis appears to be one of the characteristics common to a variety of human cancer tissues.

2. Properties—modification by phosphorylation

The enzyme preparations purified from human cancers and normal lung had the same kinetic properties and antigenicity. In the experiment on heat stability, saccharo-1, 4-lactone (a strong inhibitor) was found to have a stabilizing effect on β-glucuronidase at a concentration of 10 μM, and the effect was most prominent on the adenocarcinoma enzyme. However, after treatment of the adenocarcinoma enzyme with endoglycosidase H, the stabilizing effect on β-glucuronidase was decreased to the level of that of the enzyme from uninvolved lung enzyme. An enhanced heat stability of the tumor enzyme can be ascribed to its carbohydrate moiety which could be located in the vicinity of the active site or it could be associated with a special conformation of the enzyme.

Polyacrylamide gel isoelectric focusing of the adenocarcinoma enzyme in a pH range of 3.5 to 10 revealed a considerable charge heterogeneity (Fig. 3c), as compared to that of the normal lung enzyme which focused as a somewhat broad but almost homogenous peak of activity (Fig. 3a). Additional acidic components were also observed in the enzyme preparation from the large cell carcinoma. The main peak of the enzyme from both normal and tumor tissues had the same isoelectric point at pH 8. Treatment of the adenocarcinoma enzyme with endoglycosidase H brought about a marked change of pattern (Fig. 3d), that is, acidic charge-heterogenous components were shifted to the main component similar to that of normal lung. This result suggests that the acidic heterogeneity found in the tumor enzyme is due to heterogenous acidic carbohydrate moieties linked to the enzyme. The acidic groups in the carbohydrate chains were considered to be sialic acid residues or phosphomono- and diesters. Treatment of this enzyme with sialidase did not change the pattern. The disappearance of the most acidic components of the adenocarcinoma enzyme after treatment with alkaline phosphatase (Fig. 3e) suggests that phosphomonoester exists in these enzyme components. The less

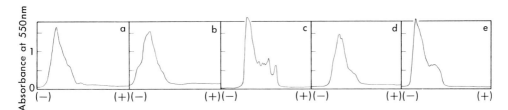

FIG. 3.   Isoelectric focusing of β-glucuronidase before and after exogenous hydrolase treatment. β-Glucuronidase from uninvolved lung without (a) or with (b) endoglycosidase H treatment, and the adenocarcinoma enzyme without (c) or with (d) endoglycosidase H or with alkaline phosphatase (e) treatment were subjected to focusing, stained for enzymic activity and scanned at 550 nm.

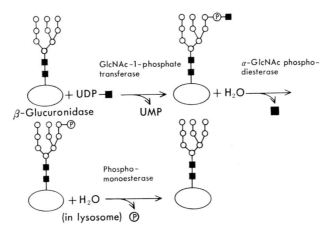

FIG. 4. Processing of β-glucuronidase on carbohydrate moiety. ■ GlcNAc; ○ mannose.

anionic shoulder components which remained after phosphatase treatment may represent the enzyme with phosphodiester groups. Treatment of the uninvolved lung enzyme with endoglycosidase H scarcely affected the pattern except that a small shoulder emerged on the cathodic side of the main peak (Fig. 3b). Indeed, the occurrence of additional acidic variants of β-glucuronidase have been noted in the change of the electrophoretic pattern of enzyme from urine and neoplastic tissues from patients with bladder cancer (27), from the basophil leukemia tumor of rat (32), and uninvolved human cells (15). However, the group responsible for the acidic variants in these tissues has not been elucidated.

β-Glucuronidase is one of the lysosomal hydrolases whose post-translational processing has been extensively investigated (17). The enzyme undergoes the processing first with formation of phosphodiester, followed by conversion to the phosphomonoester in its carbohydrate moiety and dephosphorylated mature forms (Fig. 4) (33). In light of these observations, the conspicuous appearance of acidic variants of the enzyme in lung cancer implies that there is a marked increase of immature enzyme forms resulting from an impairment at anyone of several steps. As was demonstrated in the previous section on arylsulfatase, involvement of protein phosphorylation is also not excluded.

β-Hexosaminidases

Two major types of isozymes designated as β-hexosaminidase A (Hex A) and B (Hex B) occur in vertebrates. The former is a thermolabile form with an acidic pI and the latter is a thermostable one with a basic pI. In human lung cancer, we have found that the Hex B contains a sulfhydryl group whose modification seems to be associated with the appearance of an electrophoretically distinct and heat-unstable variant in human lung adenocarcinoma (28).

1. Activity

In squamous cell carcinoma, activities of total β-hexosaminidase (16.6 ± 1.39 units/mg protein; $n=16$) and Hex A (9.96 ± 1.15; $n=15$) were significantly ($p<0.001$ and $p<0.005$, respectively) higher than those of the univolved samples. In adenocar-

cinoma the activities of total β-hexosaminidase (15.8±1.25; $n=29$) and Hex B (8.57±
0.77; $n=26$) were significantly ($p<0.005$ and $p<0.001$, respectively) higher. An increased
activity ratio of Hex B to Hex A has been reported in human colon (3) and kidney cancers (30), although the activity level remained unchanged or slightly elevated in these
tumors. However, in our study the ratio was not significantly different between the
human lung cancer and normal lung. Elevated activity of the enzyme was demonstrated
in human breast (2) and ovarian cancers (5), although the Hex B/Hex A ratio was not
higher (5).

2. Properties—modification of the sulfhydryl group

Hex B, obtained from normal lung and adenocarcinoma exhibited an optimal
activity at approximately pH 4.5. However, the enzyme from the tumor had a slightly
higher pH optimum (near pH 5.0). No significant difference of the K_m values (0.17 to
0.59 mM) with the synthetic β-GlcNAc and β-GalNAc derivatives was observed between
enzymes from normal and cancerous tissues. On the other hand, the tumor Hex B
gave two or three peaks of enzyme activity with pIs of 7.6 and 7.9, while only one peak
with pI 7.9 was observed in Hex B from normal lung (Fig. 5). The Hex A obtained either
from normal or tumor tissue lost 90% of its activity upon heating at 52° for 60 min,
while Hex B of normal tissue retained almost full activity at this temperature. However,
Hex B tumor was less stable than that from normal lung tissue. Hex B from rat colonic
cancer (4), human colonic cancer cells (23), and human hepatocarcinoma (1) has been
demonstrated to be less heat stable (1, 4, 23) and possessed acidic variant forms (4, 23).
Since Hex B is an SH-enzyme, heat-instability of the tumor Hex B was examined for
possible modification of the sulfhydryl groups. Hex B was pretreated with dithiothreitol
(DTT) at 37° for 10 min, followed by heat treatment. The pretreated tumor Hex B became more stable, similar to Hex B of normal lung, and converted to a basic form which
appeared to have a mobility similar to that of the normal lung when examined by electrophoresis. Free SH group in the purified enzymes with pIs 7.6 and 7.9 was determined
by incorporation of ^{3}H-iodoacetic acid under non-denaturing conditions. The pI 7.9
form from adenocarcinoma gave an identical value of 0.6 SH mol/mol of enzyme before
and after reduction with DTT. On the other hand, the pI 7.6 form contained 0.5 SH
mol/mol of enzyme and 0.7 SH mol/mol of enzyme before and after DTT reduction,
respectively. Therefore, it is most probable that the tumor Hex B is modified at its SH

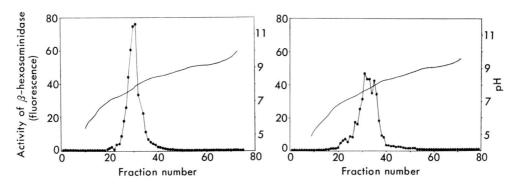

FIG. 5.   Isoelectric focusing of Hex B from normal lung (left) and lung tumor
(right).

238   A. MAKITA ET AL.

group(s). The two enzyme forms of lung cancer did not have a greatly different content of SH groups, and the conversion of the pI 7.6 form to the 7.9 form by DTT involved the reduction of only a small amount of disulfide bond (0.2 SH mol). One possible explanation for this phenomenon is that a variant form in human lung cancer involves the formation of a mixed disulfide by a reaction between the sulfhydryl group of cysteine residues of the enzyme and oxidized glutathione (GSSG), as follows:

$$\text{Enz-SH} + \text{GSSG} \xrightarrow{\qquad} \text{Enz-S-S-G} \xrightarrow{\text{DTT}} \text{Enz-SH} + \text{GSH}$$

The formation of such a mixed disulfide in the tumor enzyme could increase the one net negative charge and result in the heat-labile form. Geiger and Arnon (14) reported that the human placental β-hexosaminidase contains less SH amount by 0.1 SH mol/mol of enzyme. This type of modification has been reported in several enzymes such as carbonic anhydrase (6), and γ-glutamyl cyclotransferase (34). The formation of a mixed disulfide or other sulfhydryl modification in the enzyme is not an uncommon phenomenon. It is not clear at present whether or not the Hex B variant form involving SH groups in its structure is cancer-specific. In this regard, other modifications of tumor β-hexosaminidase such as the phosphorylation, demonstrated in previous sections, must also be considered.

Perspectives

Many lysosomal hydrolases are glycoproteins and have been demonstrated to undergo two types of post-translational processing: The one involves modification of the carbohydrate moiety and the other involves modification of the protein moiety (17). Tumor hydrolase variants phosphorylated on their carbohydrate moiety may be representative of the considerable increase or the appearance of immature stages of carbohydrate processing (Fig. 4), possibly due to the rapid proliferation of neoplastic cells or to a cancer-associated impairment. Variation of carbohydrate structure in the hydrolases of neoplastic cells seems not unusual. Modifications of protein moiety of tumor hydrolases by phosphorylation and the formation of disulfide bonds demonstrated in this article also seem to be associated with malignant transformation. It is necessary to elucidate how the alterations in a tumor described above are related to the aberrant biology of the neoplasm.

Acknowledgment

The present study was supported in part by Grants-in-Aid from the Ministries of Education, Science and Culture, and of Health and Welfare, Japan.

REFERENCES

1. Alhadeff, J. A. and Holzinger, R. T. *Biochem. J.*, **201**, 95–99 (1982).
2. Bosmann, H. B. and Hall, T. C. *Proc. Natl. Acad. Sci. U.S.*, **71**, 1833–1837 (1974).
3. Brattain, M. G., Kimball, P. M., and Pretlow, T. G., II. *Cancer Res.*, **37**, 731–734 (1977).
4. Brattain, M. G., Green, C., Kimball, P. M., Marks, M., and Khaled, M. *Cancer Res.*, **39**, 4083–4090 (1979).

5. Chatterjee, S. K., Chowdhurg, K., Bhattacharya, M., and Barlow, J. J. *Cancer*, **49**, 128–135 (1982).

6. Deutsch, H. F., Jabusch, J. R., and Lin, K.-T.D. *J. Biol. Chem.*, **252**, 555–559 (1977).

7. Dzialoszynski, L. M., Kroll, J. L., and Fröhlich, A. *Clin. Chim. Acta*, **14**, 450–453 (1966).

8. Fishman, W. H., Anlyan, A. J., and Gordon, E. *Cancer Res.*, **7**, 808–817 (1947).

9. Fujita, M., Taniguchi, N., and Makita, A. "Sapporo Cancer Seminar, the 2nd Symposium on Membrane-Associated Alterations in Cancer: Biochemical Strategies Against Cancer," July 14–17, pp. 45–46, Sapporo, Japan (1982).

10. Gasa, S., Makita, M., Hirama, M., and Kawabata, M. *J. Biochem.*, **86**, 265–267 (1979).

11. Gasa, S., Makita, A., Kameya, T., Kodama, T., Araki, E., Yoneyama, T., Hirama, M., and Hashimoto, M. *Cancer Res.*, **40**, 3804–3809 (1980).

12. Gasa, S., Makita, A., Kameya, T., Kodama, T., Koide, T., Tsumuraya, M., and Komai, T. *Eur. J. Biochem.*, **116**, 497–503 (1981).

13. Gasa, S. and Makita, A. *J. Biol. Chem.*, **258**, 5038–5039 (1983).

14. Geiger, B. and Arnon, R. *Biochemistry*, **15**, 3484–3492 (1976).

15. Glaser, J. H., Roozen, K. J., Brot, F. E., and Sly, W. S. *Arch. Biochem. Biophys.*, **166**, 536–542 (1975).

16. Hakomori, S. *Adv. Cancer Res.*, **18**, 265–315 (1973).

17. Hasilik, A. *Trends Biochem. Sci.*, **5**, 237–240 (1980).

18. Hatae, Y., Atsuta, T., and Makita, A. *Gann*, **68**, 59–63 (1977).

19. Hatae, Y., Yoda, Y., and Makita, A. *Gann*, **70**, 389–390 (1979).

20. Hoffmann, von K. D., Wagner, F., Dziambor, H., Preibsch, W., and Müller, H. J. *Zbl. Gynäkol.*, **101**, 950–952 (1979).

21. Horai, T., Nakamura, N., Tateishi, R., and Hattori, S. *Cancer*, **48**, 2016–2021 (1981).

22. Kijimoto-Ochiai, S., Makita, A., Kameya, T., Kodama, T., Araki, E., and Yoneyama, T. *Cancer Res.*, **41**, 2931–2935 (1981).

23. Kimball, P. M., Brattain, M. G., and White, W. E. *Biochem. J.*, **193**, 109–113, (1981).

24. Lippmann, H. G., Krüger, W., Elsner, G., and Wolff, W. *Arch. Geschwulstforsch.*, **47**, 703–709 (1977).

25. Mizuochi, T., Nishimura, Y., Kato, K., and Kobata, A. *Arch. Biochem. Biophys.*, **209**, 298–303 (1981).

26. Morgan, L. R., Samuels, M. S., Thomas, W., Krementz, E. T., and Meeker, W. *Cancer*, **36**, 2337–2345 (1975).

27. Motomiya, T., Yamada, K., Matsushima, S., Ijyuin, M., Iriya, K., and Okajima, E. *Urol. Res.*, **3**, 41–48 (1975).

28. Narita, M., Taniguchi, N., Makita, A., Kodama, T., Araki, E., and Oikawa, K. *Cancer Res.*, in press.

29. Natowicz, M., Baenzinger, J. U., and Sly, W. S. *J. Biol. Chem.*, **257**, 4412–4420 (1982).

30. Okochi, T., Seike, H., Higashino, K., Hada, T., Watanabe, S., Yamamura, Y., Ito, F., Matsuda, M., Osafune, M., Kotake, T., and Sonoda, T. *Cancer Res.*, **39**, 1829–1834 (1979).

31. Roy, A. B. and Trudinger, P. A. *In* "The Biochemistry of Inorganic Compounds of Sulphur," pp. 133–189 (1970). Cambridge University Press, Cambridge.

32. Schwartz, L. B. and Austen, K. F. *Biochem. J.*, **193**, 663–670 (1981).

33. Tabas, I. and Kornfeld, S. *J. Biol. Chem.*, **255**, 6633–6639 (1980).

34. Taniguchi, N. and Meister, A. *J. Biol. Chem.*, **253**, 1799–1806 (1978).

35. Taniguchi, N., Yokosawa, N., Narita, M., Mitsuyama, T., and Makita, A. *J. Natl. Cancer Inst.*, **67**, 577–583 (1981).

36. Uehara, Y., Gasa, S., Makita, A., Sakurada, K., and Miyazaki, T. *Cancer Res.*, in press.

37. Vaquero, C., Masson, C., Guigon, M., and Hewitt, J. *Eur. J. Cancer*, **11**, 739–743 (1975).
38. Warren, L., Buck, C. A., and Tuszinski, G. P. *Biochim. Biophys. Acta*, **516**, 97–127 (1978).
39. Yoda, Y., Gasa, S., Makita, A., Fujioka, Y., Kikuchi, Y., and Hashimoto, M. *J. Natl. Cancer Inst.*, **63**, 1153–1160 (1979).
40. Yoda, Y., Ishibashi, T., and Makita, A. *J. Biochem.*, **88**, 1887–1890 (1980).

VI. MEMBRANE ENZYMES IN CANCER

ALTERATION OF ARYLAMIDASE IN CANCER

Michio Niinobe and Setsuro Fujii

*Division of Regulation of Macromolecular Function, Institute for
Protein Research, Osaka University**

1. Aminopeptidase and arylamidase from human tissues were studied. The enzymes from liver were separated into three fractions on a triethylaminoethyl (TEAE)-cellulose column. Arylamidase activity of the last fraction, very low in normal liver, increased remarkably in hepatic cancer. Stomach contained three fractions. A new arylamidase peak appeared in stomach cancer. Lung contained four fractions. Arylamidase activities of the second and third fractions disappeared and a new peak appeared in lung cancer. Using antibodies against the first and second fractions purified from liver, one aminopeptidase and two arylamidases could be differentiated. All of the arylamidases different between normal and cancer tissues belonged to the same type and after neuraminidase treatment, they were eluted at the same position. These results suggest that the differences are due to the sialic acid content.

2. The specific activity of arylamidase in the extract of metaplastic mucosa of human stomach was about 10 times higher than that of normal mucosa but the same as that of small intestine. The zymogram patterns were also the same between metaplastic mucosa and small intestine. Arylamidases purified from the two tissues could not be differentiated in substrate specificity, kinetic and immunological properties, molecular weight and sensitivity to neuraminidase suggesting that the two arylamidases may be identical.

Various aminopeptidases and arylamidases have been demonstrated in most human tissues. Although their physiological functions are not clear, it has been suggested that they may participate in the amino acid transport of the intestinal tract or in the regulation of physiologically active peptides (*1, 3, 5, 6, 13*).

As to the multiplicity of arylamidase, Panveliwalla and Moss reported the separation of various forms of this enzyme from various human tissues by diethylaminoethyl (DEAE)-Sephadex column chromatography (*12*). Behal *et al.* also separated distinctive forms of arylamidase from human liver, small intestine, and pancreas by DEAE-cellulose column chromatography (*2*). Previously, we reported the various types of aminopeptidase and arylamidase in human tissues, and demonstrated the variation of substrate specificities and chromatographic patterns of these enzymes in normal and cancer tissues (*10, 17*).

On the other hand, it is well known that various enzymes such as sucrase, alkaline phosphatase, and arylamidase existing in intestinal epithelium appear in the gastric mucosa of patients demonstrating intestinal metaplasia. It has been reported that in-

* Yamada Oka 3-2, Suita, Osaka 565, Japan (新延道夫, 藤井節郎).

testinal metaplasia is frequently associated with gastric carcinoma (*4, 7–9, 14, 15*). These investigators emphasized that some cases of gastric carcinoma may arise from metaplastic mucosa. Accordingly, it has been considered to be a possible precancerous stage.

In an attempt to determine the diagnostic value of arylamidase in cancer, as a basic study, we have compared the arylamidase of human normal and cancer tissues.

Aminopeptidase and Arylamidase Activities of Various Human Tissues

The activities of aminopeptidase and arylamidase in sonically extracted suspensions of various human tissues were estimated with L-leucineamide or L-leucyl-β-naphthylamide as substrate (*16*). Preparation of the sonically extracted suspension and enzyme assay were carried out as reported previously (*16*). Aminopeptidase and arylamidase activities were found in all tissues tested, the activities being especially high in the kidney, liver, and small intestine (Table I). The enzyme activity of stomach cancer tissue was higher than that of normal stomach. On the other hand, the activity of liver cancer tissue was lower than in normal liver. Lung cancer tissue had higher L-leucineamide hydrolytic activity than that in normal lung, but had similar L-leucyl-β-naphthylamide hydrolytic activity.

TABLE I. Aminopeptidase and Arylamidase Activities of Various Human Tissues

	L-Leucineamide		L-Leucyl-β-naphthylamide	
	Specific activity[a]	Mean	Specific activity[b]	Mean
Liver	1.15, 1.50, 0.92	1.19	0.89, 1.39, 1.27	1.18
Hepatic cancer (hepatocellular carcinoma)	0.28, 1.34, 0.42	0.68	0.35, 0.42, 0.51	0.43
Stomach	0.36, 0.35, 0.19		0.41, 0.47, 0.48	
	0.43, 0.37, 0.56	0.38	0.39, 0.49, 0.36	0.43
Stomach cancer (adenocarcinoma)	1.43, 0.38, 0.45		0.67, 0.51, 0.46	
	1.06, 0.90, 0.60	0.80	0.79, 1.09, 0.68	0.70
Lung	0.47, 0.49	0.48	0.60, 0.35	0.48
Lung cancer (squamous cell carcinoma)	0.22, 0.35	0.29	0.59, 0.41	0.50
Kidney	1.58		4.54	
Ileum	1.09		3.34	
Colon	0.33		0.66	
Rectum	0.27		0.46	

[a] NH_3 formed (μmol/hr/mg protein).
[b] β-Naphthylamine formed (μmol/hr/mg protein).

Triethylaminoethyl (TEAE)-cellulose Column Chromatography of Aminopeptidases and Arylamidases from Human Normal and Cancer Tissues

Figure 1 shows the chromatographic patterns of aminopeptidases and arylamidases from human normal and cancer tissues. The enzyme solutions solubilized with bromelain treatment on the sonically extracted suspensions from each tissue were applied to a TEAE-cellulose column. In hepatic cancer arylamidase activity of Li. III increased remarkably. In stomach cancer, the new arylamidase peak (S. IV) appeared. On the other hand, in lung cancer, Lu. II and Lu. III in normal lung disappeared, and Lu. III′ was

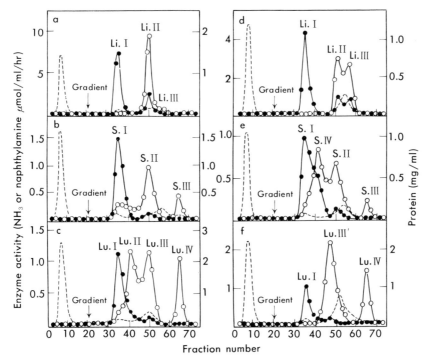

FIG. 1. TEAE-cellulose column chromatography of aminopeptidases and arylamidases from normal and cancer tissues of human liver, stomach, and lung. a and
d, normal liver and hepatic cancer; b and e, normal stomach and stomach cancer; c
and f, normal lung and lung cancer. ● activity with L-leucineamide; ○ activity
with L-leucyl-β-naphthylamide; - - - protein.

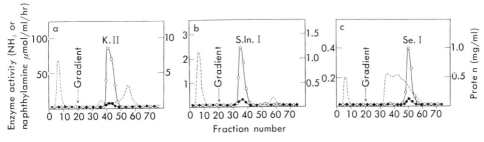

FIG. 2. TEAE-cellulose column chromatography of arylamidases from normal tissues of human kidney, small intestine, and serum. a, normal kidney; b, normal
small intestine; c, normal serum. ● activity with L-leucineamide; ○ activity with L-
leucyl-β-naphthylamide; - - - protein.

observed a few fractions earlier than Lu. III. TEAE-cellulose column chromatographies
of arylamidase from normal human kidney, small intestine, and serum were also performed. In these tissues and serum, one major peak each was observed (Fig. 2).

*Effects of Li. I and Li. II Antibodies on Aminopeptidase and Arylamidase Activities of
Various Normal and Cancer Tissues*

In order to elucidate immunological relationship among aminopeptidases and aryla-

TABLE II. Purifications of Aminopeptidase (Li. I) and Arylamidase (Li. II) from Human Normal Liver

Step	Total protein (mg)	Total activity (μmol)	Specific activity (μmol/mg)	Yield (%)
Sonication				
Li. I	5,750	11,745	2.0	100
Li. II	5,750	11,449	2.0	100
105,000×g supernatant after bromelain treatment				
Li. I	3,935	11,094	2.8	94.5
Li. II	3,935	11,038	2.8	96.4
Ammonium sulfate fractionation (40–60%)				
Li. I	902	10,429	11.6	88.8
Li. II	902	9,623	10.7	84.1
TEAE-cellulose				
Li. I	31.3	8,111	259	69.1
Li. II	36.4	7,336	202	64.1
Hydroxylapatite				
Li. I	3.2	5,984	1,870	50.9
Li. II	3.5	4,348	1,242	38.0
Sephadex G-200				
Li. I	1.3	4,116	3,165	35.0
Li. II	1.8	4,077	2,265	35.6

midases in normal and cancer tissues, Li. I (aminopeptidase) and Li. II (arylamidase) from normal liver were purified (*11*). Table II summarizes the results of a typical purification procedure on Li. I and Li. II. The final preparations of Li. I and Li. II gave a single protein band on polyacrylamide gel electrophoresis. Antibodies against the purified Li. I and Li. II were prepared using male New Zealand White rabbit. Table III shows the effects of Li. I and Li. II antibodies on activities of aminopeptidase and arylamidase from normal and cancer tissues, and from serum. As shown in Table III, aminopeptidase activities of Li. I, S. I and Lu. I in normal and cancer tissues of liver, stomach, and lung were completely inhibited by Li. I antibody. On the other hand, arylamidase activities of Li. II, Li. III, S. II, S. IV, Lu. II, Lu. III, and Lu. III′ were completely inhibited by Li. II antibody. However, arylamidase activities of S. III and Lu. IV were not affected as strongly as were Li. I, S. I, and Lu. I. Arylamidase activities of K. II, S. In. I, and Se. I were also inhibited by Li. II antibody. Accordingly, in the immunological studies using Li. I and Li. II antibodies, three immunologically different types, Li. I type, Li. II type, and the third type (Lu. IV and S. III) were shown. Li. I type is an aminopeptidase, since L-leucineamide was hydrolyzed preferentially. On the other hand, Li. II and the third types are arylamidase, since L-leucyl-β-naphthylamide was hydrolyzed preferentially.

Effect of Neuraminidase Treatment on Aminopeptidases and Arylamidases

In order to determine the cause of the differences in the column chromatographic behavior of arylamidase of Li. II type, we tried neuraminidase treatment. Treated and untreated enzyme solutions were applied to a TEAE-cellulose column. As the results of this treatment, Li. II in normal liver was converted to the type of S. IV, Lu. II,

TABLE III. Immunological Relationships between Aminopeptidases and Arylamidases from Various Normal and Cancer Tissues and from Serm

Antigen	γ-Globulin of normal rabbit, 500 μg	Antibody to Li. I				Antibody to Li. II			
		50 μg	100 μg	200 μg	500 μg	2 μg	5 μg	10 μg	150 μg
Normal liver									
Li. I	100	49.0	10.5	0	0	100	100	100	100
Li. II	100	100	100	100	100	34.0	11.3	3.0	0
Hepatic cancer									
Li. I	100	45.0	15.3	0	0	100	100	100	100
Li. II	100	100	100	100	100	33.0	13.5	0	0
Li. III	100	100	100	100	100	40.3	16.0	3.5	0
Normal stomach									
S. I	100	50.0	13.3	0	0	100	100	100	100
S. II	100	100	100	100	100	19.5	3.2	0	0
S. III	100	100	100	100	100	100	100	100	100
Stomach cancer									
S. I	100	53.5	5.0	0	0	100	100	100	100
S. IV	100	100	100	100	100	35.4	13.5	0	0
S. II	100	100	100	100	100	64.3	22.0	5.3	0
S. III	100	100	100	100	100	100	100	100	100
Normal lung									
Lu. I	100	63.0	29.5	0	0	100	100	100	100
Lu. II	100	100	100	100	100	39.5	14.0	5.1	0
Lu. III	100	100	100	100	100	51.0	19.3	0	0
Lu. IV	100	100	100	100	100	100	100	100	100
Lung cancer									
Lu. I	100	56.5	21.4	4.0	0	100	100	100	100
Lu. III'	100	100	100	100	100	43.0	16.3	0	0
Lu. IV	100	100	100	100	100	100	100	100	100
Kidney									
K. II	100	100	100	100	100	53.5	20.3	0	0
Small intestine									
S. In. I	100	100	100	100	100	40.0	21.5	7.3	0
Serum									
Se. I	100	100	100	100	100	51.9	8.0	0	0

and K. II. On the other hand, Li. II and Li. III in hepatic cancer were converted to the same type on TEAE-cellulose column chromatography. S. II in normal stomach was also converted to the cancer type (S. IV) by neuraminidase treatment, as was S. II in stomach cancer. In normal and cancer tissues of lung, neuraminidase treatment resulted in the same chromatographic behavior as did liver and stomach tissues. Namely, Lu. III and Lu. III' in normal and cancer lung were converted to Lu. II of the normal type. Li. I type (Li. I, Lu. I, and S. I) and the third type (Lu. IV and S. III) were not affected by neuraminidase treatment. Se. I in normal serum was also converted to the type of S. IV, Lu. II, and K. II. K. II and S. In. I in normal kidney and small intestine appeared to be unaltered by neuraminidase treatment. The results of neuraminidase treatment demonstrated that Li. II, Li. III, Lu. III, Lu. III', S. II, and Se. I of Li. II type were eluted in the position of Lu. II, S. IV, and K. II on TEAE-cellulose column chromatography. These converted forms may be the kidney type (K. II). Although

		Amino peptidase I	Arylamidase Ia	Ib	Ic	Arylamidase II
Liver	Normal	▲	←─── ∧			
	Cancer	▲	←── ∧ ──∧			
Lung	Normal	▲	∧──∧			∧
	Cancer	▲	←──∧	Ib		∧
Stomach	Normal	▲	←──∧			∧
	Cancer	▲	∧──∧			∧
Kidney			∧			
Small intestine		∧ Id				
Serum			←──── ∧			

FIG. 3. Summary of immunological properties and neuraminidase treatment of aminopeptidases and arylamidases from normal human and cancer tissues and serum. The new names are used in this summary: aminopeptidase I (Li. I, Lu. I, and S. I); arylamidase Ia (Lu. II, S. IV, and K. II); arylamidase Ib (Li. II, Lu. III, S. II, and Se. I); arylamidase Ib′ (Lu. III′); arylamidase Ic (L. III); arylamidase Id (S. In. I); and arylamidase II (Lu. IV and S. III). ▲ Li. I type immunologically; ∧ Li. II type immunologically; ∧ the third type immunologically. Arrows indicate the new position of arylamidases after neuraminidase treatment.

arylamidase in the small intestine is the same as Li. II type immunologically, it was eluted in the position of Li. I type. It may be due to a difference in the sugar chain.

We designed the new nomenclature of aminopeptidases and arylamidases, as shown in Fig. 3. These new names are aminopeptidase I (Li. I, Lu. I, and S. I), arylamidase Ia (Lu. II, S. IV, and K. II), arylamidase Ib (Li. II, Lu. III, S. II, and Se. I), arylamidase Ib′ (Lu. III′), arylamidase Ic (Li. III), arylamidase Id (S. In. I), and arylamidase II (Lu. IV and S. III). The immunological properties and results of conversion by neuraminidase treatment are summarized in Fig. 3. The results summarized in Fig. 3, suggest that arylamidases of Li. II type are glycoproteins which contain sialic acid. Consequently, the difference between the column chromatographic patterns on TEAE-cellulose in normal and cancer tissues may be due to the amount of sialic acid present in the enzyme molecule.

Comparative Studies of Arylamidases from Gastric Mucosa from Normal Individuals and Those with Intestinal Metaplasia, and from Small Intestine

The arylamidase activities in sonically extracted suspensions from normal and metaplastic gastric mucosas and small intestine were estimated with L-leucyl-β-naphthylamide as substrate. The specific activity of arylamidase in extracts from metaplastic areas increased about 10 times in comparison with activities in extracts from normal gastric mucosa, being almost the same as that in extracts from small intestine. Figure 4 shows the zymogram patterns of arylamidase in extracts from normal and metaplastic gastric mucosae and from small intestine. The enzyme solutions solublilized with bromelain treatment of the sonically extracted suspensions from each tissue were applied to a polyacrylamide disc gel. As can be seen, in the case of metaplasia, the new staining band appeared on the cathodic side, and the relative mobility of this band was the same

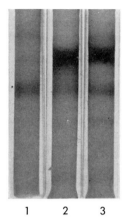

FIG. 4. Zymograms of arylamidases in extracts of normal and metaplastic gastric mucosas, and from small intestine. 1, normal gastric mucosa; 2, metaplastic gastric mucosa; 3, small intestine.

TABLE IV. Various Properties of Arylamidases Purified from Metaplastic Gastric Mucosa, Small Intestine, and Liver

	Gastric mucosa (metaplasia)	Small intestine	Liver (arylamidase Ib)
K_m values for L-leucyl-β-NA	1.0×10^{-4} M	8.0×10^{-5} M	9.4×10^{-5} M
Inhibitory effect by bestatin (K_i)	5.5×10^{-6} M	6.3×10^{-6} M	2.3×10^{-6} M
Substrate specificity (L-alanyl-β-NA/L-leucyl-β-NA)	3.3	3.3	3.7
Heat stability (residual % activity after incubation at 60° for 100 min)	78.2	87.7	54.4
Sensitivity to neuraminidase	Insensitive	Insensitive	Sensitive
Molecular weight	$180,000 \pm 5,000$	$180,000 \pm 5,000$	$170,000 \pm 5,000$
Effect of liver arylamidase antibody (arylamidase Ib)	Inhibition	Inhibition	Inhibition

NA, naphthylamide.

as that of the main band in the extract from small intestine. In order to determine whether the new arylamidase band in metaplasia is identical with that in the small intestine, these arylamidases were partially purified using columns of TEAE-cellulose and hydroxylapatite. Various properties were investigated using both arylamidase preparations. As shown in Table IV, various properties, such as K_m values for L-leucyl-β-naphthylamide, inhibitory effect of bestatin, substrate specificities employing alanyl- and leucyl-β-naphthylamide, heat stability upon incubation at 60° for 100 min, sensitivity to neuraminidase, molecular weights and the effect of antibody on hepatic arylamidase (arylamidase Ib) were similar to each other. Although both arylamidases were also similar to hepatic arylamidase (arylamidase Ib) in some characteristics, they differed in their stability upon heating and to their sensitivity to neuraminidase. Hepatic arylamidase was heat labile and neuraminidase sensitive in comparison with the other two arylamidases (Table IV).

The results suggest that arylamidases from metaplastic gastric mucosa and small intestine may be the same.

REFERENCES

1. Agar, W. T., Hird, E.J.R., and Sidhu, G. S. *J. Physiol.*, **121**, 253–263 (1953).
2. Behal, F. J., Arserson, B., Dawson, F., and Hardman, J. *Arch. Biochem. Biophys.*, **111**, 335–344 (1965).
3. Hambrook, J. M., Morgan, B. A., Rance, M. J., and Smith, C. F. *Nature*, **262**, 782–783 (1976).
4. Karpas, C. M., Payson, B. A., and Rechtschaffen, J. *N.Y. State J. Med.*, **71**, 1190–1195 (1971).
5. Knight, M. and Klee, W. A. *J. Biol. Chem.*, **253**, 3843–3847 (1978).
6. Lefkowitz, R. J., Roth, J., Pricer, W., and Pastan, I. *Proc. Natl. Acd. Sci. U.S.*, **65**, 745–752 (1970).
7. Ming, S. C., Goldman, H., and Freiman, D. G. *Cancer*, **20**, 1418–1429 (1967).
8. Morson, B. C. *Br. J. Cancer*, **9**, 365–376 (1955).
9. Nakahara, K. *J. Natl. Cancer Inst.*, **61**, 693–701 (1978).
10. Niinobe, M., Tamura, Y., Arima, T., and Fujii, S. *Cancer Res.*, **39**, 4212–4217 (1979).
11. Niinobe, M. and Fujii, S. *J. Biochem.*, **87**, 195–203 (1980).
12. Panveliwalla, D. K. and Moss, D. W. *Biochem. J.*, **99**, 501–505 (1966).
13. Simmons, W. H. and Brecher, A. S. *J. Biol. Chem.*, **248**, 5780–5784 (1973).
14. Stemmermann, G. N. and Hayashi, T. *J. Natl. Cancer Inst.*, **41**, 627–634 (1968).
15. Stemmermann, G. N. *Gann*, **68**, 525–535 (1977).
16. Tamura, Y., Niinobe, M., Arima, T., Okuda, H., and Fujii, S. *Biochim. Biphys. Acta*, **327**, 437–445 (1973).
17. Tamura, Y., Niinobe, M., Arima, T., Okuda, H., and Fujii, S. *Cancer Res.*, **35**, 1030–1034 (1975).

ALKALINE PHOSPHATASE ISOENZYMES
IN HUMAN CANCERS

Kazuya HIGASHINO

The Third Department of Medicine, Hyogo College of Medicine*

Human alkaline phosphatases (APs) are classified genetically into three types, namely term placental, early placental, and intestinal types. All of these isoenzymes are found to reappear in carcinoma and to some of them are given specific names such as Regan, Nagao, and Kasahara isoenzymes which are derived from patient's name. Other AP found in hepatoma tissue was fetal intestinal type.

Kasahara isoenzyme was L-phenylalanine sensitive, L-homoarginine insensitive, L-leucine sensitive, ethylenediamine tetraacetic acid (EDTA) sensitive, heat labile at 65° for 10 min, had pH optimum at 10.1 and reacted with anti-intestinal AP antibody. It had the fastest anodal migration among human APs. Two Kasahara variants were less migratory than Kasahara isoenzyme and seemed to differ only in neuraminic acid content.

Fetal intestinal form was the same as the adult intestinal type except insensitivity to neuraminidase reaction.

Regan and Nagao isoenzymes were L-phenylalanine sensitive, L-homoarginine insensitive, heat stable at 65° for at least 15 min, neuraminidase sensitive, and reacted with anti-placental AP antibody. Nagao isoenzyme is L-leucine and EDTA sensitive than Regan isoenzyme. Some of isoenzymes appearing in cancer seemed to differ in carbohydrate moiety from those of each original organs.

A brief discussion is made with regard to usefulness of these isoenzymes as tumor markers.

It is well documented that cancer tissues produce proteins which are different from their counterparts in the normal tissues from which they arose.

Enzymes undergo phenotypic alterations in cancer, as well and the most common type of change is the reappearance of fetal enzymes. The changes are believed to be due to the alterations of gene expression.

Alkaline phosphatase (AP) is localized in the plasma membrane of the cell like γ-glutamyl transpeptidase (γGTP). APs of humans have been studied since early this century, but real progress in the field of clinical medicine has been made since the idea of isozymes was first put forward by Markert and Møller (*34*).

In the field of cancer too, serum AP has been used as a diagnostic aid mainly for hepatobiliary and bone malignancies, since a tumor itself, the hepatobiliary obstruction effected by hepatic tumor and the osteoblastic proliferation resulted in the synthesis of the enzyme and further the rise of AP activity in serum.

---

* Mukogawa-cho 1-1, Nishinomiya, Hyogo 663, Japan (東野一彌).

In the course of extensive studies on AP in cancer, many investigators have found evidence that cancer tissues themselves produce unusual AP which is not or is only minimally present in their respective normal organs.

One example was the discovery of a unique AP in a pancreatic carcinoma which was inactivated by freezing (49). That cancer cells produced oncodevelopmental AP was first shown by Fishman *et al.* (14, 15) in 1968 by the beautiful work of proving the placental-type AP in bronchial carcinoma. Nowadays, it has become clear from experiments using cultured cancer cells that any type of AP can be produced by cancer cells (26, 53).

In this paper a brief review is made of the APs in cancers which differ from those in the original organs from where the cancer arose, in comparison with those in normal organs.

Normal Human AP

Human APs can be largely classified into three antigenically or genetically different APs (13), namely, liver-bone type, chorion, non-Regan or universal type AP (16, 37), intestinal type and placental or aminon type (Table 1).

TABLE I.   Antigenically Different Human AP in Normal and Cancer Tissues

Types of AP	Developmental tissues	Adult tissues	Cancer tissues[a]
Chorion	Early placenta (type B)	Liver, bone, lung, kidney	Early placental type including variant form
Amnion	Terminal placenta		Regan isoenzyme Nagao isoenzyme
Intestine	Fetal intestine	Intestine, liver (IL-AP)	Kasahara isoenzyme, FI-type AP
Unidentified	Early placenta (type A)		

[a] In this column, familiar names of AP that occurs in various organ carcinomas are listed for reference.

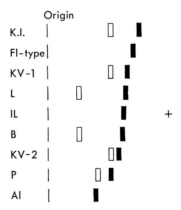

FIG. 1.   Schematic representation of electrophoretogram of human AP on poly-acrylamide gel. K. I., Kasahara isoenzyme; FI-type, FI-type AP; KV-1, KV-1 isoenzyme; L, liver AP; IL, IL-AP; B, bone AP; KV-2, KV-2 isoenzyme; P, placental AP; AI, adult intestinal AP. Open (□) and closed (■) squares denote the bands of neuraminidase treated and non-treated preparations of each isoenzyme prior to electrophoresis. FI-AP had the same mobility as FI-type AP.

1. Electrophoretic patterns of AP isoenzymes

A schematic representation of the electrophoretogram of all AP isoenzymes is shown in Fig. 1. Among normal APs, liver AP migrates the fastest, followed by isoenzymes of bone, placenta, and adult intestine in the order of decreasing mobility. Neuraminidase treatment of these isoenzymes prior to electrophoresis produces the decrease in mobility. Intestine-like liver AP (IL-AP) and adult intestinal AP (AI-AP) are not sensitive to the treatment (25, 44), while liver and bone type AP come to have the same mobility after neuraminidase treatment (Fig. 1).

2. Liver-bone type AP

This type of isoenzyme seems to originate from early placenta (6–10 weeks gestation) or chorion. In adult, it is distributed widely in many tissues including liver, bone, and kidney. These isoenzymes cannot be differentiated from each other by the conventional immunological method but can be by electrophoretic mobility (Fig. 1) and, to some extent, by heat stability.

As shown in Table II, the common properties of liver-bone type AP are L-homoarginine sensitive, L-phenylalanine insensitive, heat labile, and neuraminidase sensitive. Its pH optimum is at pH 10.1. The detailed structure of the enzyme is not yet clearly understood.

Liver AP is usually found in normal serum, and bone AP in serum of children and early adolescence.

According to the report by Fishman et al. (16), there were two types of AP, A and B, in human placenta of 6–10 weeks of gestation. AP-A was antigenically different from any human AP and AP-B was the same as liver-bone type AP. The latter also had the same antigenicity as AP in the lung and kidney. Fishman et al. (16) called this enzyme "non Regan" AP and Miki et al. (37) called it the "universal" type AP since it was present in all tissues.

3. Placental AP

Placental AP usually means AP occurring in the serum of women 11 weeks after gestation and disappearing 3–4 days after delivery. Although the phenotypes of placental

TABLE II. Comparative Enzymic Properties of Human Normal AP

	Liver AP	Bone AP	Placental AP	Intestinal AP	Intestine-like liver AP
Inhibition (5 mM)					
L-Phenylalanine	±	±	⧺	⧺	⧺
L-Homoarginine	⧺	⧺	±	±	±
Heat inactivation					
56°, 15 min	⧺	⧺	−	⧺	⧺
65°, 10 min	c.i	c.i	−	c.i	c.i
Optimal pH	10.1	10.1	10.6	10.1	10.1
Sensitivity to neuraminidase	+	+	+	−	−
Reactivity with					
Anti-liver AP antibody	⧺	+	−	−	−
Anti-placental AP antibody	−	−	⧺	+	+
Anti-intestinal AP antibody	−	−	+	⧺	⧺

c.i, completely inactivated.

AP are plentiful in 2% of the cases, there are three common electrophoretic types with fast, intermediate, and slow mobilities (10). Among rare variants, the D-variant AP appears in 0.4% of the placentas (28) but recently it has also occurred in testes at low activity (0.4–4.6% of total activity) (6).

The term placental AP applies to one which is L-phenylalanine sensitive and is rather L-homoarginine insensitive. It is heat stable at 65° for 15 min, has pH optimum at 10.6 and is neuraminidase sensitive. It reacts with anti-placental AP antibody. AP from some placenta also reacts with anti-intestinal AP antibody.

4 Intestinal AP

Intestinal AP is more frequently present in the serum of persons of salivary secretor and B or O blood type than in serum of persons of non-secretors and A blood type. This phenomenon has been explained by a genetic association between the occurrence of intestinal isoenzyme in serum and the blood group system and secretor status (33). But a report appearing recently (3) stated that the intestinal isoenzymes bound with erythrocytes of blood type A and, as a result, the soluble intestinal isoenzyme level became low. Since this binding occurred with erythrocytes of only blood type A, the soluble isoenzyme level was unchanged in persons of B or O blood group.

IL-AP is an AP of an intestinal type occurring as a minor component in normal liver (44). The properties of intestinal AP and IL-AP are almost the same, except for a little difference in electrophoretic mobility and heat stability. They are thus L-phenyl-alanine sensitive, L-homoarginine resistant, neuraminidase insensitive, react with anti-intestinal AP antibody, and have pH optimum at 10.1. It is generally recognized that there is immunologically some cross reactivity between placental and intestinal AP. Though these two isoenzymes are normally occurring ones, IL-AP has not yet been found in serum.

In serum of normal persons, then, there may occur four kinds of APs, namely, liver, bone, placental, and intestinal (Table II).

APs in Human Cancers

In many carcinoma cases, an elevation of AP activity is observed. In cases with primary hepatoma, the elevated AP is often of the liver type, mainly because production of this type is induced by partial or complete obstruction of the biliary tract and possibly also by tumor production. In cases of liver metastasis, serum AP activity contributes to the diagnosis. For example, an unreasonable incerase in serum AP and high activity remaining after removal of a primary carcinoma would suggest metastasis in the liver and other organs. If the increased isoenzymes are identified, this will contribute more than only activity.

Total activity of liver AP increases in hepatobiliary carcinoma, bone type AP increases in bone metastasis and multiple myeloma and occasionally in lung carcinoma with hyperparathyroidism, and intestinal AP increases in liver cirrhosis. AP of high molecular weight reported as a membrane fragment or complex with lipoprotein appears in biliary obstruction (7, 21, 45, 50, 60).

It has long been suggested that cancer tissues produce APs which are not in the original tissues from which cancers arise. For instance, Gault et al. (17), and Nichols et al. (43) reported respectively that high serum AP activity in patients with lung carcinoma or adrenal carcinoma returned to normal after removal of the carcinoma. Schlang and McHenry (*49*) also showed a unique AP in serum of a patient with pancreatic carcinomas, as stated previously. Now it is clear that human cancer tissues produce Regan and Nagao isoenzymes or Kasahara isoenzyme and fetal intestinal (FI)-type AP or early placental AP; these isoenzymes are listed in Table I. Not called by a specific name are some forms of early placental APs which differed slightly from their corresponding form (liver, bone, kidney AP, *etc.*) only in electrophoretic mobility. An electrophoretogram of these cancer associated APs is also shown in Fig. 1.

1. *Liver-bone type AP in lung carcinoma*

In cancer, chorion or early placental type AP occurs. In the carcinoma tissues and serum of a patient with lung adenocarcinoma which had invaded the entire lung and looked radiologically like alveolar cell carcinoma, we found this type of AP. In this patinet serum AP activity was constantly more than 100 K.A.U. but serum γGTP remained within normal range. The specific activity in the lung carcinoma tissue was 2.1 U/mg protein and was about 70 times as high as the average activity in normal lung tissue (0.033 U/mg protein). Enzymic properties were like those of liver-bone type or early placental type AP (Tables II and III). Timperley (*55*) has reported this type of AP in bronchial carcinoma tissue.

TABLE III. Comparative Properties of AP in Cancer Tissues

	Placental AP		Kasahara I and its variants	FI-type AP	Early placental B type AP
	Regan I	Nagao I			
Electrophoretic mobility on 5% PAG	α_2-β globulin		K I: fast α_2-globulin KV-1: between K.I and liver AP KV-2: equal or slightly cathodic to liver AP	Slightly anodal to liver AP	Equal to bone AP (α_2-β globulin)
Inhibition					
L-Phenylalanine (5 mM)	+++	+++	+++	+++	+
L-Leucine (5 mM)	+	+++	++	+	+
L-Homoarginine (5 mM)	±	±	±	±	++
EDTA (0.1 mM)	±	+++	+	++	+
Heat inactivation					
56°, 30 min	−	−	++	+ ~ ++	+++
65°, 4 min	−	−	+++	+++	+++
Optimal pH	10.6	10.6	10.1	10.1	10.1
Sensitivity to neuraminidase	+	+	+	−	−
Reactivity with					
Anti-liver AP antibody	−	−	−	−	+
Anti-placental AP antibody	+++	+++	− or +[a]	Not examined	−
Anti-intestinal AP antibody	+	+	++	++	−
Anti-Kasahara AP antibody	+	+	+++	++	−

[a] Depending on lot of antigen used for preparation of the antibody.

2. *Kasahara isoenzyme and FI-type AP*

We found and designated Kasahara isoenzyme and its variants and FI-type AP and these are described in more detail.

Kasahara isoenzyme and FI-type AP extracted by Morton's modified procedures from the hepatoma tissue were partially purified by acetone fractionation, diethylamino-ethyl (DEAE)-cellulose and Sephadex G-200 chromatography (*25*). Initially, hepatoma extract contained both Kasahara isoenzyme and liver AP plus FI-type AP. First, Kasahara isoenzyme was separated from FI-type plus liver AP by DEAE-cellulose and thereafter FI-type AP was separated from liver AP by DEAE-cellulose chromatography after treatment of the latter fraction with neuraminidase. Liver AP was neuraminidase sensitive while FI-type AP was insensitive, thus enabling to give difference in negative charge between the two.

Kasahara isoenzyme had the fastest anodal migration. There were two Kasahara variants, one (KV-1) migrated between Kasahara isoenzyme and liver AP positions and the other (KV-2) electrophoresed to the position between liver and placental APs (Fig. 1). FI-AP electrophoresed just ahead of liver AP. Kasahara isoenzyme and its two variants were neuraminidase sensitive and the mobilities were retarded but had the same mobility following treatment; the FI-AP and FI-type, however, were neur-aminidase resistant and their mobilities were not changed. Kasahara isoenzyme and its variants seemed to differ only in neuraminic acid content (*19, 20*).

The properties of Kasahara isoenzyme and its variants were almost the same: L-phenylalanine sensitive, L-leucine sensitive, L-homoarginine insensitive, ethylenedi-amine tetraacetic acid (EDTA) sensitive, slightly heat labile at 56° for 30 min, heat labile at 65° for 10 min, with pH optimum at 10.1, reacted with both anti-Kasahara isoenzyme antibody and anti-AI-AP antibody (Table III and Fig. 2). Kasahara isoenzyme and the variant AP by Warnock and Reisman (*58*) are very alike in terms of certain properties examined.

FI-type AP which occurred in some hepatoma tissues having Kasahara isoenzyme was also just like a molecular form of FI-AP and AI-AP in properties except for elec-trophoretic mobility and heat stability. FI-type AP variant isoenzyme found in cirrhotic liver (*31*) differed from FI-type AP in electrophoretic mobility (not shown in Fig. 1).

No differences were found among these isoenzymes, in sensitivity to inhibition by

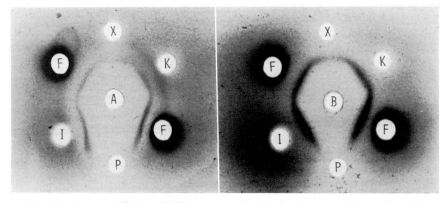

FIG. 2. Immunodiffusion of AP isoenzymes by Ouchterlony's technique. A, anti-intestinal AP antibody; B, anti-Kasahara isoenzyme antibody; F, FI-AP; I, AI-AP; P, placental AP; K, Kasahara isoenzyme; X, FI-type AP.

TABLE IV. Some Properties of AP

	Kasahara I	FI-type AP	FI-AP	AI-AP
Inhibition by K_2HPO_4 (10 mM)	+	+	+	+
Michaelis constant for phenyl phosphate	1.1	0.9	1.2	1.2
Effect of SDS (0.5%)[a]	−	−	−	−
Urea 2 M	╫	╫	╫	╫
8 M	╫╫	╫╫	╫╫	╫╫
Effect of Con A	Reactive	Non-reactive	Reactive	Non-reactive

[a] At this concentration, placental AP was inactivated almost completely.
 Grade of inhibition: − ± 10%; + 10-30%; ╫ 30-50%; ╫╫ 50-70%; ╫╫ 70-90%.

inorganic phosphate, K_m value for phenyl phosphate or the effect of sodium dodecylsulfate (SDS) on AP activity (Table IV). Reactivity of these isoenzymes to concanavalin A (Con A) was also examined by the change of electrophoretic mobility after binding with Con A. Kasahara isoenzyme and FI-type AP were reacted with Con A, while FI-AP and AI-AP were not, suggesting the difference of carbohydrate moiety of the glycoprotein between these two groups of enzymes. Neither isoenzyme was affected by SDS. On the contrary, at this concentration placental AP was completely inactivated by SDS (not shown in the table).

The Kasahara isoenzyme was found only in cell lines like FL-amnion cells (23), CCL6 fetal intestinal cells (32), and lines established from maxillary carcinoma (53) and hepatoblastoma (54).

These isoenzymes from both normal and cancer tissues, namely, FI-AP, AI-AP, IL-AP, Kasahara isoenzyme and its two variants, and FI-type AP would be classified into a family of intestinal origin.

In summary, an intestinal AP family shares common enzymic and immunologic properties, but is different in electrophoretic mobility, heat stability, the effect of SDS, sensitivity to neuraminidase, and reactivity with Con A.

3. Regan and Nagao isoenzymes

Regan and Nagao isoenzymes are recognized as the placental type AP emerging in cancer tissue. Since the discovery of the Regan isoenzyme by Fishman *et al.* (14, 15), it has been the subject of many studies.

With respect to the identity between Regan and placental isoenzymes, it was reported that they do not differ in usual enzymic and immunologic properties (15) as shown in Table III. Thus a Regan isoenzyme is L-phenylalanine sensitive, L-homoarginine insensitive, heat stable at 65°, for more than 15 min, neuraminidase sensitive, and is reactive with anti-placental AP antibody. The optimal pH is 10.6 (15).

Greene and Sussman (18) reported Regan and the placental isoenzyme are identical in terms of molecular weight of the subunit, isoelectric point, N-terminal amino acid, and the constituting peptides by fingerprinting method. On the contrary, Benham *et al.* (2) found placental type AP in 5 patients with ovarian carcinoma, but their electrophoretic mobilities were not the same as a usual AP type. They suggested the expression of AP genes in cancer is different from that of the usual genes of AP.

Another placental type AP associated with a carcinomatous lesion is the Nagao iso-

258   K. HIGASHINO

enzyme (39). This isoenzyme is much more sensitive to L-leucine and EDTA than the Regan isoenzyme, but its other properties are indistinguishable. Inglis et al. (28) suggested that the Nagao isoenzyme was identical to the D-variant form of placental AP. But Nakayama et al. (40, 41) argued against this opinion, since they found the mobility of Nagao isoenzyme differed from case to case. Doellgast and Fishman (9) showed that D-variant and Nagao isoenzymes behave differently against inhibition by L-leucine and L-leucine peptides (L-leucinamide, L-Leu-L-Leu-L-Leu, and L-Leu-Gly-Gly) and suggested a difference in primary structure.

Prevalence of Cancer Associated AP

1. Prevalence of Kasahara isoenzyme and FI-type AP

The prevalence of Kasahara isoenzyme in hepatoma tissue was 27.3% according to our investigation (58).

Warnock and Reisman found the prevalence of their variant AP in hepatoma was 80% (8 of 10 patients) (58). This percentage seems to be so high comparing with ours if the variant enzyme is identical with Kasahara isoenzyme. The percentage of isoenzyme in the tissue is higher than in the seurm in agreement with our results (22). With regard to the relevance of Kasahara isoenzyme prevalence to grading of differentiation of hepatoma by Edmondson and Steiner (11), almost all cases in our studies fell into grade III. Kasahara isoenzyme also occurred in massive and nodular types of hepatoma (22) and was found in other carcinoma tissues such as stomach, pancreatic, maxillary, prostatic, and urinary bladder carcinomas (8, 24, 35). Nevertheless its prevalence and high activity in serum are often seen specifically in hepatocellular carcinoma. The prevalence of Kasahara isoenzyme in the serum of patients with hepatoma was about 15%. But Miyazaki et al. (38) and Sawabu et al. (48) reported recently respective values of 27% and 18%. It is very interesting that Regan isoenzyme seldom occurred in hepatoma in contrast with the high prevalence of Kasahara isoenzyme. Accordingly, the latter could be a hepatoma marker. Kasahara isoenzyme seldom occurred in benign diseases, but exceptional cases were a cirrhotic liver patient (one of 300 benign disease cases) (22), a uremic patient (one of 1,000 cases) (52), and a fatty liver patient (one of 50 cases) (58).

Our recent observations on the occurrence of FI-type AP in hepatoma revealed that it emerged in 4 of 12 hepatoma tissues and all cases were also noted to have Kasahara isoenzyme (25). Miki et al. found a very similar enzyme in stomach and colonic carcinomas (36).

2. Prevalence of Regan and Nagao isoenzymes

Regan and Nagao isoenzymes seem to occur not only in lung carcinoma of various cell types (15, 29) but also in many of malignant tumors such as stomach, colonic, pancreatic, and maxillary carcinomas and so on (41, 42, 52). The prevalence of both heat stable isoenzymes in the serum of patients with a carcinoma varies from 0.6 to 21% depending on the reporters (4, 40–42, 46, 51, 52, 57).

Radioimmunological methods enabled the determination of very small amounts of these isoenzymes and, using this, Usategui-Gomez found that about 90% of patients with malignant tumors had these isoenzymes, although in 90% activities were not elevated (57). A recent report states that the Regan isoenzyme was found at a relatively high incidence in genitourinary carcinomas (12). It was found that 90% of the seminoma was stained for this isoenzyme located at the tumor cell membrane (56). This high prevalence of Regan isoenzyme is in contrast to its absence in embryonal carcinoma.

There was a positive correlation between the stage of disease and the enzyme prevalence in ovarian carcinoma but not in uterus carcinoma (30). With regard to the diagnosis of early stage of ovarian carcinoma, however, Cantarow et al. suggested that difficulty in the use of tumor markers including Regan isoenzyme for this purpose, because no excellent marker had yet been found (5).

Regan isoenzyme was more frequently positive in the advanced stage (phase IV) of hematopoietic tumors, including lymphoma and leukemia, but the specific activity was not always high (1).

3. Early placental type AP

As stated previously, non-Regan AP was found to emerge in various organ carcinomas. This could be regarded as an altered form of each organ-specific AP and occurred in lung carcinoma (55), liver carcinoma (27), and renal cell carcinoma (59). The prevalence has not yet been reported, though in renal cell carcinoma up to 32% of abnormally increased serum AP activity originating in a primary tumor was contributed by non-Regan type AP (59).

Diagnosis of Cancer by Combined Use of Tumor Markers

With regard to hepatocellular carcinoma, many tumor markers are available as a means for diagnosis. Use of only a single marker is not common. Whether or not the diagnostic ratio for hepatocellular carcinoma increases with plural tumor markers is important and interesting. Sawabu et al. (47) used there markers, namely, α-fetoprotein, variant AP which is almost equal to Kasahara isoenzyme, and hepatoma specific novel γGTP and compared each prevalence. It was found that there was no association between the occurrence of one marker and any other. In 31 cases with α-fetoprotein below 400 ng/ml (not indicative of hepatocellular carcinoma) Kasahara isoenzyme was positive in 8 cases (26%) and novel γGTP was positive in 15 cases (58%). Consequently, 19 cases (61%) with hepatocellular carcinoma which were negative for α-fetoprotein could be detected by combined usage of the two additional markers. Totally, 73 out of 85 hepatocellular carcinoma cases examined (86%) were diagnosed by combined use of these markers.

Therefore use of plural tumor markers is evidently beneficial in the diagnosis of hepatoma. This may also be true with other organ carcinomas.

It may become possible in the near future to diagnose each organ carcinoma with each specific antibody against each carcinoma cell protein and/or its specific isoenzyme. It has already been shown that AP isoenzyme can be separated into more molecular forms than we knew by the reactivity with monoclonal antibody produced using a hybridoma cell between the mouse spleen cell which had been sensitized specifically against each AP isoenzyme and mouse myeloma cell.

Acknowledgment

This work was supported by Grant-in-Aid for Cancer Research from the Ministry of Education, Science and Culture.

REFERENCES

1. Belliveau, R. E., Yamamoto, L. A., Wassell, A. R., and Wiernik, P. H. *J. Clin. Pathol.*, **62**, 329–334 (1974).
2. Benham, F. J., Povey, M. S., and Harris, H. *Clin. Chim. Acta*, **86**, 201–215 (1978).
3. Bayer, P. M., Hotschek, H., and Knoth, E. *Clin. Chim. Acta*, **108**, 81–87 (1980).
4. Cadeau, B. J., Blackstein, M. E., and Malkin, A. *Cancer Res.*, **34**, 729–732 (1974).
5. Cantarow, W. D., Stolbach, L. L., Bhattacharya, M., Chatterjee, S. K., and Barlon, J. J. *Int. J. Radiat. Oncol. Biol. Phys.*, **7**, 1095–1098 (1981).
6. Chang, C. H., Angellis, D., and Fishman, W. H. *Cancer Res.*, **40**, 1506–1510 (1980).
7. Crofton, P. M., Elton, R. A., and Smith, A. F. *Clin. Chim. Acta*, **98**, 263–275 (1979).
8. Dingjan, P. G., Postma, T., and Stroes, J.A.P. *Clin. Chim. Acta*, **60**, 169–183 (1975).
9. Doellgast, G. J. and Fishman, W. H. *Clin. Chim. Acta*, **75**, 449–454 (1977).
10. Donald, L. J. and Robson, E. B. *Ann. Human Genet.*, **37**, 303–313 (1974).
11. Edmondson, H. A. and Steiner, P. E. *Cancer*, **7**, 462–503 (1954).
12. Fishman, W. H. *Prostate*, **1**, 399–410 (1980).
13. Fishman, W. H. and Ghosh, N. K. *Adv. Clin. Chem.*, **10**, 255–370 (1967).
14. Fishman, W. H., Inglis, N. R., Stolbach, L. L., and Krant, M. J. *Cancer Res.*, **28**, 150–154 (1968).
15. Fishman, W. H., Inglis, N. R., Green, S., Anstiss, C. L., Gosh, N. K., Reif, A. E., Rustigian, R., Krant, M. J., and Stolbach, L. L. *Nature*, **219**, 697–699 (1968).
16. Fishman, L., Miyayama, H., Driscoll, S. G., and Fishman, W. H. *Cancer Res.*, **36**, 2268–2273 (1976).
17. Gault, M. H., Cohen, M. W., Kahana, L. K., Leelin, F. T., Meakins, J. F., and Aronovitch, M. O. *Can. Med. J.*, **96**, 87–94 (1962).
18. Greene, P. J. and Sussman, H. H. *Proc. Natl. Acad. Sci. U.S.*, **70**, 2936–2940 (1973).
19. Hada, T., Higashino, K., Okochi, T., and Yamamura, Y. *Clin. Chim. Acta*, **89**, 311–316 (1978).
20. Hada, T., Higashino, K., Okochi, T., Yamamura, Y., Matsuda, M., Osafune, M., Kotake, T., and Sonoda, T. *Gann*, **70**, 503–508 (1979).
21. Hattori, N., Murayama, H., Kitsui, H., and Arima, M. *Acta Hepatol. Japon.*, **10**, 40–44 (1969) (in Japanese).
22. Higashino, K., Ohtani, R., Kudo, S., Hashinotsume, M., Kang, K., Hada, T., Okochi, T., Takahashi, Y., and Yamamura, Y. *Ann. Intern. Med.*, **83**, 74–78 (1975).
23. Higashino, K., Kudo, S., Ohtani, R., Yamamura, Y., Honda, T., and Sakurai, J. *Ann. N.Y. Acad. Sci.*, **259**, 337–346 (1975).
24. Higashino, K., Kudo, S., Ohtani, R., and Yamamura, Y. *Gann*, **67**, 909–911 (1976).
25. Higashino, K., Otani, R., Kudo, S., and Yamamura, Y. *Clin. Chem.*, **23**, 1615–1623 (1977).
26. Higashino, K., Otani, R., and Hada, T. *Metabolism*, **17**, 229–241 (1980) (in Japanese).
27. Higashino, K., Ohtani, R., Kudo, S., and Hada, T. Unpublished observation.
28. Inglis, N. R., Kirley, S., Stolbach, L. L., and Fishman, W. H. *Cancer Res.*, **33**, 1657–1661 (1973).
29. Kang, K.-Y., Higashino, K., Hashinotsume, M., Takahashi, Y., Aoki, T., Tsubura, E., and Yamamura, Y. *Gann*, **63**, 217–224 (1972).
30. Kellen, J .A., Bush, R. S., and Malkin, A. *Cancer Res.*, **36**, 269–271 (1976).
31. Kudo, S., Higashino, K., and Yamamura, Y. *Gann*, **70**, 15–19 (1979).
32. Kudo, S., Seike, H., Higashino, K., Otani, R., Yamamura, Y., Takeuchi, T., and Hirohashi, Y. *In* "Carcino-Embryonic Proteins, Chemistry, Biololgy and Clinical Application," Vol. II, ed. F-G. Lehman, pp. 665–672 (1979). Elsevier / North Holland Biomedical Press, Amsterdam, New York, and Oxford.

33. Langman, M.J.S., Constantinopoulos, A. P., and Bouchier, I.A.D. *Nature*, **217**, 863–865 (1968).
34. Markert, C. L. and Møller, F. *Proc. Natl. Acad. Sci. U.S.*, **45**, 753–763 (1959).
35. Miki, K., Suzuki, H., Iino, S., Niwa, H., Oda, T., Sugiura, M., and Hirano, K. *Japan. J. Gastroenterol.*, **73**, 162–168 (1976) (in Japanese).
36. Miki, K., Oda, T., Suzuki, H., Iino, S., and Niwa, H. *Scand. J. Immunol.*, **8** (Suppl. 8), 563–570 (1978).
37. Miki, K., Oda, T., Suzuki, H., Niwa, H., Iino, S., and Miyazaki, J. *In* "Carcino-Embryonic Proteins, Chemistry, Biology and Clinical Application," Vol. I, ed. F.-G. Lehmann, pp. 403–410 (1979). Elsevier / North Holland Biomedical Press, Amsterdam, New York, and Oxford.
38. Miyazaki, J., Iino, S., Miki, K., and Endo, Y. *Saishin Igaku*, **36**, 867–872 (1981) (in Japanese).
39. Nakayama, T., Yoshida, M., and Kitamura, M. *Clin. Chim. Acta*, **30**, 546–548 (1970).
40. Nakayama, T. and Kitamura, M. *Ann. N.Y. Acad. Sci.*, **259**, 325–336 (1975).
41. Nakayama, T. and Kitamura, M. *Rinshobyori*, **23**, 338–345 (1975) (in Japanese).
42. Nathanson, L. and Fishman, W. H. *Cancer*, **27**, 1388–1397 (1971).
43. Nichols, F., Bower, B., Williams, H., and Martin, R. *In* "Programs of the 48th Annu. Meet. Endocrine Soc.", p. 107, Chicago, June (1966).
44. Otani, R., Higashino, K., and Yamamura, Y. *Clin. Chim. Acta*, **82**, 249–258 (1978).
45. Read, D. R. and Hambrick, E. *Dis. Colon. Rectum*, **20**, 101–107 (1977).
46. Sawabu, N. *In* "From Viral Hepatitis to Hepatocellular Carcinoma," ed. N. Hattori, pp. 248–259 (1982). Gan to kagakurhohosha, Tokyo (in Japanese).
47. Sawabu, N., Nakagen, M., Ozaki, K., Wakabayashi, T., Toya, D., Hattori, N., and Ishii, M. *Ann. Acad. Med.*, **9**, 206–209 (1980).
48. Sawabu, N., Nakagen, M., Sendai, H., Takahashi, H., Tanaka, N., and Hattori, N. *Sogorinsho*, **30**, 291–296 (1981) (in Japanese).
49. Schlang, H. A. and McHenry, L. E., Jr. *N.Y. State J. Med.*, **62**, 3811–3813 (1962).
50. Shinkai, K. and Akedo, H. *Cancer Res.*, **32**, 2307–2313 (1972).
51. Stolbach, L. L. *Ann. N.Y. Acad. Sci.*, **166**, 760–774 (1969).
52. Suzuki, K., Iino, S., and Oda, T. *Naika*, **29**, 838–843 (1972) (in Japanese).
53. Tanaka, M., Kudo, S., Higashino, K., and Kishimoto, S. *Oncodev. Biol. Med.*, in press.
54. Tanaka, M., Yamamoto, H., Kishimoto, S., and Higashino, K. Unpublished observations.
55. Timperley, W. R. *Lancet*, **ii**, 356 (1968).
56. Uchida, T., Shimoda, T., Miyata, H., Shikata, T., Iino, S., Suzuki, H., Oda, T., Hirano, K., and Sugiura, M. *Cancer*, **48**, 1455–1462 (1981).
57. Usategui-Gomez, M., Yeager, F. M., and Fernandez de Castro, A. *Cancer Res.*, **33**, 1574–1577 (1973).
58. Warnock, M. L. and Reisman, R. *Clin. Chim. Acta*, **24**, 5–11 (1969).
59. Whitaker, K. B., Eckland, D., Hodgson, H.J.F., Saverymuttu, S., Williams, G., and Moss, D. W. *Clin. Chim.*, **28**, 374–377 (1982).
60. White, D. R., Maloney, J. J., III, Muss, H. B., Vance, R. P., Barnes, P., Howard, V., Rhyne, L., and Cowan, R. J. *J. Am. Med. Assoc.*, **242**, 1147–1149 (1979).

γ-GLUTAMYL TRANSPEPTIDASE FROM TUMOR TISSUES—CHEMICAL, ENZYMATIC, AND BIOLOGICAL PROPERTIES

Naoyuki Taniguchi,[*1] Noriko Yokosawa,[*1] Susumu Iizuka,[*1]
Yutaka Tsukada,[*2] Fumiyo Sako,[*1] and
Nobuko Miyazawa[*1]

*Biochemistry Laboratory, Cancer Institute[*1] and Department of
Biochemistry, Hokkaido University School of Medicine[*2]*

γ-Glutamyl transpeptidase (γGTP) purified from rat ascites hepatoma (AH-66) and yolk sac tumor cells was found to be immunochemically identical to those of normal rat liver and kidney. The protein moiety was solely responsible for the immunological properties of the γGTP. This conclusion was further supported by the fact that the amino acid compositions of the enzymes were very similar. However, the carbohydrate content of the enzyme from tumor cells differed from that of kidney enzyme in having a higher content of hexose and hexosamine. The differences in carbohydrate content appeared to result in differences in these enzymes in molecular weight, peptide mapping and several kinetic properties.

An immunoassay of the enzyme showed that the increased enzymatic activity in neoplastic or preneoplastic tissues is associated with the increased level of immunoreactive enzyme protein.

In cultured cell lines of rat yolk sac tumor the enzyme is initially synthesized in the form of a large molecular weight precursor which is rapidly converted to the size of the final enzyme molecule. These studies will make it possible to investigate the processing mechanisms of the protein as well as the carbohydrate portions of the tumor enzymes. Much evidence has accumulated in recent years to support the idea that the γGTP is one of the oncofetal proteins and one of the best markers for the preneoplastic lesion.

γ-Glutamyl transpeptidase (γGTP) is a membrane-associated enzyme that catalyzes the initial step in the breakdown of glutathione in tissues (*23–25*). The enzyme is widely distributed in various mammalian tissues (*23*) among which kidney shows the highest activity.

The fetal liver and hepatoma contain very high levels of the enzyme, whereas the adult rat liver contains a very low level (*12, 31–34*). During the process of azo dye-induced hepatocarcinogenesis in rats, the enzyme activity increased 10 to 100-fold (*10, 11, 34, 40*). The enzyme is now considered to be one of the best markers for the preneoplastic lesion of experimental hepatoma (*3, 7–9, 15–17*) and is now employed as a tumor marker for the hepatoma patients (*28, 29*). Studies on the γGTP prompted us to investigate whether or not there is any difference between the enzymes from normal and

[*1,*2] Kita 15, Nishi 7, Kita-ku, Sapporo 060, Japan (谷口直之, 横沢紀子, 飯塚　進, 塚田　裕, 酒向史代, 宮沢伸子).

tumor tissues with respect to antigenicity, physicochemical properties, and kinetic properties.

In our previous studies, the enzyme was purified to a homogeneous state from azo dye-induced hepatoma (34) and was found to be immunochemically similar to fetal enzyme (36). We recently purified the enzyme from yolk sac tumor of rats and found it to be identical to that of kidney and the AH-66 hepatoma with respect to antigenicity and amino acid composition (43). These results indicate that the γGTPs from various tissues are very similar. This review is concerned with studies on the physicochemical, enzymatic, and biological properties of γGTP in relation to tumor tissues.

Physicochemical Studies on γGTP from Various Tumor Tissues

1. Purification and molecular weight

γGTP was highly purified from the yolk sac tumor and AH66 cells (43) by procedures that included extraction with non-ionic detergent, ammonium sulfate and acetone fractionations followed by digestion with bromelain and chromatography on diethylaminoethyl (DEAE)-cellulose and Sephadex G-100. The purity of the enzyme was examined by disc gel electrophoresis under non-denaturating conditions. On the gel, the samples showed a broad band. However the localization of enzyme activity was identical to that found for protein in each preparation. Treatment of these preparations with sodium dodecyl sulfate (SDS) in the presence of 2-mercaptoethanol gave two non-identical subunits of molecular weight 68,000 and 45,000 for yolk sac tumor γGTP and 66,000 and 37,000 for AH-66 cell γGTP.

2. Amino acid and carbohydrate analysis

The amino acid and carbohydrate compositions of yolk sac tumor, AH-66, kidney and azo dye-induced hepatoma enzymes were analyzed (38, 43). There was a statistically significant similarity in amino acid composition between four different preparations. However the enzymes from yolk sac tumor and AH-66 cells had high contents of carbohydrate and higher amounts of hexose and hexosamine as compared to the kidney enzyme. No significant differences were observed in their sialic acid content. Glucosamine was the only amino sugar found in the three enzyme preparations, suggesting that the carbohydrate chains are linked to protein through the N-glycoside type N-acetylglucosaminyl asparagine bond. Quite recently Yamashita *et al.* (42) analyzed the carbohydrate structure of AH-66 γGTP and normal rat liver and found that the total number of asparagine-linked sugar chains in one molecule of AH-66 γGTP was four times that of liver γGTP. These differences found in carbohydrate analysis reflect the differences found in the molecular weight of the three preparations (38, 43).

3. Peptide mapping of chymotryptic peptides of γGTP

γGTP was labeled with ^{125}I and subjected to chymotryptic digestion. The digested peptides were spotted on a silica gel-coated thin layer gel plate and the sample peptides were resolved by electrophoresis in the first dimension and thin layer chromatography in the second dimension in order to compare the several γGTPs prepared from tumor and normal tissues. Since the enzyme is a typical glycoprotein, therefore the carbohydrate moiety of the enzyme might affect the proteolytic digestion. However, very interestingly, the mapping patterns of the γGTPs from yolk sac tumor and AH-66 cells were found

A)   B)   C)

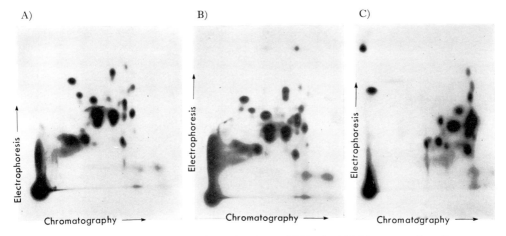

FIG. 1. Pepetide mapping analysis of various γGTPs. A, AH-66 enzyme; B, yolk sac tumor (YST) enzyme; C, normal rat kidney enzyme. γGTPs were radioiodinated with ^{125}I and digested with chymotrypsin. Two dimensional separation of the enzymes on thin layer plates were carried out. Digestion mixture was resolved by electrophoresis in the first dimension and ascending chromatography in the second dimension.

to be very similar (Fig. 1A, B), whereas the enzyme from normal rat kidney was quite different (Fig. 1C). This and several catalytic properties indicate that the carbohydrate moieties are very different while it is possible that the protein portion of these enzymes do not differ greatly from one another. These data also indicate that the enzymes from tumor tissues are very similar with respect to carbohydrate and protein structure.

4. Immunological properties

Both antibodies against enzymes from the kidney and AH-66 raised in the goat were found to be monospecific by immunodiffusion (Fig. 2). Only one precipitin line between anti-kidney γGTP antibody and the three purified γGTPs was observed. The lines were completely fused with each other without spur formation. Similarly, the fused line between the anti-AH-66 enzyme antibody and the three enzymes indicated that the latter three were immunologically identical. These data were also confirmed by an inhibition study of the enzyme activity by antibody (38). Previous studies have indicated that the transpeptidases from azo dye-induced hepatoma and fetal liver are immunologically identical (36). Quite recently a highly purified γGTP was obtained from normal rat liver and it also cross-reacted with various γGTPs (Yokosawa et al., unpublished). These results and the present study indicated that the protein moiety is solely responsible for the immunological properties of the transpeptidase. This conclusion was further supported by the fact that the amino acid compositions of the enzymes from yolk sac tumor, AH-66 cells, azo dye-induced hepatoma, normal rat kidney and liver are quite similar as described.

5. Heterogeneity and isoelectric focusing experiment

The final preparation of the transpeptidase from kidney AH-66 and yolk sac tumor showed a diffuse band on disc gel electrophoresis. This diffuseness might, in part, reflect the microheterogeneity of the transpeptidase arising from the differences in sialic acid

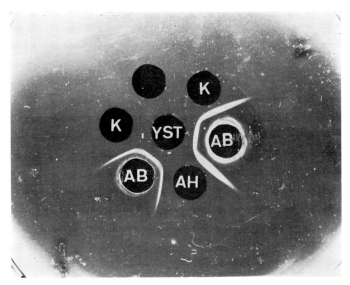

Fig. 2. Specificity and cross-reactivity of γGTPs from various sources on a double immunodiffusion in agar. AB well contains antibody against rat kidney γGTP; yolk sac tumor (YST), AH-66, K wells contain γGTPs from YST cells, AH-66 cells, and rat kidney, respectively.

content. On isoelectric fractionation, these three enzymes showed a similar charge heterogeneity. Each of the three purified enzymes was subjected to isoelectric focusing. They exhibited multiple peaks of activity at pH 4.8 to 7. When the enzymes from AH-66 and the yolk sac tumor were treated with neuraminidase and then focused, a peak of activity was obtained at pH 7.4. However, when the kidney enzyme was extensively treated with neuraminidase, it showed a heterogeneous distribution of activity ranging from pH 6 to 8, even though the peaks at lower pH values were greatly reduced. One of the fractions from the yolk sac tumor enzyme, which was bound to the DEAE-cellulose designated as "bound form," exhibited a peak of activity at pH 4.8. This peak was also shifted to a form having a pI value of 7.4 after neuraminidase treatment. The findings described above are consistent with the view that much of the heterogeneity observed previously on isoelectric focusing of the transpeptidase preparations is related to the state of sialylation of the enzyme molecules. The kidney enzyme was electrofocused in the presence of 10 mM dithiothreitol to inhibit the occurrence of heterogeneity due to sulfhydryl modifications. This phenomenon had been reported earlier in the other γ-glutamyl cycle enzyme, γ-glutamyl cyclotransferase (37). No effect of dithiothreitol on the charge heterogeneity of the desialylated enzyme was observed. These results have led us to conclude that the presence of charge heterogeneity in the γGTP molecule, observed by isoelectric focusing before neuraminidase treatment, is entirely due to differences in sialylation. On the other hand, the charge difference in the kidney enzyme after neuraminidase treatment, is due to other structural and conformational differences including carbohydrate moiety.

6. Kinetic properties

An apparent K_m value for γ-glutamyl-p-nitroanilide and a K_i value for anthglutin, a specific inhibitor of the enzyme (26), were determined for the three enzymes with respect to the transpeptidation reaction. The K_m value using γ-glutamyl-p-nitroanilide as substrate were very similar, whereas the pattern of inhibition by anthglutin differed among the three enzymes. The kidney enzymes had an inhibition pattern of a mixed type whereas the other two enzymes from tumor cells revealed a competitive pattern. The K_m values for the hydrolysis of GSH and GSSG were not significantly different from each other among the three preparations. The rates of hydrolysis of glutathione and γ-glutamyl alanine by the purified enzymes were examined over various pH ranges (38) according to the method described by McIntyre and Curthoys (22). The hydrolytic rate of glutathione by the kidney enzyme was maximal at pH 7.4 and decreased sharply as the pH changed. In contrast, the rate of hydrolysis catalyzed by the other two enzymes from tumor cells had rather broad pH optima. This tendency was also observed when γ-glutamyl alanine was used as a substrate. The purified enzymes were incubated with 50 μM γ-glutamyl-p-nitroanilide in the presence and absence of a mixture of 18 amino acids. A study was also carried out in which a single amino acid (L-alanine) was added. In these experiments, the rates of formation of p-nitroaniline found in the presence of amino acids were corrected by subtracting the p-nitroaniline which had formed due to hydrolysis. This provides an approximation of the amount of transpeptidation that occurs under these conditions (2). Since the presence of amino acids inhibits hydrolysis, the actual values for transpeptidation would be expected to be somewhat high. The extent of transpeptidation in the presence of 0.5 mM alanine alone may be estimated from these data to be about 10% of the total γ-glutamyl donor utilized at pH 7.4. In the presence of an amino acid mixture, with a higher concentration of alanine (5 mM), about 50% of the total γ-glutamyl donor utilized was involved in transpeptidation. At pH 7.5 the rates of utilization of γ-glutamyl donor by hydrolysis and by transpeptidation were similar, and the extent of transpeptidation was substantial at a physiological pH range. These results indicate that the relative contributions of the transpeptidation and hydrolytic reactions of these enzymes are almost equal under physiological conditions as described previously (2, 38). The extent of transpeptidation relative to hydrolysis of the tumor enzymes seems to be even higher *in vivo*.

γGTP in the Experimental Hepatoma

During azo dye-induced hepatocarcinogenesis, the activity increases after the onset of feeding of azo dye, then decreases to a normal level and again increases to a high level in the developed hepatoma (33). The transient increase of the activity is coincident with the appearance of oval cells which have been characterized as a bile duct cells (5). The oval cell is believed to differentiate into small hepatocytes which then became mature hepatocytes (9, 15–17).

Immunoreactive γGTP Levels in Fetal and Adult Rat Livers, Hyperplastic Foci and Hepatoma

A specific and sensitive enzyme immunoassay method for rat γGTP was developed (39), making it possible to determine the levels of immunoreactive enzyme protein in various liver tissues. Normal adult liver contains a very low concentration of γGTP, while fetal liver contains much higher levels. Kidney and small intestine contain large amounts of γGTP. Azo dye-induced hepatoma and hyperplastic nodules also have higher levels of this enzyme. Utilizing our enzyme immunoassay, the mean amount of normal rat liver γGTP was found to be 1.43 ng/mg protein. When the enzyme was determined in 20 normal rat livers, there was a mean activity of 74.4 nmol/min/mg protein. By dividing the observed enzyme specific activity by enzyme concentration, a calculated mean specific activity of 52 units/mg protein was obtained. This calculated value for normal rat liver compares well with the amount of protein which can be purified from normal rat liver (unpublished data). This close agreement in absolute specific activity provides assurance for the accuracy of the enzyme immunoassay used in the experiment.

γGTP activity and the enzyme content of 30 samples of rat liver and hepatoma tissues were compared (39). A significant positive correlation was observed between the amount of enzyme detected by both methods ($p < 0.01$). In the hepatoma tissue, the increase in enzyme content was not always associated with an increased amount of enzyme activity, indicating that the enzymatic assay might not reflect the true concentration of γGTP in certain hepatoma tissues. At enzyme levels below 10 ng/ml a correlation between the two assay methods did not appear to exist.

γGTP Content during Azo Dye Hepatocarcinogenesis

The γGTP content was determined by enzyme immunoassay during the process of hepatocarcinogenesis induced by 3'-methyl-4-dimethyl-aminoazobenzene (3'-Me-DAB). During chemical carcinogenesis in rats, an elevated γGTP content was first observed 4 weeks after commencement of 3'-Me-DAB feeding. After 6 to 8 weeks the enzyme content decreased to the original level and this was followed by a sustained increase in the enzyme levels after 18 weeks. At the time of the first peak, the γGTP content ranged from 55–360 ng/g wet weight of tissue. The γGTP content prior to the carcinogen treatment ranged from 5 to 30 ng/g wet weight of tissues.

Perspective

1. Significance of γGTP as a tumor marker enzyme
1) γGTP as an oncofetal protein

In some respects, the property of glutathione metabolism in tumor tissues resembles that in fetal organs (35). The activation of γGTP in hepatoma tissue indicates the expression of a "fetal gene." However, the enzyme activity is distributed in various normal tissues except normal adult liver in which a very low activity is found. There is therefore some controversy about whether or not the enzyme is one of the oncofetal proteins. Among fetal tissues, liver, colon, lung, and skin contain substantially high activities of γGTP. The high activities found in the corresponding tumor tissues are a result of gene derepression or ontogenic reversion of the enzyme. The gene expression of α-fetoprotein and γGTP are observed independently, because histochemical stainings do not reveal the same localization of the two proteins in the same section of the hepatoma tissues (14). These observations do not exclude the possibility that γGTP is an oncofetal protein, since even α-fetoprotein is present in trace amounts in normal adult liver. The antigenic and enzymatic properties of the enzymes from fetal liver and hepatoma are identical, and the enzyme activity is very low in the adult rat hepatocyte, suggesting that the γGTP may be considered a typical oncofetal protein in the rat and possibly in the human.

2)   Preneoplastic hepatocyte and γGTP as a marker for preneoplastic lesion

The preneoplastic lesion also contains increased activity, which may reflect the appearance of oval cells. In general, a single administration of carcinogen to rats brings about 2 to 5-fold increase of activity and then at 1 to 2 days the activity increases to a plateau, the level of which is almost equal to that of fetal liver. These changes are found using several carcinogens such as 2-acetoaminofluorene (AFF), N-nitrosodiethylamine, N-nitrosomorpholine, 3'-Me-DAB, aflatoxin B_1, and thioacetamide. In experimental tumors of the liver, Farber and his group (8, 9) reported a model of a single administration experiment using AFF. The experiment was initiated with a single administration of carcinogen which was later followed by a partial hepatectomy or by further administration of AFF. In some cases after a single administration of hepatocarcinogen, promotion was carried out by treatment with phenobarbital. In this method, initiation with a powerful hepatocarcinogen was followed by selective proliferation as seen in local areas of hepatocytes. Proliferation of normal hepatocytes was inhibited by administration of AFF, while partial hepatectomy brings about proliferation of "altered hepatocytes" resistant to the cytotoxic effect of AFF (3). In this experiment neoplastic lesions were observed in which high γGTP activity was found. Neoplastic or hyperplastic nodules observed during the process of hepatocarcinogenesis had a high activity of γGTP. In these nodules G-6-Pase and ATPase activities were nearly eliminated while a positive marker of these foci was considered to be γGTP activity. Transplantable hepatomas with different rates of growth or differentiation were examined relative to γGTP activity. No correlation was found between the γGTP activity and the degree or differentiation or the growth rate (11).

Tsuchida *et al.* (41) reported that the antigenicity of γGTP from hyperplastic nodules is identical to that of rat kidney even though they did not determine the amino acid and sugar composition. It is of diagnostic value to identify the preneoplastic lesion of human serum or human liver by means of γGTP.

3)   γGTP in tumor cells and the detoxification process

It seems quite reasonable that γGTP functions in the detoxification process of tumor cells. Normal adult hepatocytes have GSH-S transferase and cysteinyl glycinase but lack γGTP activity. However, in tumor tissues these three enzymes exist, suggesting that the capacity for detoxification may be much better than that found in normal hepatocyte. Quite recently Deml (7) reported that GSH is stained in the same sites as γGTP. Laishes (19) reported that γGTP positive cells are found when cultured in the presence of a chemical carcinogen; life span is much longer than that of the normal hepatocytes. This indicates that the cells in the preneoplastic lesions which have a γGTP positive phenotype proliferate in the liver during the feeding of AFF. This proliferation could be explained by the fact that the detoxification process of preneoplastic cells (γGTP positive cells) is more active than that of normal hepatocytes.

Chasseud (2) reported that the process of mercapturic acid conjugation is involved in the detoxification of a highly reactive electrophile such as a proximate carcinogen. The carcinogen which is activated by drug metabolizing enzymes in microsomes, is conjugated initially with GSH by GSH-S transferase. GSH-S transferase has a very strict specificity for the sulfhydryl moiety of glutathione but has a broad specificity for electrophiles. Most of the GSH and GSH-S-transferases are located in hepatic parenchymatous cells. Topological studies of γGTP have revealed that the enzyme is localized on the outer surface of the cell membrane (13), while the substrate of γGTP, glutathione, is distributed intra-cellularly. It is therefore necessary that glutathione translocates from inside to the outside of the cell. There must be present a translocation system for intra-cellular glutathione. In erythrocytes and liver, GSH is oxidized to GSSG which is translocated from the inside to the outside of the cell. This efflux phenomenon is ATP dependent. Sies's group (1) and ours (18) demonstrated that the efflux of GSSG is competitively inhibited by glutathione-S-conjugates in inside out vesicles and in liver cells. These results suggests that the translocase plays an important role in the efflux of the glutathione or the glutathione-S-conjugate system. These studies clarify the mechanism by which glutathione translocates to the outside of the cells. A specific antiserum against kidney γGTP has provided useful information in studies on the im-munohistochemical localization of the γGTP (20, 39). By light microscopy the enzyme was seen on the luminal surface of the proximal tubules of the kidney, and by electron microscopy it was seen in the cell membrane of hepatocytes (39). Quite recently Spater et al. (30) clearly demonstrated that γGTP is localized in the proximal convoluted renal tubules. These observations indicate that mercapturic acid conjugation should take place effectively in these organs.

4) Enzyme immunoassay and the content of γGTP protein in various normal and tumor tissues

Normal rat liver contains a very small amount of the enzyme and therefore con-ventional enzymatic assays are not a reliable way of measuring it. In the present study we employed a specific enzyme immunoassay to quantitate the very low amount of the enzyme protein in normal rat liver. We found a positive correlation between results derived from the enzyme immunoassay and the enzymatic assay. Increased activity was accompanied by an increased amout of immunoreactive protein.

During azo dye hepatocarcinogenesis increased immunoreactive γGTP was ob-served at early and late stages, observations are in good agreement with previous data obtained which using the enzymatic assay. The metabolic significance of the increased γGTP content still remains a mystery. The first increase observed in the early stage and the second increase at a late stage may have a different metabolic significance. The first increase of the enzyme protein may reflect of the appearance of renewed small hepatocytes derived from oval cells or preneoplastic lesions as observed in aflatoxin-induced hepato-carcinogenesis (15–17). The second increase of protein may be due to the production of the enzyme by hepatoma cells. Sakamoto et al. (27) explained these phenomena by their different responses toward cyclic AMP. High levels of γGTP observed in hepatoma tissues may be important in the metabolism of glutathione which is related to the me-tabolism of several xenobiotic compounds including hepatocarcinogens.

5) Processing of γGTP as an experimental model for cancer-associated alterations of the carbohydrate moiety

As described above, the characteristics of γGTP from tumor tissue are not in the protein but in the carbohydrate moiety of the enzyme. The "novel type" of γGTP fre-quently found in the hepatoma patient (28, 29) is probably expressed by an alteration in the processing of the bound carbohydrate component of the enzyme. Sawabu et al. reported that the novel type of γGTP has a different affinity for several lectins as com-pared to other forms of γGTP molecules (29). Quite recently in our laboratory γGTP was biosynthesized in cultured cell lines of yolk sac tumor (44). The cells were pulse-labeled with ^{14}C-leucine, ^{35}S-methionine, and ^{3}H-glucosamine. After the extraction with 1% Triton X-100, the γGTP-related products were isolated from the other products of translation by immunoprecipitation with specific anti-γGTP antibody. The antigen-antibody complex was subjected to SDS-polyacrylamide gel electrophoresis. After electrophoresis three major components were discerned. Two of these polypeptides are identical to the H- and L-subunits of γGTP purified from normal kidney. The molecular weight of the third component is approximately 80–100 K, and this component is only found in the experiment with short-pulse time experiment. A high molecular weight component was not seen in the experiments with longer labeling periods such as 45 min. These data suggest that the γGTP in tumor cells is synthesized initially as a precursor form with a large molecular weight which is then rapidly processed to a mature γGTP. This observation is consistent with the data on rat kidney enzyme (21). Utilizing these systems we may be able to clarify the mechanisms by which cancer-associated alterations of carbohydrate moiety occur.

Yamashita et al. (42) analyzed the carbohydrate structures of γGTPs from AH-66 cell lines and from normal rat liver and found that AH-66 γGTP contains bisecting-N-acetylglucosamine residues whereas normal rat liver lack this residue. The glycosyl-transferase responsible for bisecting-N-acetylglucosamine residue on the carbohydrate moiety of γGTP is induced in the malignant cells. Cummings and Kornfeld (6) recently reported that the bisecting-N-acetylglucosamine residue has an affinity for the erythro-agglutinating phytohemagglutinin lectins from red kidney beans. Knowledge of the structural properties of γGTP will be important in the study of specific antibodies against the carbohydrate moiety and the antibodies themselves will be useful as a tool for the diagnosis and treatment of cancer.

Acknowledgment

This work was supported in part by Grants in-Aid for Cancer Research from the Ministry of Education, Science and Culture, and of Health and Welfare, Japan, and Princess Takamatsu Cancer Research Fund.

REFERENCES

1. Akerboom, T.P.M., Bilzer, M., and Sies, H. FEBS Lett., **140**, 73–76 (1982).
2. Allison, D. R. and Meister, A. J. Biol. Chem., **256**, 2988–2992 (1981).
3. Cameron, R., Kellen, J., Kollin, A., Malkin, A., and Farber, E. Cancer Res., **38**, 823–829 (1978).
4. Chasseud, L. F. Adv. Cancer Res., **29**, 175–275 (1979).
5. Chisaka, N., Kaneko, A., and Dempo, K. Sapporo Med. J., **51**, 91–104 (1982) (in Japanese).
6. Cummings, R. D. and Kornfeld, S. J. Biol. Chem., **257**, 44235–44240 (1982).
7. Deml, E. and Osterle, D. Cancer Res., **40**, 490–491 (1980).
8. Farber, E. and Solt, D. Carcinogenesis, **2**, 443–448 (1978).
9. Farber, E., Ross, G., Laishes, B., Lin, J., Medline, A., Ogawa, K., and Solt, D. In "Carcinogens: Identification and Mechanism of Actions," ed. A. C. Griffin and C. R. Shaw, pp. 319–335 (1979). Raven Press, New York.
10. Fiala, S. and Fiala, E. S. J. Natl. Cancer Inst., **57**, 591–598 (1976).
11. Fiala, S., Fiala, A. E., and Dixon, B. J. Natl. Cancer Inst., **48**, 1393–1401 (1976).
12. Fleming, N., Groscurth, P., and Kistler, G. Histochemistry, **51**, 209–218 (1977).
13. Horiuchi, S., Inoue, M., and Morino, Y. Eur. J. Biochem., **87**, 429–437 (1978).
14. Jalanko, H. and Ruoslahti, E. Cancer Res., **39**, 3495–3501 (1979).
15. Kalengayi, M.M.R. and Desmet, V. J. Cancer Res., **35**, 2845–2852 (1975).

16. Kalengayi, M.M.R. and Desmet, V. J. *Cancer Res.*, **35**, 2836–2844 (1975).
17. Kalengayi, M.M.R. and Desmet, V.J. *In* "Primary Liver Tumors," ed. H. Remmer, H. M. Bolt, P. Bannasch, and H. Popper, pp. 467–483 (1980). Univ. Park Press, Baltimore.
18. Kondo, T., Murao, M., and Taniguchi, N. *Eur. J. Biochem.*, **125**, 551–554 (1982).
19. Laishes, B. A., Ogawa, K., Roberts, E., and Farber, E. *J. Natl. Cancer Inst.*, **60**, 1009–1015 (1978).
20. Marathe, G. V., Nash, B., Haschemeyer, R. H., and Tate, S. S. *FEBS Lett.*, **107**, 436–440 (1979).
21. Matsuda, Y., Tsuji, A., and Katunuma, N. *Adv. Enzyme Regul.*, **21**, in press.
22. McIntyre, T. M. and Curthoys, N. P. *J. Biol. Chem.*, **250**, 6499–6504 (1979).
23. Meister, A., Tate, S. S., and Griffith, O. W. *Methods Enzymol.*, **77**, 237–253 (1981).
24. Meister, A. *Science*, **180**, 33–39 (1973).
25. Meister, A. and Tate, S. S. *Annu. Rev. Biochem.*, **45**, 559–640 (1976).
26. Minato, S. *Arch. Biochem. Biophys.*, **192**, 235–242 (1979).
27. Sakamoto, Y., Higashi, T., and Tateishi, N. This volume, pp. 281–289.
28. Sawabu, N., Nakagen, M., Ozaki, K., Wakabayashi, T., Toya, D., Hattori, S., and Ishii, M. *Ann. Acad. Med.*, **9**, 206–209 (1980).
29. Sawabu, N., Hattori, S., Toya, D., Ozaki, K., and Wakabayashi, T. "Sapporo Cancer Seminar, the 2nd Symposium on Membrane-Associated Alterations in Cancer: Biochemical Strategies against Cancer," July 14–17, Sapporo, Japan (1982) (Abstr.).
30. Spater, H. W., Poruchynsky, M. S., Quintana, N., Inoue, M., and Novikoff, A. B. *Proc. Natl. Acad. Sci. U.S.*, **79**, 3547–3550 (1982).
31. Szewczuk, A. and Albert, Z. *Folia Histochem. Cytochem.*, **11**, 75–82 (1973).
32. Szewczuk, A., Milnerowicz, H., and Sobiech, K. A. *Neoplasma*, **25**, 297–308 (1978).
33. Taniguchi, N., Tsukada, Y., Mukuo, K., and Hirai, H. *Gann*, **65**, 381–387 (1974).
34. Taniguchi, N. *J. Biochem.*, **75**, 473–480 (1974).
35. Taniguchi, N., Tsukada, Y., and Hirai, H. *Biochim. Biophys. Acta*, **354**, 161–167 (1974).
36. Taniguchi, N., Saito, K., and Takakuwa, E. *Biochim. Biophys. Acta*, **391**, 265–271 (1975).
37. Taniguchi, N. and Meister, A. *J. Biol. Chem.*, **253**, 1799–1806 (1978).
38. Taniguchi, N., Yokosawa, N., Tsukada, Y., Minato, S., and Makita, A. *In* "Glutathione—Storage, Transport and Turnover in Mammals," ed. Y. Sakamoto, T. Higashi, and N. Tateishi, pp. 153–166 (1983). Japan Sci. Soc. Press, Tokyo.
39. Taniguchi, N., Yokosawa, N., Iizuka, S., Sako, F., Tsukada, Y., Sato, M., Dempo, K., and Makita, A. *Ann. N.Y. Acad. Sci.*, in press.
40. Tateishi, N., Higashi, T., Nomura, T., Naruse, A., Nakashima, K., Shiozaki, H., and Sakamoto, Y. *Gann*, **67**, 215–222 (1976).
41. Tsuchida, S., Hoshino, K., Sato, T., Ito, N., and Sato, K. *Cancer Res.*, **39**, 4200–4205 (1979).
42. Yamashita, K., Hitoi, A., Taniguchi, N., Yokosawa, N., Tsukada, Y., and Kobata, A. *Cancer Res.*, in press.
43. Yokosawa, N., Taniguchi, N., Tsukada, Y., and Makita, A. *Oncodev. Biol. Med.*, **2**, 165–177 (1981).
44. Yokosawa, N., Taniguchi, N., Tsukada, Y., and Makita, A. *Oncodev. Biol. Med.*, in press.

γ-GLUTAMYL TRANSPEPTIDASE IN RATS WITH MORRIS HEPATOMA

Apolinary SZEWCZUK

*Biochemical Laboratory, Institute of Immunology and Experimental Therapy, Polish Academy of Sciences**

A rapid increase of γ-glutamyl transpeptidase (γGTP) activity was noted in serum during growth of transplantable Morris hepatoma 5123D in Buffalo rats. Elevated γGTP activity was also observed in the tumor, urine and some organs of these rats. The increased serum γGTP originated from the hepatoma. Treatment with stilbestrol and with Sustanon or castration of the hepatoma-bearing rats diminished the increase of the serum γGTP. When the hepatoma was passaged in F_1 rats (Buffalo× Wistar), a new hepatoma variant was obtained which was faster in growth rate than the original hepatoma. γGTP activity was not elevated in serum, urine, or some organs of this variant. By immunological techniques, elevated amounts of the enzyme were demonstrated in the hepatoma variant. On zymograms of serum γGTP of rats bearing the hepatoma, a fraction II was elevated and a light form of hepatoma γGTP appeared in addition to the five γGTP fractions present in normal rat serum. Only the two fractions reacted with antibody to hepatoma γGTP. Heavy (molecular weight (Mr) 108,000) and light (Mr 70,000) forms of γGTP purified from the hepatoma 5123D after solubilization with deoxycholate and bromelain, respectively, contained sialic acid. The hepatoma enzyme was inhibited competitively by anthglutin and its isomers, while the kidney enzyme was inhibited non-competitively.

The activity of γ-glutamyl transpeptidase (γGTP) in human serum is markedly increased during growth of some tumors such as those of the liver, and therefore its assay is a good marker of primary and secondary cancer of that organ. A considerable increase of γGTP activity is also observed in rat liver after long time administration of certain chemical carcinogens or aflatoxins.

Among activities of five different enzymes tested in our laboratory (two acylases, arylamidase, γGTP, and pyrrolidonecarboxylylpeptidase), only γGTP activity was markedly increased in the liver of Buffalo rats during growth of transplantable Morris hepatoma 5123D (7). Its activity was increased also in some other organs of the hepatoma-bearing rats. Elevated γGTP activity was also noted in Albert hepatoma of mouse, spontaneous mammary cancer of mouse, Kirkman-Robbins hamster hepatoma and Yoshida sercoma of Wistar rats (7).

In Morris hepatoma 5123D grown in Buffalo rats, the specific activity was much higher than that in normal rat liver (7). γGTP activity in rat serum was consistently increased during growth of the hepatoma, and after 9 weeks, its mean value was about

---

* 53-114 Wroclaw, Poland.

50-times that in serum of control rats (7). Similarly, elevated γGTP activity in the serum and tumors has been observed in Buffalo rats with Morris hepatoma 7777.

Effect of the Size of the Hepatoma and Hormones on γGTP Activity in Serum (1, 2)

The specific activity (mU/mg) in the tumor does not depend on the age and size of the Morris hepatoma 5123D. It is almost constant during the growth of the hepatoma. But the total γGTP activity in the tumor as well as in the serum increases during the growth of the hepatoma. A correlation was observed between the enzyme activity and the size of the hepatoma (2) which is illustrated in Table I. Elevated γGTP activity was also observed in the urine of hepatoma-bearing rats; the total enzyme activity excreted daily in the urine was 3–4 times higher than that of control rats (Table I). An increasing tendency toward formation of metastases in the rat lung was observed during growth of the hepatoma. γGTP activity was histochemically observed almost exclusively in the bile canaliculi of the hepatoma and in its metastases (2).

When the leg implanted with the hepatoma was amputated 10 day after implantation, γGTP activity in serum and urine was decreased rapidly and maintained at the normal level for months; metastases of the hepatoma to the lungs were not observed 10 days after the implantation, but occurred after more than 20 days (2). No change of serum or urinary γGTP was observed, 2 days after operation, in rats from which the healthy leg was amputated while the tumor-bearing leg was left intact (2). On the other hand, partial (three-fourths) hepatectomy and pancreatectomy of rats with the hepatoma (3 to 4 weeks after implantation) did not bring about effect on serum and urinary γGTP activity and on metastases in the lungs. These results support the notion that serum γGTP and part of the urinary γGTP in the hepatoma-bearing rats are synthesized by the hepatoma and not by the liver.

Recently M. Albert has demonstrated that treatment of the 5123D hepatoma-bearing rats for a few days with stilbestrol decreased γGTP activity in the serum, tumor, and liver to the level of control rats (1). When the treatment with stilbestrol was stopped, enzyme activity slowly increased. A much weaker effect on γGTP activity in the serum

TABLE I. γGTP Activity in Rats with Morris Hepatoma 5123D (2)

Days after implantation[a]	Size of tumor (cm³)	γGTP activity[b] in			
		Hepatoma		Serum (mean±S.D. mU/mg)	Urine (mean±S.D. mU/day)
		Specific (mU/mg)	Total (mU/tumor)		
10				1.7±0.5	
17	2.3	2.8	840	5.2±1.1	
20			1,860		1,400±420
23	5.5	2.6	1,860	12.9±3.9	
24					1,700±550
28			3,130		1,800±550
30	12.7	2.5	3,130	16.5±4.1	
Control rats				0.81±0.23	

[a] Thirty mg finely minced hepatoma was implanted intramusculary into one hind leg of 2-month-old rats.

[b] Determined at pH 8.6 with γ-L-glutamyl-α-naphthylamide as substrate.

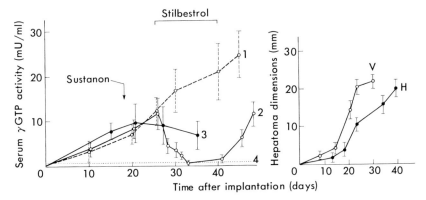

Fig. 1. (left) Effect of treatment with sex hormones on γGTP activity in serum of Buffalo rats with implanted Morris hepatoma 5123D. 1, untreated; 2, treated intramuscularly with stilbestrol (daily 40 μg/kg); 3, treated with Sustanon at 18th day; 4, treated with Sustanon at 2nd day.

Fig. 2. (right) Growth rate of Morris hepatoma 5123D in Buffalo rats (H) and of its variant in F_1 (Buffalo×Wistar) rats (V).

of hepatoma-bearing rats was exerted by Sustanon (product of Organon, Holland) (Fig. 1), but no effect was noted when the rats were treated with testosterone. The increase of serum γGTP activity in male rats with the hepatoma was faster than in females. Castration of male rats significantly inhibited the rate of increase of the serum enzyme (1). These results suggest that some sex hormones exert an influence on the synthesis of γGTP in hepatoma and on the passage of the enzyme to the blood stream.

γGTP in an F_1 on Line of Rats with Hepatoma (3)

Morris hepatoma 5123D does not take in Wistar rats, but take readily and grows in F_1 (Buffalo×Wistar) rats. In the first passage of the hepatoma in the F_1 hybrids, a much lower increase of serum γGTP activity was observed, than in Buffalo rats. The second passage in F_1 rats yielded a new hepatoma variant, named by us hepatoma 5123D/AS (3). The growth rate of this hepatoma was much faster than that of Morris hepatoma 5123D in Buffalo rats (Fig. 2). Enzyme activity in the liver, brain, pancreas, spleen, and lung of rats bearing hepatoma 5123D was much higher than that in F_1 hybrids bearing hepatoma 5123D/AS (Table II). No significant differences were noted in γGTP activity in organs of the hepatoma variant bearers and that of control rats (3). Activity of γGTP,

TABLE II. γGTP Activity in Some Organs of Control and Hepatoma-bearing Rats (3)

Organ	Activity (mU/mg±S.D.)		
	Control	With Morris hepatoma 5123D	
	Buffalo rats	In Buffalo rats	Passaged in F_1
Kidney	180±30	226±25	191±30
Liver	0.45±0.10	2.45±0.95	0.36±0.11
Brain	0.80±0.25	2.00±0.70	0.70±0.22
Spleen	0.95±0.30	3.50±1.05	0.85±0.25
Lung	1.00±0.25	2.90±0.65	1.00±0.15

TABLE III. Enzyme Activities in Morris Hepatoma 5123D (3)

Enzyme	Activity (mU/mg ± S.D.)	
	In Buffalo rats	In F_1 rats
γGTP	5.4 ± 0.80	0.54 ± 0.21
Acylase	5.1 ± 1.9	3.0 ± 1.0
Aminopeptidases tested with following β-naphthylamides:		
L-pyroglutamyl-	0.12 ± 0.02	0.12 ± 0.02
L-alanyl-	17.0 ± 5.6	22.9 ± 4.1
L-leucyl-	7.9 ± 3.1	8.1 ± 3.0
glycyl-	5.2 ± 1.5	3.9 ± 1.9
α-aspartyl-	3.1 ± 1.4	3.8 ± 1.1
α-glutamyl	6.0 ± 2.2	4.4 ± 1.4
L-lysyl-	19.2 ± 4.2	19.0 ± 4.1
L-arginyl-	15.0 ± 3.9	22.6 ± 5.0
L-histidyl-	8.0 ± 3.4	5.9 ± 2.5
L-phenylalanyl-	14.2 ± 3.1	11.4 ± 3.1
L-tyrosyl-	6.3 ± 1.9	6.4 ± 2.1

acylase and amino peptidases tested toward 10 different amino acid naphthylamides was also assayed in homogenates from both hepatomas taken 4 weeks after tumor implantation (Table III). Only in γGTP activity a large and significant difference was noted between the hepatoma 5123D and its variant. The enzyme activity in the first tumor was markedly increased but that in hepatoma 5123D/AS was as low as in liver of control rats (3). No increase of the enzyme activity was also noted in the serum of F_1 rats during growth of the hepatoma variant (Fig. 3). At the same time γGTP activity constantly increased in the serum of Buffalo rats bearing Morris hepatoma 5123D. In the urine of rats 31 days after implantation of hepatoma 5123D/AS, the mean daily output

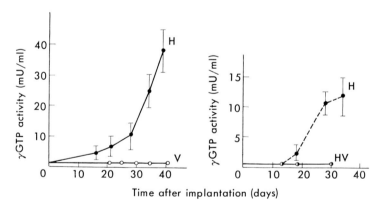

Time after implantation (days)

FIG. 3. (left) γGTP activity in serum of rats with the hepatoma 5123D (H) and of F_1 rats with the hepatoma variant (V). Each point on the figure represents the mean value from determinations in 6–8 animals.

FIG. 4. (right) Behavior of serum γGTP activity in Buffalo rats implanted hepatoma 5123D in one hind leg and simultaneously the hepatoma variant in the other leg. On the 13th day the legs with hepatoma variant were removed from rats in one group but the other hepatoma remained intact (H). In the second group of rats, the legs with both hepatomas were left intact (HV).

of γGTP activity was 550 ± 250 mU. In the urine of control rats the activity was 650 mU while that of Buffalo rats with hepatoma 5123D was $1,700 \pm 60$ mU (3).

γGTP in Rats with Both Hepatomas (3)

Two groups of Buffalo rats were implanted simultaneously with hepatoma 5123D in one leg and the hepatoma variant in the other leg. On the 13th day, the rats were divided in two groups, and in one group the legs with the hepatoma variant were surgically amputated and the other group was left intact. Serum γGTP activities were assayed in both groups of rats at intervals of several days (Fig. 4). The enzyme activity in rats with both hepatomas remained at a low level equal to the mean activity in the serum of control rats. A marked increase of serum γGTP activity took place in rats whose leg with the hepatoma variant had been amputated (3). In other experiments the hepatoma variant was implanted in rats on the 15th days after implantation of hepatoma 5123D, and after several days a distinct decrease of γGTP activity was observed in the serum of these rats. The effect of the hepatoma variant on the decrease of γGTP activity in rats with hepatoma 5123D was observed only in in vivo experiments. Preincubation for a few hours of mixtures consisting of equal volumes of hepatoma homogenates or sera obtained from rats with hepatoma 5123D and from the hepatoma variant bearers did not change the γGTP activity. Also, dialysis for many hours of the homogenate or serum from rats with the hepatoma variant did not affect γGTP activity. This proves that hepatoma 5123D/AS does not possess an inhibitor of γGTP, but probably produces a factor which inhibits synthesis of the enzyme in hepatoma 5123D.

Immunological Studies of γGTP in Hepatomas (8)

In a double immunodiffusion test, the antibody directed against γGTP from Morris hepatoma 5123D gave a single precipitin line with γGTP purified from hepatoma 5123D; similarly with the enzyme purified from variant hepatoma grown in F_1 rats. The intensities of these two lines were identical when the protein concentration of γGTP from hepatoma 5123D was 8-times lower than the concentration of the enzyme preparation from the hepatoma variant. The specific γGTP activity of the first γGTP preparation was about 10-times higher than that of the second; the respective values were 1.95 U/mg and 0.2 U/mg. By the single radial immunodiffusion method, the content of γGTP in the hepatoma 5123D was 7.7-times higher than in the hepatoma variant. Both γGTP preparations gave immunological cross-reaction in double immunodiffusion test (8).

Direct and indirect immunofluorescence methods for localization of γGTP in microscopic sections of hepatomas were used. In hepatoma 5123D sections, strong immunofluorescence was observed in the plasma membranes and cytoplasm of tumor cells when antibody to γGTP from hepatoma 5123D and fluorescein isothiocyanate goat antirabbit immunoglobulin were used. In sections of the variant hepatoma, fluorescence was much weaker. The fluorescence intensity of both hepatomas was however the same when 16-times diluted antibody was used for staining of hepatoma 5123D sections. Similar results were noted when an indirect tecnhique was used. It should be added that the hepatoma 5123D studied by immunofluorescence showed about 20-times higher γGTP activity than did the hepatoma variant (8).

These immunological results will imply that in the hepatoma variant the synthesis of γGTP is inhibited.

γGTP Fractions in Serum and Binding with Antibody (9)

Recently a new fluorescence method for localization of γGTP fractions after electrophoresis in polyacrylamide gel was elaborated (5). The method employs 7(γ-L-glutamyl)-4-methyl-coumarlylamide as a fluorogenic substrate and glycylglycine as acceptor of γ-glutamyl groups. The liberated 7-amino-4-methyl-coumarin is intensively fluorescent.

On γGTP zymograms of control rat serum (0.5 mU γGTP/ml) five γGTP fractions were observed. Two (fractions I and II) of them migrated rapidly and were located in the α-globulin region. Another two (fractions III and IV) were slowly migrating and located between the β- and γ-globulins. The last fraction (fraction V) did not migrate. All γGTP fractions of control serum were not visualized when the gel was stained by a histochemical method employing γ-L-glutamyl-α-naphtylamide. In the serum of Buffalo rats with hepatoma 5123D (7 mU/ml), besides the above mentioned five fractions there was also an enhanced activity of fraction II. Also a new fraction appeared with an electrophoretic mobility identical to that of the light γGTP form (L) from hepatoma. On zymograms of serum from rats with hepatoma 7777, the same γGTP fractions were observed as in the serum of rats with hepatoma 5123D, except that there was a seventh fraction (L-2), migrating more slowly than the L form (9). After preincubation of control serum with anti-hepatoma γGTP, all γGTP fractions remained on the zymogram. It was also demonstrated that preincubation of serum from hepatoma-bearing rats with antibody causes the disappearance of fractions L and L-2 and a decrease of fraction II activity. However the non-migrating fraction increased (Fig. 5). This strongly suggests that only hepatoma γGTP fractions can bind with the antibody, but the enzyme fractions in control serum are immunologically distinguishable. On zymograms of serum from rats with the hepatoma variant, all six γGTP fractions, identical with the fractions from serum of the hepatoma-bearing rats were found but the intensities of fractions II and L were very weak (Fig. 5). Both fractions bound antibody to hepatoma γGTP. These results show that in sera of rats with transplanted hepatoma, new γGTP fractions appear which are immunologically indistinguishable from the hepatoma enzyme. However they differ from the enzyme fractions present in control serum.

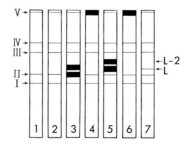

FIG. 5. γGTP zymograms of rat sera and effect of antibody to hepatoma γGTP (9). 1, serum of control Buffalo rat; 2, as 1 but preincubated with antibody; 3, serum of Buffalo rat with Morris hepatoma 5123D; 4, as 3 but preincubated with antibody; 5, serum of Buffalo rat with hepatoma 7777; 6, as 5 but preincubated with antibody; 7, serum from F_1 with hepatoma variant.

Isolation of the Enzyme Molecular Forms

In the homogenate from Morris hepatoma, over 95% of the total γGTP activity is bound to the sedimented fractions. The relative percent of enzyme activity in nuclear, mitochondrial, microsomal, and cytoplasmic fractions was found to be 32, 5, 60, and 3%, respectively (10). On zymograms of the hepatoma homogenate as well as of cytoplasmic fraction, only two γGTP bands were observed; a very slowly migrating band corresponding to the heavy γGTP molecular form and a fast migrating band corresponding to the light form of the enzyme. After treatment of the homogenate with sodium deoxycholate, the γGTP activity increased in the $100,000 \times g$ supernatant while the heavy form decreased. Digestion of the microsomal fraction with bromelain caused almost complete solubilization of the hepatoma γGTP and production of the light enzyme form (9). These observations were useful for isolation of both γGTP molecular forms.

Properties of γGTP Molecular Forms

The heavy form of γGTP was prepared from hepatoma 5123D (10). The heavy γGTP form migrated very slowly upon polyacrylamide gel electrophoresis at pH 8.3, but its electrophoretic mobility was markedly increased in the gel containing Triton X-100. This and other observations prove that the heavy γGTP form shows a great tendency to aggregate and detergent diminishes the tendency. The sedimentation coefficient determined by centrifugation in a sucrose gradient with Triton X-100 was calculated to be 5.6 S and the molecular weight (Mr) 108,000 (10). This value is similar to that of γGTP from azo dye-induced rat hepatoma described by Taniguchi (11).

The light γGTP form from the hepatoma migrates much faster in polyacrylamide gel electrophoresis than does the heavy form and does not show a tendency to aggregate. Its Mr was determined to be 70,000 (9) which is very close to that of the light form of rat kidney γGTP (12).

Both hepatoma γGTP forms and rat kidney γGTP are similarly inactivated by 5 mM phenylmethanesulfonylfluoride in the presence of 1 M maleate and by 6-diazo-5-oxo-L-norleucine (9). They are similarly activated by glycylglycine and inhibited by L-serine and borate (9, 10). Both hepatoma and kidney γGTPs contain sialic acid and bind to concanavalin A (Con A)-Sepharose (9). Both hepatoma γGTP forms cross-react immunologically with antibodies to hepatoma γGTP (heavy form) and rat kidney γGTP (light form) (9), confirming earlier observations of Taniguchi et al. that other rat tumor γGTPs are indistingushable from rat kidney γGTP (11, 13).

Inhibition of γGTP by Anthglutin and Its Isomers (9)

Several years ago Minato (4) isolated γ-L-glutamyl(O-carboxy)phenylhydrazide from a strain of Penicillium oxalicum. This substance, anthglutin, was found to be a strong inhibitor of various γGTP. We synthesized chemically this compound and the derivatives (9). Synthetic anthglutin was a very potent inhibitor for the light form of γGTP from Morris hepatoma 5123D with a K_i 18 μM. The D-enantiomer of anthglutin was a little less effective inhibitor. The K_i value for γ-L-glutamyl(m-carboxy)phenylhydrazide was about 10 times higher and the K_i for γ-L-glutamyl(p-carboxy)phenylhydrazide was 100 times higher than that for anthglutin. Similar K_i values were noted

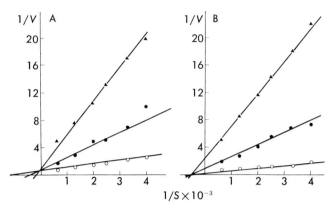

FIG. 6.   Lineweaver-Burk plots of inhibition of Morris hepatoma 5123D and rat kidney γGTPs by anthglutin. A, hepatoma-γGTP; B, kidney-γGTP. ▲ 400 μM; ● 80 μM; ○ no inhibitor.

for these hydrazides for the light form of γGTP from rat kidney. The Lineweaver-Burk plots for inhibition revealed that anthglutin inhibits the hepatoma enzyme competitively and the kidney enzyme non-competitively (Fig. 6).

The difference in the type of inhibition by anthglutin and its isomers is an interesting feature distinguishing hepatoma γGTP from kidney γGTP.

REFERENCES

1.   Albert, M. *Folia Histochem. Cytochemi.*, **17**, 365–379 (1979).
2.   Albert, W. *Folia Histochem. Cytochem.*, **14**, 181–188 (1976).
3.   Albert, Z., Szewczuk, A., and Albert, W. *Neoplasma*, **24**, 49–55 (1977).
4.   Minato, S. *Arch. Biochem. Biophys.*, **192**, 235–240 (1979).
5.   Prusak, E., Siewinski, M., and Szewczuk, A. *Clin. Chim. Acta*, **107**, 21–26 (1980).
6.   Szewczuk, A. *In* "Gamma-glutamyltransferases: Avances in Biochemical Pharmacology," 3rd series, ed. G. Siest and C. Heusghen, pp. 55–60 (1982). Masson, Paris Publ.
7.   Szewczuk, A. and Albert, Z. *Folia Histochem. Cytochem.*, **11**, 75–82 (1973).
8.   Szewczuk, A., Milnerowicz, H., Albert, Z., and Richter, R. *Neoplasma*, **27**, 241–245 (1980).
9.   Szewczuk, A., Milnerowicz, H., Prusak, E., and Albert, Z. *Folia Histochem. Cytochem.*, **20**, 25–33 (1982).
10. Szewczuk, A., Milnerowicz, H., and Sobiech, K. A. *Neoplasma*, **25**, 297–308 (1978).
11. Taniguchi, N. *J. Biochem.*, **75**, 473–480 (1974).
12. Tate, S. S. and Meister, A. *J. Biol. Chem.*, **250**, 4619–4627 (1975).
13. Yokosawa, N., Taniguchi, N., Tsukada, Y., and Makita, A. *Oncodev. Biol. Med.*, **2**, 165–177 (1981).

GANN Monograph on Cancer Research 29, 1983

FACTORS INVOLVED IN THE APPEARANCE AND SWITCH-OFF OF HEPATIC γ-GLUTAMYL TRANSPEPTIDASE

Yukiya SAKAMOTO, Taneaki HIGASHI, and Noriko TATEISHI

*Department of Biochemistry, Institute for Cancer Research,
Osaka University Medical School**

In mice and rats, γ-glutamyl transpeptidase (γGTP) activity in the liver increases greatly in late fetal life reaching a maximum at birth and then decreasing within 10 days to a low level in adult liver. In late fetal life, the concentration of plasma corticosterone is high, and exogenous glucocorticoid causes increase in γGTP activity in the liver, indicating that endogenous corticosterone induces γGTP. The hepatic response to the hormone disappears within a week after birth. The hepatic level of adenosine 3′,5′-monophosphate (cAMP) increases in fetuses before parturition and is maintained at a high level for 5 days after birth. Since the injection of dibutyryl cAMP accelerates the decay of γGTP activity after birth, cAMP appears to stimulate degradation of the enzyme.

A diet containing 0.06% 3′-methyl-4-dimethylaminoazobenzene (3′-MeDAB) increases hepatic γGTP activity in adult rats within 4–7 weeks. When rats are given the same diet for a longer period the enzyme activity decreases, and then increases again until tumors developed. The first activity rise is reversed by keeping the animals on a basal diet, but after the second rise begin the high activity persists even when the carcinogen is omitted from the diet. Injection of hydrocortisone elevates the enzyme activity in rats given diet containing 3′-MeDAB for 2 weeks or longer. As the plasma corticosterone level remains within the normal range during exposure to 3′-MeDAB, the liver seems to acquire the ability to express γGTP in response to the hormone. When rats are given a diet containing 3′-MeDAB, hepatic cAMP increases once and then decreased; the period of the rise of cAMP coincides with that of the first rise of γGTP activity. Therefore, the first rise of γGTP activity during hepatocarcinogenesis is probably reduced by the high level of cAMP. A lower concentration of cAMP in the late phase of carcinogenesis may have contributed to the continuous rise of γGTP activity.

Changes on the cell surface during malignant transformation are a current topic of interest in relation to cancer. Special attention has been paid to some functional proteins, and the structures and functions of isozymes of ecto-enzymes associated with the plasma membranes of normal and malignant tissues have been compared (24, 34–36, 43, 44). Among these enzymes, γ-glutamyl transpeptidase (γGTP) has been studied mostly, because it is a (pre) neoplastic marker in the liver (4, 10, 18, 21, 22) and is postulated to have a physiological role in transport and metabolism of amino acids (5,

---

* Fukushima 1-1-50, Fukushima-ku, Osaka 553, Japan (坂本幸哉, 東　胤昭, 立石紀子).

28, 42). The metabolic turnover and biosynthesis of γGTP in several tissues has also been investigated (19, 23, 27, 45). In the liver, γGTP usually shows low activity but a high turnover rate (19) and seems to be an adaptive enzyme. One of the most critical problems to be solved in relation to carcinogenesis is the mechanism of expression of γGTP and its regulation in liver tissues. During normal differentiation hepatic γGTP is usually induced in the liver during the late fetal period and decreases abruptly after birth (36, 43). In contrast, during hepatocarcinogenesis hepatic γGTP is induced within a few weeks by azo-dye and other carcinogens (4, 6, 11, 18, 22). With prolonged treatment with carcinogens the elevated activity decreases once and then increases again, and the second rise of γGTP activity is not reversed. Therefore, comparison of the factors involved in the induction and switch-off of hepatic γGTP during normal differentiation and during carcinogenesis should provide significant information regarding carcinogenesis.

Induction of Hepatic γGTP in Late Fetal Life and Its Decay in Newborn Animals

1. Transient changes in hepatic γGTP activity in the perinatal period

In adult rats and mice, γGTP activity in the liver is much lower than in the kidney (14, 36, 43). During normal development of mice, however, hepatic γGTP activity increases greatly in the late fetal period, reaching a maximum at birth and then decreasing to the adult level within 10 days (36). γGTP, therefore, belongs to the "late fetal cluster" according to the classification by Greengard (16), although its transient induction is unusual. We have proposed that this temporary increase in γGTP activity plays a role in releasing cysteine from glutathione for protein synthesis at this critical period of life (42). Histochemical examination of γGTP in fetal and neonatal liver has shown that it is located in the periphery of hepatocytes in whole liver lobules. Positive areas have a random (or uniform) distribution and no positive islands (4) are found (41).

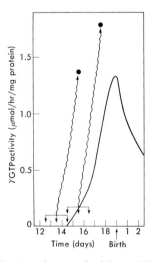

FIG. 1. Precocious induction of mouse fetal liver γGTP activity by multiple injections of hydrocortisone into pregnant mice. JCR/Jcl mice were used. ● γGTP activity in fetal liver attained by three consecutive injections of hydrocortisone (see text for other conditions). Curve shows change of liver γGTP activity in pups during natural development.

2. Involvement of glucocorticoid in the increase of liver γGTP activity in the late fetal period

In the late fetal period the liver responds to various endocrine stimuli. Hepatic glycogen, for example, accumulates precociously in response to glucocorticoid (*15*). We injected hydrocortisone-21-acetate (25 μg/g body weight) subcutaneously into pregnant mice once a day for three consecutive days (days 12–14, or days 14–16), and measured γGTP activity in the fetal liver 24 hr after the last injection. Results showed that the activity was elevated precociously to a level comparable to, or higher than, the maximum naturally attained at birth (Fig. 1). Studies with tritiated hydrocortisone showed that transfer of hydrocortisone from the mother to the pups corresponded quantitatively to γGTP induction (Tateishi *et al.*, unpublished results). The response of the pups to glucocorticoid injection (elevation of γGTP activity) lasted until one week after birth (*39*). Similar change of hepatic γGTP activity and its response to glucocorticoid were also observed in perinatal rats (*37*). In normal adult mice (ICR/Jcl, female) and rats (Donryu, male), liver γGTP activity was not affected by injection of hydrocortisone or by adrenalectomy (*39, 41*), although Billon *et al.* reported that in female Wistar rats γGTP activity decreased 50% after adrenalectomy and was restored by hydrocortisone injection (*1*).

As mouse plasma contained five times more corticosterone on days 17 and 18 in fetal life than on day 7 after birth (*37, 39*), corticosterone probably induced liver γGTP in the late fetal period during normal development. The corticosterone level in the plasma decreased abruptly half a day before birth and continued to decrease gradually for a week after birth (*40*). There is no doubt that the decrease of corticosterone triggered a rapid decrease of hepatic γGTP after birth (*38*).

3. Stimulation by adenosine 3′, 5′-monophosphate (cAMP) of decrease of hepatic γGTP after birth

cAMP and glucocorticoid act cooperatively in induction of some catabolic enzymes such as tyrosine aminotransferase and serine dehydratase (*9, 15*). As shown in Table I, decrease of hepatic γGTP activity was prevented by injection of hydrocortisone at phys-

TABLE I.   Effects of Hydrocortisone and dbcAMP on the Decrease of Hepatic γGTP Activity in Neonatal Mice (ICR/Jcl)

Injection		γGTP activity (nmol/hr/mg proteins)	
		Days after birth	
1st	2nd	2	4
Saline[a]	Saline	950	491
Saline	dbcAMP[b]	924	213
Hydrocortisone[c]	Saline	1,204	—[e]
Hydrocortisone[d]	Saline	1,273	730
Hydrocortisone[c]	dbcAMP[b]	1,063	—[e]
Hydrocortisone[d]	dbcAMP[b]	1,154	352

The second injection was given 24 hr after the first and animals were killed 90 min later.
[a] An equivalent volume of saline was injected.
[b] dbcAMP 25 μg/g body weight (i. p.).
[c] Hydrocortisone-21-acetate, 1 μg/g body weight (s. c.).
[d] Hydrocortisone-21-acetate, 25 μg/g body weight (s. c.).
[e] Not determined.

iological or pharmacological doses. Unexpectedly, the intraperitoneal injection of N^6, $O^{2'}$-dibutyryl adenosine 3′, 5′-monophosphate (dbcAMP) resulted in a decrease of hepatic γGTP activity in mice pretreated with hydrocortisone. Without exogenous hydrocortisone, dbcAMP also accelerated the natural decrease of γGTP activity (38). These results suggest that a high level (twice that in adults) of hepatic cAMP in neonates stimulate a decrease of γGTP activity. A proteolytic mechanism seems to be operative, because actinomycin D inhibited the decrease of γGTP and 'super induction' (13) of γGTP was observed (40). There is some evidence that glucagon or dbcAMP stimulates protein breakdown in hepatocytes (7, 20, 32), although it is uncertain whether these agents act in the same way in neonatal liver.

Biphasic Changes in Hepatic γGTP Activity in Rats under the Influence of Carcinogens

1. Change of hepatic γGTP activity in rats on a diet containing 3′-methyl-4-dimethyl-aminoazobenzene (3′-MeDAB)

High activity of γGTP appears transiently in liver tissue at a specific period in normal development of mice and rats (11, 36, 43), indicating the possible usefulness of γGTP as a marker of this specific stage of differentiation. γGTP activity is high in precancerous liver tissues induced by a variety of hepatic carcinogens (6, 11, 18, 22, 33). If induction of γGTP is an obligatory step in carcinogenesis, or is closely related to carcinogenesis, comparison of the inductions of γGTP in normal development and during carcinogenesis should be important in understanding how "abnormal differentiation" differs from normal differentiation. The former is often irreversible and the latter reversible with regard to change in γGTP activity. In the experiment shown in Fig. 2, a group of Donryu rats 8–9 weeks of age was grown on a diet containing 0.06% 3′-MeDAB. Hepatic γGTP activity increased after 4–7 weeks on this diet, then decreased and then increased again. The first peak of activity tended to appear earlier when younger rats were used (Tateishi *et al.*, unpublished results). In control animals fed for 16 weeks on a basal diet of the same composition but without 3′-MeDAB, there was no significant change in hepatic γGTP activity. Next, we examined the reversibility of the changes in γGTP activity. When a group of rats was given a diet containing 3′-MeDAB for 6 weeks and then maintained

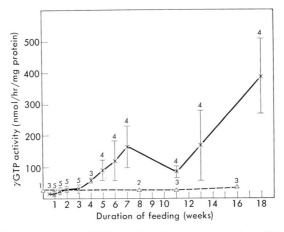

FIG. 2.   Change in hepatic γGTP activity of rats maintained on 3′-MeDAB-containing diet.   × 3′-MeDAB-containing diet; △ basal diet.

on a basal diet for the next 5 weeks, the enzyme activity fell to the normal adult level. But when rats were given a diet containg 3'-MeDAB for 13 weeks, the γGTP activity did not decrease on withdrawal of the carcinogen. These results confirm the Fialas' finding (11, 12) that after pretreatment of rats with 3'-MeDAB for a certain period high γGTP activity persists irrespective of further administration of the carcinogen.

2. Restoration of responsiveness to glucocorticoid in the livers of rats fed a diet containing 3'-MeDAB

At the perinatal period in normal development, the responsiveness of the liver to glucocorticoid and the high concentration of corticosterone result in an increase of γGTP activity. We examined the responsiveness of the liver to exogenous hydrocortisone after azo-dye feeding. As already described, adult rats maintained on a basal diet did not respond to hydrocortisone injected subcutaneouly. But in rats maintained on a diet containing 3'-MeDAB for 2 weeks, hepatic γGTP activity increased in response to hydrocortisone. When the period on the diet was extended to 8 weeks, stimulation of the enzyme activity by glucocorticoid was demonstrated more clearly (Table II). Dependency of γGTP activity on glucocorticoid was confirmed in bilaterally adrenalectomized rats.

TABLE II.   Effect of Hydrocortisone on Hepatic γGTP Activity in Rats Maintained on Diet Containing 3'-MeDAB

Diet	Period (weeks)	Injection	γGTP activity (nmol/hr/mg protein)
3'-MeDAB	2	Saline[a]	72± 1[b] (4)[c]
		Hydrocortisone	111±20 (4)
3'-MeDAB	8	Saline	180±38 (4)
		Hydrocortisone	349±51 (5)
Normal	8	Saline	38± 5 (4)
		Hydrocortisone	40± 6 (5)

Five mg/100 g body weight of hydrocortisone-21-acetate suspended in saline was injected subcutaneously and 24 hr later γGTP activity was measured.
[a] An equivalent volume of saline was injected.
[b] Mean±S. D.
[c] Number of rats used.

TABLE III. Effect of Bilateral Adrenalectomy on the Induction of Liver γGTP in Rats Given a Diet Containing 3'-MeDAB

Group	Treatment		γGTP activity (nmol/hr/mg protein)
1		3'-MeDAB diet 8W	155± 9[a] (3)[b]
2	1W↑Adx	3'-MeDAB diet 8W	49±36 (3)
3		3'-MeDAB diet 9.5W	160±27 (4)
4		3'-MeDAB diet 9.5W ↑Adx 1.5W	86± 8 (4)

[a] Mean±S.D.
[b] Number of rats used.
Adx, adrenalectomy;   W, week.

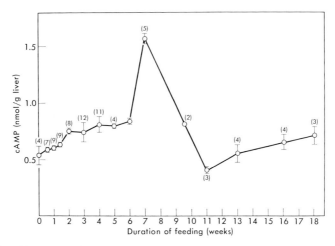

FIG. 3. Alteration of hepatic cAMP level of rats (male Donryu strain) grown on a
diet containing 3'-MeDAB.

When these rats were maintained on a diet containing 3'-MeDAB for 8 weeks hepatic
γGTP did not increase, confirming the results described by Fiala and Fiala (*11*) on
hypophysectomized and adrenalectomized rats. Adrenalectomy of rats, *after* 8 weeks on
this diet reduced the elevated activity significantly in 2 weeks, suggesting that the presence of endogenous glucocorticoid is necessary for maintaining a high activity of γGTP
(Table III). However, the plasma corticosterone level in rats given a diet containing
3'-MeDAB for 18 weeks remained within the normal range (*41*). So, at least in the first
phase, an increase of γGTP activity must have resulted from revival of responsiveness
of the liver to glucocorticoid caused by administration of the azo-dye. As induction of
tyrosine aminotransferase by hydrocortisone was partially suppressed in rats fed a diet
containing 3'-MeDAB (Higashi *et al.*, unpublished results), a specific alteration in
chromatin probably took place that led to increased expression of γGTP in the liver.

3. Alteration of the hepatic cAMP level in rats grown on a diet containing 3'-MeDAB

Another factor that modulated the level of liver γGTP in the perinatal period was
cAMP. Continuous administration of 3'-MeDAB to rats as a constituent of their diet led
to a gradual increase of cAMP in the liver, and after the first increase of γGTP activity
cAMP also increased greatly after 6 weeks on the diet, reaching a maximum after 7
weeks. Then it decreased until week 11 and again increased very slowly (Fig. 3). Like
the decrease of γGTP in the postnatal period, the transient fall of γGTP activity after
the first peak may be explained by the action of cAMP in stimulating the breakdown of
γGTP.

The second continuous rise of γGTP during carcinogenesis possibly occurred when
the breakdown of γGTP slowed down in the presence of a reduced concentration of
cAMP. We are now studying the mechanism of action of cAMP in causing the degradation of γGTP.

DISCUSSION AND CONCLUSIONS

For a long time, attempts have been made to find out characteristics of enzymes specific for malignant tumor cells. These studies have revealed a particular aspect of the enzyme pattern—fetalism in a variety of tumor cells, which was comprehensively described by Greenstein in his book (*17*). Knox (*25*) reanalyzed the data compiled by Greenstein and extended his analysis to data accumulated later in his own and other laboratories, especially on hepatic tissues. He concluded that "there were quantitative family resemblances between the composition of fetal liver and hepatoma and between regenerating liver and (adult) liver, but little similarity between these pairs of hepatic tissues" (*25*). This means that there are resemblances between fetal liver and hepatoma other than those common to growing tissues. Hepatic γGTP is unique in showing a tremendous but transient increase in the perinatal period in mice and rats. This type of increase of γGTP is not found in any other tissue (*2*) except the small intestine (*26*). High activity of γGTP was also found in many rat hepatomas induced by various carcinogens (*6, 10, 18, 21, 22, 30*), although there was no correlation between the enzyme activity and cell proliferation. Several investigators clearly demonstrated that the activity of hepatic γGTP increased in the preneoplastic phases of carcinogenesis (*4, 6, 11, 22, 37*). The present studies indicate that the first rise, but not the second rise, of liver γGTP activity in rats given 3'-MeDAB resembles the transient rise in the late fetal period. Probably the same mechanism initiated by glucocorticoid acts in inducing γGTP under these two conditions. Although hepatocarcinomas may exhibit various γGTP activities representing various arrested stages in ontogeny (*29*), it appears that liver cells must pass through a stage corresponding to perinatal liver during chemical carcinogenesis.

Responsiveness to glucocorticoid resulting in increase of hepatic γGTP was not observed in normal male rats, and adrenalectomy did not affect the enzyme activity (*41*). Billon *et al.* reported that in female rats, bilateral adrenalectomy caused partial decrease of hepatic γGTP, which was restored by injecting hydrocortisone (*1*). The effect of glucocorticoid on γGTP activity of hepatocytes in primary culture is still controversial (*3, 8, 31*), but it is noteworthy that γGTP activity was elevated by cultivating hepatocytes *in vitro*. It is possible that in adult rats, especially male rats, hepatic γGTP is prevented from being fully expressed by unknown factors *in vivo*, but that under some conditions in: (1) the perinatal period, (2) the early stage of chemical carcinogenesis, and (3) culture *in vitro*, liver cells may be partially relieved from, or less sensitive to, suppressive factors, probably including cAMP. During the second rise of γGTP observed in the late stage of carcinogenesis, high γGTP activity probably becomes constitutive.

Acknowledgment

This work was supported by Grants-in-Aid for Scientific Research (301043 and 501008) from the Ministry of Education, Science and Culture of Japan, from Society for Promotion of Cancer Research, and from the Osaka Anti-Cancer Association of Japan.

REFERENCES

1. Billon, M. C., Dupre, G., and Hanoune, J. *Mol. Cell. Endocrinol.*, **18**, 99–108 (1980).
2. Braun, J.-P., Rico, A., and Benard, P. *C. R. Acad. Sci. Paris*, **286**, 1483–1485 (1978).
3. Coloma, J., Gómez-Lechón, M. J., Garcia, M. D., Felíu, J. E., and Báguena, J. *Experientia*, **37**, 941–943 (1981).
4. Cameron, R., Kellen, J., Kolin, A., and Farber, E. *Cancer Res.*, **38**, 823–829 (1978).
5. Curthoys, N. and Hughey, R. P. *Enzyme*, **24**, 383–403 (1979).
6. Deml, E. and Oesterle, D. *Cancer Res.*, **40**, 490–491 (1980).

7. Deter, R. L., Baudhuin, P., and deDuve, C. *J. Cell Biol.*, **35**, C11–C16 (1967).

8. Edwards, A. M. *Cancer Res.*, **42**, 1107–1115 (1982).

9. Ernest, M. J., Chen, C.-L., and Feigelson, P. *J. Biol. Chem.*, **252**, 6783–6791 (1977).

10. Fiala, S., Fiala, A. E., and Dixon, B. *J. Natl. Cancer Inst.*, **48**, 1393–1401 (1972).

11. Fiala, S. and Fiala, E. S. *J. Natl. Cancer Inst.*, **51**, 151–158 (1973).

12. Fiala, S., Mohindru, A., Kettering, W. G., Fiala, A. E., and Morris, H. P. *J. Natl. Cancer Inst.*, **57**, 591–598 (1976).

13. Garren, L. D., Howell, R. R., Tomkins, G. M., and Crocco, R. M. *Proc. Natl. Acad. Sci. U.S.*, **52**, 1121–1129 (1964).

14. Goldbarg, J. A., Friedman, O. M., Pineda, E. P., Smith, E. E., Chatterji, R., Stein, E. H., and Rutenberg, A. M. *Arch. Biochem. Biophys.*, **91**, 61–70 (1960).

15. Greengard, O. and Dewey, H. K. *J. Biol. Chem.*, **242**, 2986–2991 (1967).

16. Greengard, O. *In* "Essays in Biochemistry," Vol. 7, ed. P. N. Campbell and F. Dickens, pp. 159–205 (1971). Academic Press, London.

17. Greenstein, J. P. "Biochemistry of Cancer," 2nd Ed. (1954). Academic Press, New York.

18. Harada, M., Okabe, K., Shibata, K., Masuda, H., Miyata, K., and Enomoto, M. *Acta Histochem. Cytochem.*, **9**, 168–179 (1976).

19. Higashi, T., Tateishi, N., Naruse, A., and Sakamoto, Y. *Biochem. Biophys. Res. Commun.*, **68**, 1280–1286 (1976).

20. Hopgood, M. F., Clark, M. G., and Ballard E. J. *Biochem. J.*, **186**, 71–79 (1980).

21. Huberman, E., Montesano, R., Drevon, C., Kuroki, T., St. Vincent, L., Pugh, T. D., and Goldfarb, S. *Cancer Res.*, **39**, 269–272 (1976).

22. Kalengayi, M.M.R., Ronchi, G., and Desmet, V. J. *J. Natl. Cancer Inst.*, **55**, 579–588 (1975).

23. Katunuma, N. and Matsuda, K. *Seikagaku*, **54**, 513 (1982) (in Japanese).

24. Kawahara, S., Ogata, S., and Ikehara, Y. *J. Biochem.*, **91**, 201–210 (1982).

25. Knox, W. E. "Enzyme Patterns in Fetal, Adult and Neoplastic Tissues," 2nd Ed. (1976). S. Karger, Basel.

26. Menard, C., Malo, C., and Calvert, R. *Biol. Neonate*, **40**, 70–77 (1981).

27. Nash, B. and Tate, S. S. *J. Biol. Chem.*, **257**, 585–588 (1982).

28. Orlowski, M. and Meister, A. *Proc. Natl. Acad. Sci. U.S.*, **67**, 1248–1255 (1970).

29. Potter, V. R. *Cancer Res.*, **28**, 1901–1907 (1968).

30. Richards, W. L., Tsukada, Y., and Potter, V. R. *Cancer Res.*, **42**, 1374–1381 (1982).

31. Sirica, A. E., Richards, W., Tsukada, Y., Sattler, G. A., and Pitot, H. C. *Proc. Natl. Acad. Sci. U.S.*, **76**, 283–287 (1979).

32. Shelburne, J. D., Arstile, A. U., and Trump, B. F. *Am. J. Pathol.*, **72**, 521–540 (1973).

33. Taniguchi, N., Tsukada, Y., Mukuo, K., and Hirai, H. *Gann*, **65**, 381–387 (1974).

34. Taniguchi, N., Saito, K., and Takakuwa, E. *Biochim. Biophys. Acta*, **391**, 265–271 (1975).

35. Tateishi, N., Higashi, T., Nakashima, K., Naruse, A., Shiozaki, H., Miyazaki, K., and Sakamoto, Y. *In* "Proc. Japan. Cancer Assoc., 35th Annu. Meet," p. 164, Tokyo (1976) (in Japanese).

36. Tateishi, N., Higashi, T., Nomura, T., Naruse, A., Nakashima, K., Shiozaki, H., and Sakamoto, Y. *Gann*, **67**, 215–222 (1976).

37. Tateishi, N., Higashi, T., Naruse, A., Kim, K., Nakashima, K., and Sakamoto, Y. *In* "Proc. Japan. Cancer Assoc., 36th Annu. Meet." p. 184, Tokyo (1977) (in Japanese).

38. Tateishi, N., Higashi, T., Hikita, K., Ohno, Y., Furukawa, M., and Sakamoto, Y. *In* "Proc. Japan. Cancer Assoc., 37th Annu. Meet.," p. 186, Tokyo (1978) (in Japanese).

39. Tateishi, N., Higashi, T., Ohno, T., Furukawa, M., Nakashima, K., and Sakamoto, Y. *Seikagaku*, **50**, 917 (1978) (in Japanese).

40. Tateishi, N., Higashi, T., and Sakamoto, Y. *In* "Proc. XIth IUB Congress (Abstr. No. 07-1-H 90)," p. 484, Toronto (1979).

41. Tateishi, N., Higashi, T., Matsuda, H., Furukawa, M., Ohno, T., Sekii, K., and Sakamoto, Y. *In* "Proc. Japan. Cancer Assoc., 38th Annu. Meet., p. 226, Tokyo (1979) (in Japanese).
42. Tateishi, N., Higashi, T., Nakashima, K., and Sakamoto, Y. *J. Nutr.*, **110**, 409–415 (1980).
43. Tsuchida, S., Hoshino, K., Sato, T., Ito, N., and Sato, K. *Cancer Res.*, **39**, 4200–4205 (1979).
44. Yokosawa, N., Taniguchi, N., Tsukada, Y., and Makita, A. *Oncodev. Biol. Med.*, **2**, 165–177 (1981).
45. Yokosawa, N., Taniguchi, N., Tsukada, Y. *Seikagaku*, **54**, 720 (1982) (in Japanese).

GANN Monograph on Cancer Research 29, 1983

CLINICAL VALUE AND SOME PROPERTIES OF NOVEL γ-GLUTAMYL TRANSPEPTIDASE ISOENZYME SPECIFIC TO SERA OF HEPATOCELLULAR CARCINOMA

Norio Sawabu,[*1],[*2] Daishu Toya,[*1] Kenji Ozaki,[*1] Tokio Wakabayashi,[*1] Masatoshi Nakagen,[*1] and Nobu Hattori[*1]

The First Department of Internal Medicine, School of Medicine, Kanazawa University[*1]

One or more specific bands (novel γ-glutamyl transpeptidase (γGTP)), such as bands II, II', and I' were electrophoretically detectable in 109 (55%) of 200 patients with hepatocellular carcinoma (HCC), but only in 3% of 279 patients with other hepatobiliary diseases. Novel γGTP was found in 38% of the HCC patients with α-fetoprotein (AFP) levels below 400 ng/ml. The incidence of novel γGTP was independent of the clinical stage as classified by liver scanning. Even in Stage I, where filling defects were not seen, the incidence was 52%. It is concluded that novel γGTP is useful in diagnosis of HCC patients with low levels of AFP or at a relatively early stage.

Some properties of γGTP purified from HCC tissues were investigated and compared with those of the normal kidney enzyme. Specific bands separated from sera of HCC patients and the enzyme from kidney were identical in enzymatic and immunological properties, whereas a considerable difference was observed in electrophoresis, concanavalin A (Con A) affinity, effect of neuraminidase and isoelectric point. Respective bands II, II', and I' could be differentiated in Con A affinity and neuraminidase reaction. These results support the possibility that novel γGTP in sera of HCC patients is largely due to a difference in carbohydrate moiety of γGTP.

Histological and biochemical studies showed that the activity of γ-glutamyl transpeptidase (γGTP) was high in the liver of fetal and neonatal rats, but decreased rapidly after birth so that the activity of this enzyme in adult rat liver may be approximately 1/30 to 1/100 lower than that in fetal rat liver (*1, 4*).

Studies on experimental cancer in mice and rats showed that γGTP was significantly increased in the liver cells both during the precancerous stage and in the liver cell carcinomas (*3, 5, 9, 13–15, 17, 25, 31, 32*). Similarity in the kinetic and immunological properties of γGTP between the azo dye-induced hepatoma and fetal rat liver was also observed by Taniguchi *et al.* (*28, 29*). This enzyme activity of human serum is markedly elevated not only in hepatocellular carcinoma (HCC) but also in the metastatic carcinoma, irrespective of the presence or absence of obstructive jaundice as shown in Fig. 1. Intensive

---

[*1] Takaramachi 13-1, Kanazawa 920, Japan (沢武紀雄, 登谷大修, 尾崎監治, 若林時夫, 中源雅俊, 服部信).

[*2] Present address: Cancer Institute Hospital, Kanazawa University, Yoneizumi 4-86, Kanazawa 920, Japan.

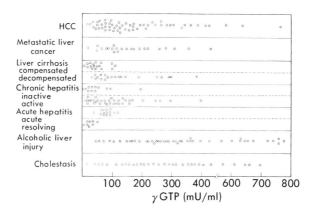

FIG. 1.   Serum γGTP activity in various hepatobiliary diseases.

staining of γGTP activity is observed in most HCC cells, while the activity is not noted in the metastatic tumor cells but only in the bile canaliculi and sinusoidal wall adjacent to the tumor (30). These facts strongly suggest that the fetal activity of γGTP resurges in HCC cells, and fetal isoenzyme of γGTP might be detectable in sera of patients with HCC as well as α-fetoprotein (AFP). With these points in mind, we previously reported the presence of a γGTP isoenzyme specifically present in sera of HCC (22–24).

This paper deals with the clinical value and certain properties of this isoenzyme chiefly as found in work performed by the authors.

Fractionation of γGTP Isoenzyme and HCC Specific Bands

There have been some methods for fractionations of the γGTP isoenzyme (8, 12, 20, 21, 27). However to distinguish specific bands in HCC, polyacrylamide gradient gel electrophoresis is most useful. Figure 2 shows the γGTP zymograms of sera from hepatobiliary diseases. By this method, which was described in detail in our previous publications (22, 24), γGTP isoenzymes in sera were separated into thirteen bands. No bands other than II, II′, and I′ were characteristic of any group of patients so far studied. On the other hand, band II which was seen in the region near ceruloplasmin, and band II′ which appeared between bands II and III, were found specifically in the sera of patients with HCC. In addition to these two bands, band I′ which was located just at the cathodic side of band I, had high specificity for HCC. We have referred to these bands as HCC specific novel γGTP isoenzyme (novel γGTP). Band I′ is not obvious because of its overlapping with band I. As will be shown later in detail, band I′ is un-bound to concanavalin A (Con A). By this lectin-binding property, band I′ can be clearly distinguished from band I.

Bands II, II′, and I′ could be detected in 97, 93, and 95 of 200 patients with HCC, respectively. They were rarely detected in patients with a disease other than HCC, that is, cholangioma (none of 8 cases), metastatic cancer to liver (3/52), biliary carcinoma (0/16), pancreatic carcinoma (0/11), liver cirrhosis (1/57), chronic hepatitis (1/43), acute and subacute hepatitis (0/14), alcoholic liver injury (2/36), intrahepatic cholestasis (0/16), and cholelithiasis (0/26). The concomitant appearance of all three bands was observed in 72% of 109 patients with HCC in whom one or more of these bands was found. Frequency of other combinations was variable. At least one or more of these bands was

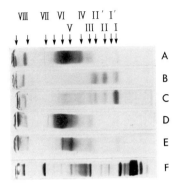

FIG. 2.   Serum γGTP isoenzymograms. A, alcoholic liver injury; B and C, HCC;
D, obstructive jaundice due to choledocholithiasis; E, metastatic liver cancer; F,
normal serum protein stained with Amido Black.

detectable in 109 (55%) out of 200 patients with HCC. Moreover, this figure was 63% in 100 patients with HCC in whom the γGTP isoenzyme was more recently examined. On the other hand, of 279 patients with hepatobiliary diseases other than HCC, one or more of these bands was found in three with metastatic liver cancer, two with alcoholic liver injury, one with liver cirrhosis, and one with chronic hepatitis. In all, the prevalence of novel γGTP was about 3% among patients with other hepatobiliary diseases.

The detection of human AFP in adult serum was initially considered to be virtually diagnostic of HCC or teratoblastoma containing yolk sac cell elements (2). However, increased levels of AFP were found in some patients with various types of liver disease other than HCC when a much more sensitive method for AFP detection such as radioim- munoassay was employed. Nevertheless, it has been widely accepted that AFP is a highly specific indicator for HCC in the various serological tests (11). The same may be said of the novel γGTP. Recently, Kojima et al. (16), who used the same method for electro- phoretic fractionation of γGTP in sera of HCC as we did, reported similar results to those we observed.

Clinical Significance of Novel γGTP

Figure 3 compares the serum activity of γGTP in patients of HCC with and without novel γGTP. Novel γGTP could not be detected in patients whose serum γGTP activity was less than 80 mU/ml. On the other hand, patients without novel γGTP were seen in whose serum γGTP activity remarkably increased. All of these patients had some com- plication such as obstructive jaundice which could raise the level of serum γGTP activi- ty. Although the prevalence of novel γGTP was only 55% among all HCC patients, it was 72% in patients whose serum γGTP activity was above 100 mU/ml. No significant difference in serum activity of alkaline phosphatase, one of the ductal enzymes, was observed in patients with and without novel γGTP.

For AFP, the same comparison is shown in Fig. 4. Novel γGTP was seen more frequently in patients with higher AFP levels. However, it was found in 29 (38%) of 76 patients with AFP levels lower than 400 ng/ml. Furthermore, 11 patients with novel γGTP were seen even among 41 with levels of AFP below 100 ng/ml. In general, about 35% of the patients with HCC showed AFP at a concentration less than 400 ng/ml,

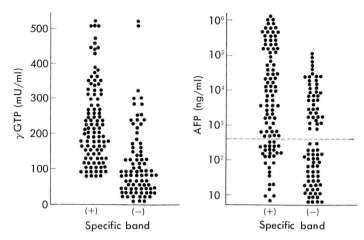

FIG. 3 (left).   Correlation with positivity of novel γGTP isoenzyme and serum γGTP activity.

FIG. 4 (right).   Correlation with positivity of novel γGTP isoenzyme and serum levels of AFP. Dotted line indicates AFP levels of 400 ng/ml.

which is typical of the sera of patients with hepatic diseases other than HCC. Thus, a specific diagnosis cannot be made for about one-third of HCC patients using the AFP test. With these points in mind, the novel γGTP can be especially useful for diagnosis of patients with HCC in whom serum AFP is low or negative.

We compared the incidence of novel γGTP in the four stages of HCC classified by liver scanning according to criteria proposed by the Japanese Association for the Study of HCC. These criteria are as follows: Stage I, no detectable filling defect on anterioposterior view; Stage II, filling defect is less than 20% in proportion to the whole hepatogram; Stage III, 20–70%; and Stage IV, more than 70%. The incidence of novel γGTP in each stage of 156 patients with HCC in whom liver scanning findings could be evaluated, was as follows:

Stage	I	II	III	IV
Total patients	17	50	82	7
Positive patients	9	26	48	3
Incidence (%)	53	52	59	43

The incidence of novel γGTP was independent of stage. As far as the carcinoembryonic antigens (CEA) and AFP which are now employed as tumor markers, there is an obvious correlation between tumor mass and CEA blood concentration, while the value of AFP is not necessarily parallel to the size and stage of tumors. Novel γGTP in our study does not increase in parallel with advancement of the stage as classified by liver scan. Moreover, even in Stage I in which the filling defect was undetectable on liver scanning, the incidence of novel γGTP was 53%, almost as much as the 55% in the total HCC patients. Accordingly, novel γGTP is expected to be a useful marker for relatively early detection of HCC.

Characterization of Novel γGTP Isoenzyme

1. γGTP from HCC tissue in comparison with the enzyme from normal kidney

γGTP was purified from HCC tissues of patients with novel γGTP according to the method described by Orlowski and Meister (19) and its physicochemical and immunological properties were compared with those of the normal adult human kidney enzyme. The procedure for purification includes solubilization of the enzyme from membranes using deoxycholate and bromelain, and treatment with acetone. Furthermore, after fractionation by ammonium sulfate, the pooled sample was subjected to Ultrogel ACA-34 gel chromatography and diethylaminoethyl (DEAE) cellulose ion exchangeable chromatography. A purification of about 1,500-fold was achieved, with an overall yield of about 5%. Because of the difficulties in obtaining a sufficient amount of the purified enzyme from normal liver in which the activity of γGTP was quite low, we compared various properties of the enzyme from HCC with those of normal adult kidney enzyme obtained by the same procedures.

The enzymes from HCC and kidney were found to be similar or identical with respect to the K_m values (1.44 to 1.55 mM), pH optimum (7.9), thermostability, effect of various amino acids as acceptors and behavior to cations or ethylenediamine tetraacetic acid (EDTA), except for molecular weight, isoelectric points, Con A affinity and neuraminidase reaction. The respective molecular weights of HCC and kidney enzyme were estimated to be about 92,000 and 81,000 by plotting the relative elution value using Ultrogel ACA-34 gel filtration.

A large proportion of HCC enzyme bound to Con A, although the ratio of bound to unbound fraction was different in every HCC. On the other hand, more than 80% of normal kidney enzyme passed through Con A-Sepharose. After neuraminidase treatment, the proportion of binding fraction to Con A-Sepharose was increased in kidney enzyme, but not in HCC enzyme. Figure 5 exhibits zymograms of preparations from Con A affinity chromatography. Con A-bound fraction from HCC enzyme was seen at band I designed in serum γGTP zymogram, and Con A-unbound fraction from it was located at the cathodic side just in the former band, so that the former could be distinguished from the latter in electrophoretic mobility. On the other hand, Con A-bound and un-

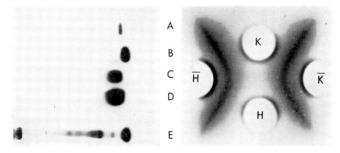

FIG. 5 (left). γGTP isoenzymogram after Con A affinity chromatography. A and B, Con A-unbound and bound fractions from HCC, respectively; C and D, Con A-unbound and bound fractions from normal kidney, respectively; E, serum of an HCC patient.

FIG. 6 (right). Double immunodiffusion in agarose gel stained with γGTP activity. γGTPs purified from HCC (H) and kidney (K). Antisera against the γGTPs purified from HCC (H̄) and from kidney (K̄).

bound fractions from kidney enzyme were identical with respect to electrophoretic mobility, corresponding to almost the same region as band II. After neuraminidase treatment, both Con A-unbound and bound fractions electrophoresed more slowly than the corresponding forms of the HCC enzymes, and had almost the same mobility. Contrarily, there was no difference in the electrophoretic mobility between Con A-unbound and bound fractions of the normal kidney enzyme unrelated neuraminidase treatment.

On isoelectric focusing in density gradients using an ampholite electrofocusing column, the main peak of kidney γGTP had a pI value of 4.4, whereas that of HCC γGTP exhibited a pI value of 4.0. After neuraminidase treatment, the bands of both enzymes were shifted to a more alkaline range, and neuraminidase treatment reduced the difference of pI value between γGTP of HCC and that of kidney.

By a technique of immunoabsorption using normal human serum, rabbit antisera against γGTP from HCC and kidney respectively were obtained. In an Ouchterlony double diffusion, γGTP from HCC and normal kidney were fused to antisera against HCC and against normal kidney to form a continuous line as exhibited in Fig. 6; the enzymes from HCC and kidney were indistinguishable in antigenicity. Also, in the test on activity inhibition the inhibition pattern of HCC enzymes by anti-normal kidney γGTP and anti-HCC γGTP were essentially identical.

2. Some properties of subfractions of novel γGTP

Mention will be made of the study on purified fractions from sera of HCC patients in order to clarify the difference in properties among bands II, II′, and I′, subfractions of novel γGTP. After fractionation by ammonium sulfate, novel γGTP-positive sera of HCC patients were subjected to gel chromatography using Ultrogel ACA-34 and then to electrophoresis on 4–30% polyacrylamide gradient gel slabs. After electrophoresis, the gel containing each fraction was cut out and eluted. Furthermore, bands I and I′ were separated by Con A affinity chromatography.

Comparison of the properties among the subbands is summarized in Table I. Band I, the nonspecific band, had the highest sensitivity to neuraminidase followed by I′, II, and II′ in a descending order. Band II′ showed little change in electrophoresis even after treatment with neuraminidase. To Con A, band II showed high affinity not too inferior to band I which was completely bound, while band I′ had no affinity and band II′ exhibited a weak affinity. Thus, there is considerable difference among the subbands when only neuraminidase reaction and Con A affinity are examined.

After treatment with bromelain, most of the activity of bands II and II′ showed a shift in electrophoretic mobility to a region consistent with bands I and I′, but bands I and I′ showed no reaction whatever to bromelain. γGTP in the tissue is mostly present

TABLE I. Some Properties of Each Band of γGTP Isoenzyme

	I	I′	II	II′
Neuraminidase	++	+	±	−
Bromelain	−	−	++	++
Con A	++	−	+	±
Anti-HCC	++	++	++	++
Anti-kidney	++	++	++	++

++ very sensitive; + sensitive; ± slightly sensitive; − non-sensitive.

in a membrane-bound form, and the isolation of γGTP from the tissue requires dissolution by bromelain or deoxycholate.

When immunological properties of these subbands were examined in inhibition tests and tests on cross-reactivity using two antisera against γGTPs from HCC and kidney, antigenicity of all the subbands including the nonspecific band I was identical.

Experimental liver cancer studies suggested that γGTP with carcinofetal characters produced by HCC cells may be released into the blood. However, we do not know the pathophysiological mechanism responsible for the appearance of novel γGTP in the sera of HCC patient. Tsuchida *et al.* (*32*) reported that the γGTP of HCC and the precancerous rat liver tissues was immunologically indistinguishable from γGTP of the normal rat kidney, but could differ from it at least in sialic acid content. Similarly, γGTP preparations from different organs within a mammalian species are immunologically identical, but differ significantly not only in sialic acid content but also some other carbohydrate components (*10, 18, 26*). In our studies too, the enzymes from human HCC and kidney were found to be similar or identical in enzymatic and immunologic properties, whereas a considerable difference was observed in electrophoresis, Con A affinity, effect of neuraminidase and isoelectric point. Moreover, specific γGTP isoenzyme subbands in sera of HCC patients were immunologically indistinguishable not only from each other but also from band I, the nonspecific band and kidney γGTP. These results will support that novel serum γGTP in HCC patients is largely due to a modification in the carbohydrate moiety which may occur in the altered posttranslational processing of the glycoprotein.

Hada *et al.* (*6, 7*) noted that γGTP from renal carcinoma does not differ from γGTP from adult kidney in enzymatic and immunological properties but it moves more to the anode on electrophoresis compared with adult kidney γGTP. Moreover, they have demonstrated that it differs from the latter at least in its contents of sialic acid and other carbohydrate components. This γGTP may be of little clinical use since it does not flow out into the blood, however, it seems to fall into the same category as novel γGTP in HCC.

Novel γGTP does not conform to the definition of isoenzyme in the classic sense, *e.g.*, an enzyme consisting of a protein which is coded to a different gene and has a different primary structure. However, in the light of the present situation in which a synzyme or allozyme not conforming to such a definition is interpreted broadly and regarded as isoenzyme, novel γGTP is also considered to be in this category.

Whether or not the carbohydrate structure of bands II, II', and I' enzymes is specific to HCC or how they are related to one another remains to be resolved. If a specific carbohydrate structure and the formation mechanism of such structure are elucidated, a specific antibody recognizing glycolinkage will be developed, which, in turn, will pave the way for new clinical applications.

Acknowledgment

This work was supported in part by grants-in-aid from the Ministry of Education, Science and Culture and the Ministry of Health and Welfare, Japan.

REFERENCES

1. Albert, Z., Rzucidlo, Z., and Starzyk, H. *Acta Histochem.*, **37**, 34–39 (1970).

2. Alpert, E., Uriel, J., and deNechaud, B. *N. Engl. J. Med.*, **278**, 984–986 (1968).
3. Cameron, R., Kellen, J., Malkin, A., and Farber, E. *Cancer Res.*, **38**, 823–829 (1978).
4. Fiala, S., Fiala, A. E., and Dixon, B. *J. Natl. Cancer Inst.*, **48**, 1393–1401 (1972).
5. Fiala, S. and Fiala, E. S. *J. Natl. Cancer Inst.*, **51**, 151–158 (1973).
6. Hada, T., Higashino, K., Yamamoto, H., Yamamura, Y., Matsuda, M., Osafune, M., Kotake, T., and Sonoda, T. *Clin. Chim. Acta*, **85**, 267–277 (1978).
7. Hada, T., Higashino, K., Yamamoto, H., Okochi, T., Sumikawa, K., and Yamamura, Y. *Clin. Chim. Acta*, **112**, 135–140 (1981).
8. Hetland, Ö., Andersson, T. R., and Gerner, T. *Clin. Chim. Acta*, **62**, 425–431 (1975).
9. Huberman, E., Montesano, R., Drevon, C., Kurok, T., Vincent, L. St., and Pugh, T. D. *Cancer Res.*, **39**, 269–272 (1979).
10. Huseby, N.E. *Clin. Chim. Acta*, **111**, 39–45 (1981).
11. Ishii, M. *GANN Monogr. Cancer Res.*, **14**, 89–98 (1973).
12. Iguarta, E. B., Domecq, R., and Findor, J. *Klin. Wochenschr.*, **51**, 272–274 (1973).
13. Jalanko, H. and Ruoslahti, E. *Cancer Res.*, **39**, 3495–3501 (1979).
14. Kalengayi, M.M.R., Ronchi, G., and Desmet, V. J. *J. Natl. Cancer Inst.*, **55**, 579–582 (1975).
15. Kitagawa, T., Watanabe, R., and Sugano, H. *Gann*, **71**, 536–542 (1980).
16. Kojima, J., Kanatani, M., Nakamura, N., Kashiwagi, T., Tohjoh, F., and Akiyama, M. *Clin. Chim. Acta*, **106**, 165–172 (1980).
17. Laishes, B. A., Ogawa, K., Roberts, E., and Farber, E. *J. Natl. Cancer Inst.*, **60**, 1009–1016 (1978).
18. Miura, T., Matsuda, Y., Tsuji, A., and Katunuma, N. *J. Biochem.*, **89**, 217–222 (1981).
19. Orlowski, M. and Meister, A. *J. Biol. Chem.*, **240**, 338–347 (1965).
20. Orlowski, M. and Szewczuk, A. *Clin. Chim. Acta*, **15**, 387–391 (1967).
21. Patel, S. and O'Gorman, P. *Clin. Chim. Acta*, **49**, 11–17 (1973).
22. Sawabu, N., Nakagen, M., Yoneda, M., Makino, H., Kameda, S., Kobayashi, K., Hattori, N., and Ishii, M. *Gann*, **69**, 601–604 (1978).
23. Sawabu, N., Nakagen, M., Ozaki, K., Wakabayashi, T., Toya, D., Hattori, N., and Ishii, M. *Ann. Acad. Med.*, **9**, 206–209 (1980).
24. Sawabu, N., Nakagen, M., Ozaki, K., Wakabayashi, T., Toya, D., Hattori, N., and Ishii, M. *Cancer*, **51**, 327–331 (1983).
25. Sells, M. A., Katyal, S. L., Sell, S., Shinozuka, H., and Lombardi, B. *Br. J. Cancer*, **40**, 274–283 (1979).
26. Shaw, L. M., Peterson-Archer, L., London, J. W., and Marsh, E. *Clin. Chem.*, **26**, 1523–1527 (1980).
27. Staeffen, J., Ballan, P., Ferrer, J., Beylot, J., Series, C., and Terme, R. *Pathol. Biol.*, **23**, 615–622 (1975).
28. Taniguchi, N. *J. Biochem.*, **75**, 473–480 (1974).
29. Taniguchi, N., Saito, K., and Takakuwa, E. *Biochim. Biophys. Acta*, **391**, 265–271 (1975).
30. Tanaka, M. *Acta Pathol. Japon.*, **24**, 651–665 (1974).
31. Tateishi, N., Higashi, T., Nomura, T., Naruse, A., Nakashima, K., Shinozuka, H., and Sakamoto, Y. *Gann*, **67**, 215–222 (1976).
32. Tsuchida, S., Hoshino, K., Sato, T., Ito, N., and Sato, K. *Cancer Res.*, **39**, 4200–4205 (1979).

AUTHOR INDEX

SUBJECT INDEX